Textbook on Professional Trends and Adjustments in Nursing

For General Nursing and Midwifery (GNM)

Textbook on Professional Trends and Adjustments in Nursing

For General Nursing and Midwifery (GNM)

I Clement
MSc(N) MSc (Psy) MA (Sociol)
MA (Childcare and Edu) PhD (N) PGDHA
Professor and Principal
VSS College of Nursing
Bengaluru, Karnataka, India

Professional Life Member
PhD Society of India, Chennai, Tamil Nadu
Nursing Research Society of India, New Delhi
Trained Nurses' Association of India, New Delhi
Christian Medical Association of India, New Delhi
Indian Society of Psychiatric Nurses, Bengaluru, Karnataka
Medical Surgical Nursing Society of India, Chennai
Indian Society of Neuroscience Nursing, New Delhi
Asian Association of Cardiac Nurses, Kolkata, West Bengal

Health Organization Member
Indian Red Cross Society
St John's Ambulance Association
General Secretary-Indian Society of Medical Surgical Nurses
Bengaluru, Karnataka, India

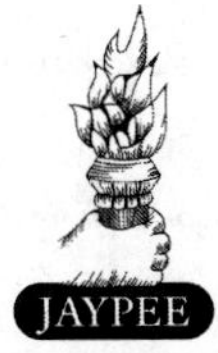

JAYPEE

JAYPEE BROTHERS MEDICAL PUBLISHERS

The Health Sciences Publisher

New Delhi | London

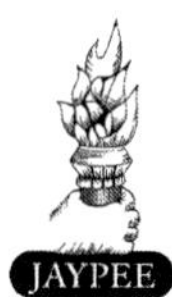

Jaypee Brothers Medical Publishers (P) Ltd

Headquarters
EMCA House
23/23-B, Ansari Road, Daryaganj
New Delhi - 110 002, India
Landline: +91-11-23272143, +91-11-23272703
+91-11-23282021, +91-11-23245672
E-mail: jaypee@jaypeebrothers.com

Corporate Office
4838/24, Ansari Road, Daryaganj
New Delhi - 110 002, India
Phone: +91-11-43574357
Fax: +91-11-43574314
E-mail: jaypee@jaypeebrothers.com

Overseas Office
J.P. Medical Ltd
83 Victoria Street, London
SW1H 0HW (UK)
Phone: +44 20 3170 8910
E-mail: info@jpmedpub.com

EU GPSR Authorised Representative
Logos Europe, 9 rue Nicolas Poussin
17000, La Rochelle, France
Phone: +33 (0) 6 67 93 73 78
E-mail: contact@logoseurope.eu

Website: www.jaypeebrothers.com
Website: www.jaypeedigital.com

Inquiries for bulk sales may be solicited at: jaypee@jaypeebrothers.com

Textbook on Professional Trends and Adjustments in Nursing for General Nursing and Midwifery (GNM)

First Edition: 2016, Reprint: **2026**

ISBN 978-93-85891-10-6

Printed at: Samrat Offset Pvt. Ltd.

Dedicated to

Smt KS Geetha
Founder and Chairman
JK College of Nursing and Paramedical
KSG Group of Institutions
Coimbatore, Tamil Nadu
India

Preface

It gives me immense pleasure to present this *Textbook on Professional Trends and Adjustments in Nursing.* First of all, I thank my Lord Almighty who blessed me with strength to complete this book. Nursing profession is noble profession where every nursing student is molded to meet the future legal and ethical issues, they are well prepared to adapt and inculcate professional adjustments in their nursing voyage as per the trends in nursing. Every nurse needs to learn and update his/her knowledge to meet the increasing and challenging demands of trending nursing care. Today's health scenario and the awareness towards concept healthcare among the public has increased and every patient expects good quality care. Therefore, every nurse needs to be responsible towards the concept of Professional Trends and Adjustments in Nursing.

This book is essential for student of all years in nursing, especially for the first year nursing students to ground this knowledge on professional trends and adjustments and also it will be useful reference for nursing teachers and postgraduate students, which will throw light on concepts in nursing, different roles in nursing profession, nursing ethics and ethical principles, legal issues, trends and issues in nursing, quality assurance in nursing care, nursing theories, nursing informatics, and about professional organizations. This book has fourteen sections incorporated in sixty-eight chapters illustrated in simple English. Each chapter has adequate diagrams and tables; it also has the glossary explained at the end of the book. This book is designed as per Indian Nursing Council requirements, that every nurse should have knowledge and good attitude towards professional trends and adjustments to become a complete nurse.

I wish all the best to nurse community.

I Clement

Acknowledgments

I am thankful to the Lord Almighty who strengthens me with His abundant blessings through innumerable means, helping me in all my accomplishments.

My heartfelt thanks to Shri Sommana, Former Minister of Karnataka and Chairman of VSS Group of Institutions for his constant support and encouragement.

My sincere thanks to my Guru, Dr BT Basavanthappa, Principal, Rajarajeshwari College of Nursing, Bengaluru, Karnataka, India; Professor PV Ramachandran, Chairman, College of Nursing, Sri Ramachandra University, Chennai, Tamil Nadu, India, a great philosopher and internationally renowned teacher of nursing, who helped me in discovering the world of knowledge. I am thankful to Ms Shylaja Sommana, Managing Directors; Dr BS Naveen, Dr BS Arun and Ms Divya from VSS Group of Institutions, Bengaluru, Karnataka, India, for their support and encouragement.

I am also grateful to Dr BC Bhagavan, Syndicate Member of RGUHS, Bengaluru, Professor, Department of Surgery, Kempegowda Institute of Medical Sciences, Bengaluru, Karnataka, India, and Dr Aswathnarayanan, MLA, Chairman, Padmashree Group of Institutions, Bengaluru, Karnataka, India.

Special thanks to Dr TV Ramakrishnan, Professor, Department of Anesthesiology and Head, Department of Clinical Services, and Accident and Emergency Medicine, Sri Ramachandra University, Chennai, Tamil Nadu, India; Dr Jeyaseelan Manickam Devadasan Syndicate Member, The Tamil Nadu Dr MGR Medical University, Chennai, and Dean and Professor, Annai JKK Sampoorani Ammal College of Nursing, Erode, Tamil Nadu, India; Dr Tamilmani, Principal, Annai JKK Sampoorani Ammal College of Nursing, Erode, Tamil Nadu, India; Professor (Mrs) Jessie Sudarsanum, Head, Department of Medical Surgical Nursing, Annai JKK Sampoorani Ammal College of Nursing, Erode, Tamil Nadu, India, and all my teachers and students.

I convey my sincere thanks to my beloved parents, brothers and sisters and my wife Nisha Clement for her continuous support and constant encouragement in each step of my life. I take this opportunity to thank my little ones, Cibin, Cynthia and Cavin. I extend thanks to my beloved friend and brother Mr Regi T Kurien, USA.

Special thanks to Shri Jitendar P Vij (Group Chairman), Mr Ankit Vij (Group President), Mr Tarun Duneja (Director–Publishing), Mr KK Raman (Production Manager) and Mr Rajesh Sharma (Production Coordinator) of M/s Jaypee Brothers Medical Publishers (P) Ltd, New Delhi, India, and also Mr Venugopal V (Associate Director—South), Mr Santhosh Kumar (Author Coordinator), Ms Sajini SV (Team Head) and other staff members of M/s Jaypee Brothers Medical Publisher (P) Ltd, Bengaluru branch.

Contents

Section-1: Concept of Nursing

Section-2: Nursing as a Profession

Section-3: Ethical Issues

Section-4: Legal Issues

Section-5: Professional Adjustments

Section-8: Advanced Nursing Skills

Section-11: Advancement in Nursing

Section-12: Staff Welfare

Section-13: Professional Organizations

Section-14: Alterative Therapies

Section-1

Concept of Nursing

1 Introduction to Nursing

1.1 INTRODUCTION

Nursing has been called the oldest of the arts and the youngest of the profession. The word nurse evolved from the Latin word nutritious, which means nourishing. The roots of medicine and nursing are intertwining and found in mythology, ancient eastern and western cultures and religion. Nursing, besides being a honorable profession, is one of the oldest arts and an essential modern occupation. Nursing is one of the greatest of humanitarian services and all people whether ill or well, rich or poor, literate or illiterate, young or old, at work or at play, in or out of hospital, are in some way or other, directly or indirectly closely associated with it. Nursing has its own body of knowledge scientifically based and humanitarianism that promises expanded benefits to people and society. It assists the individual or family to achieve their potential for self-direction for health.

1.2 DEFINITION

Nursing is defined by various authors at various times. Hansderson says "nursing is primarily assisting the individuals (sick or well) in the performances of those activities, contributing or its recovery (or to a peaceful death) that he would perform unaided, if he had the necessary strength, will or knowledge.

The unique contribution of nursing is to help the individual to be independent or such assistance as soon as possible.

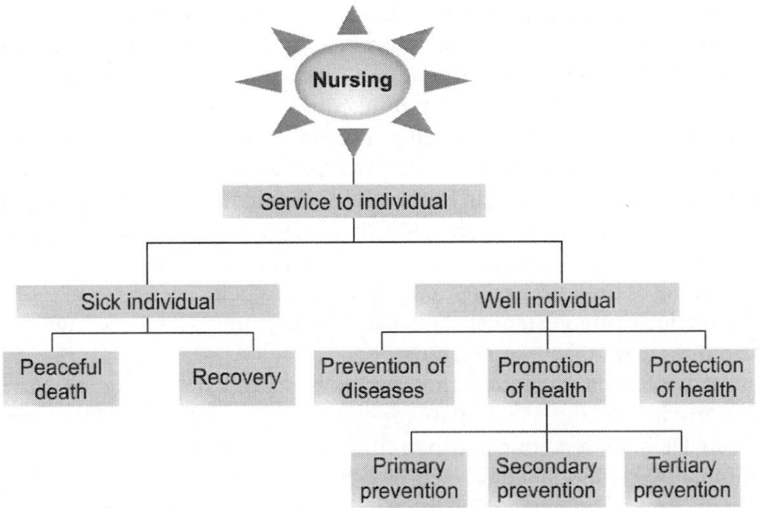

Fig. 1.1: Henderson's definition of nursing

1. **The International Council of Nurses** defines "Nursing is to assist the individual, sick or well in the performance of those activities contributing to health or to its recovery (or to peaceful death) that he would perform unaided if he had the necessary strength, will or knowledge".
2. **Florence Nightingale:** Nursing defined as the act of utilizing the environment of the patient to assist him in his recovery.
3. **Canadian Nurses Association-1987:** Nursing practice as a dynamic, caring and helping relationship in which the nurse assists the client to achieve and obtain optimal health.
4. **American Nurses Association:** Nursing practice as direct goal oriented and adaptable to service the needs of the individual, the family and community during health and illness.

1.3 HISTORICAL DEVELOPMENT OF NURSING IN INDIA

1905: Association of Nursing Superintendents was constituted/formed.

1908: Trained Nurses Association of India was established/formed.

1909: Bombay Presidency Nursing Association was formed. Missionary Nurses North India Board, set up under Medical Missionary Association of India.

1911: The South Indian Board was established Indian Nursing Association of Illinois (INAI) affiliated to International Council of Nurses.

1912: The First Nurses, Registration Act was enacted in Madras Presidency.

1930: The Christian Nurses Auxiliary formed by the missionary nurses.

1934: The Bengal Nurses Act was enacted for the nurses, midwives and Health vistor (HV) of undivided Bengal.

1936: The Mid India Board of Education affiliated to Christian Nurses league, Christian Nurses Auxiliary Association was affiliated to Trained Nurse Association of India (TNAI).

1941: Standardized pay scales and terms of services were established in Madras. State nursing superintendent, appointed at state level (Madras).

1942: The Auxiliary Nursing Service (ANS) was established. One nursing superintendent was appointed as nursing advisor at Directorate General of Health Services (DGHS), Government of India, to organize nursing services.

1943: Establishment of School of Nursing Administration for Military Nursing Services Health Survey and Development Committees (Bhore) constituted by Government of India. Study groups worked on proposal for university education in nursing in India. Christian Medical College (CMC) Vellore and Madras General Hospital started courses to train nursing tutors. Commissioned rank was given to the Indian Military Nursing sisters.

1946: Bhore Committee submitted report, recommendations made on improvement of various aspects of nursing profession: Nursing education, working conditions, nursing services in hospital and community and deputing nurses for higher education to abroad, etc. Establishment of the College of Nursing at Delhi (now Rajkumari Amrit Kaur College of Nursing) under the Union Ministry of Health to start university nursing education programme for the first time in India leading to Bachelor's degree in nursing, i.e., BSc (Hons.) Nursing.

1947: Indian Nursing Council Act was passed (31.12.1947) on the basis of recommendations of Bhore Committee. Degree programme for nursing started in Vellore.

1948: The first meeting of Indian Nursing Council (INC) was held.

1950: The INC took decision to establish Auxilliary Nursing and Midwifery (ANM) programme to meet the requirement of workers in nursing.

1951: Establishment of urbanfield teaching center is started at College of Nursing, Delhi in collaboration with existing. Municipal Corporation of Hyderabad (MCH) centers of Municipal Corporation, Delhi for teaching of urban community health nursing.

1952: Establishment of residential field teaching center for teaching community health nursing in the rural area under College of Nursing, Delhi in collaboration with primary health centre, Najafgarh.

1953: Ms Edith Buchanan, vice principal, Rajkumari Amrit Kaur (RAKCON) College of Nursing, New Delhi was sent to Columbia University to earn her Doctorate in Education (DEd) through World Health Organization (WHO) fellowship.

1954: Government of India constituted committee to review conditions of services, emoluments; etc. of nursing profession (Shetty committee). Shetty Committee Report was published, recommended nursing staff norms of hospital community and other improvements in nursing.

1955: Establishment of child guidance clinic at RAK College of Nursing for providing services and strengthening community health nursing and pediatric nursing. Ms Margareta Craig, principal, College of Nursing, Delhi attended ICN meeting in France, to present a paper on the need for nursing research in India.

1959: Dr Edith M Buchanan, succeeded in establishing the long cherished "Master of Nursing" degree programme at RAK College of Nursing, New Delhi under University of Delhi (October 1959). Healthy Survey and Planning Committee (Dr LN Mudaliar) was constituted by Government of India to review the progress made in health since, Bhore committee recommendation.

1961: Mudaliar Committee report published made some recommendations to improve nursing profession.

1963: A WHO assisted technical project was undertaken at the INC to revise the General Nursing and Midwifery (GNM) course. Dr Buchanan, succeeded in sending Mrs Sulochana Krishnan, one of the first graduates of this newly established, MN degree programme, to earn the DEd degree from Columbia University.

1964: Dr Marie Ferguson, a public health nurse came to the College of Nursing, New Delhi was able to create greater appreciation and understanding of the need and value of research in planning nursing administration and education with senior leaders of the country conducted "Activity studies to define the nursing and non-nursing functions of nursing personnel".

1965: A WHO publication on 'Guide for School of Nursing' in India was published.

1966: Trained Nurse Association of India (TNAI) established research section under the Chairmanship of Ms Margareta Craig. TNAI conducted 'Time study' with the co-operation of Ms Anna Gupta, principal, RAKCON, under the supervision of Dr Sulochana Krishnan.

1969-71: INAI and VHAI, CHAP conducted study on survey on the socioeconomic status of nurses in India.

1973: Kartar Singh Committee report on multipurpose workers and Health and family planning department published and recommended ANM and Lady health visitors (LHVs) were redesignated and health workers (F) and health assistant (F) to cover the required population at rural area for providing proper health services.

1975: Srivastav Committee report on 3 tier-plan of health care delivery system to rural area was recommended.

1976: Dr Marie Farell and Dr Aparna Bhaduri of RAKCON, New Delhi, conducted seminars on nursing research for educationists at Delhi, Mussoorie (Uttarakhand) and Yarcaid to strength the nursing research in India.

1978: Government Nurses Association of Karnataka established.

1981: Dr Farrell and Dr Bhaduri's book 'Health Research'—A Community based Approach' published by World Health Organization.

1986: The Nursing Research Society of India (NRSI) was established to promote research within and around nursing environment. Dr (Mrs) Inderjit Walia was founder president. Mrs Uma Handa was its secretary. MPhil in nursing programme started at RAKCON, under Delhi University.

1987: Reports of the expert committee on health and manpower planning, production and management (Bajaj Committee) published. This committee also dealt with nursing service conditions norms and nurse's emoluments, etc.

1988: RAKCON, New Delhi was designated as World Health Collaboration Centre for Nursing Developments reports of the high power committee on nursing and nursing profession published. Dr Ruth Hurner book "Nursing Education in India" published on the basis of survey.
1991: Author registered PhD in nursing at Bangalore University.
1992: PhD in nursing programme started at RAKCON, under Delhi University. Mrs Asha Sharma got registered for the Doctoral course.

1.4 SCOPE OF NURSING

There was a time when professional nurses had very little choice of service because nursing was centered in the hospital and bedside nursing. Career opportunities are more varied now for a numbers of reasons. The list of opportunities available is given under:

1. **Staff nurse** provides direct patient care to one patient or a group of patients. Assists ward management and supervision. She is directly responsible to the ward supervisor.
2. **Ward sister or Nursing supervisor:** She is responsible to the nursing superintendent for the nursing care management of a ward or unit. Takes full charge of the ward. Assigns work to nursing and non-nursing personnel working in the ward. Responsible for safety and comfort of patients in the ward. Provides teaching sessions if it is a teaching hospital.
3. **Department supervisor/Assistant nursing superintendent:** She is responsible to the nursing superintendent and deputy nursing superintendent for the nursing care and management of more than one ward or unit, e.g. surgical department and out-patient department.
4. **Deputy nursing superintendent:** She is responsible to the nursing superintendent and assists in the nursing administration of the hospital.
5. **Nursing superintendent:** She is responsible to the medical superintendent for safe and efficient management of hospital nursing services.
6. **Director of nursing:** She is responsible for both nursing service and nursing educations within a teaching hospital.
7. **Community Health Nurse (CHN)** services rendered mainly focusing Reproductive Child Health programme.
8. **Teaching in nursing:** The functions and responsibilities of the teacher in nursing are planning, teaching and supervising the learning experiences for the students. Positions in nursing education are clinical instructor, tutor, senior tutor, lecturer, and associate professor, Reader in nursing and Professor in nursing.
9. **Industrial nurses:** They are providing first aid, care during illness, health educations about industrial hazards and prevention of accidents.
10. **Military nurse:** Military Nursing service became a part of the Indian Army by which means nurses became commissioned officers who are given rank from lieutenant to major general.
11. **Nursing service abroad:** Attractive salaries and promising professional opportunities, which cause a major increase for nursing service in abroad.
12. **Nursing service administrative positions:** At the state level the Deputy Director of Nursing at the state health directorate. The highest administrative position on a national level is the Nursing Advisor to the Government of India.

CONCLUSION

Nursing is defined as providing care to the healthy or sick individuals for preventive, promotive, curative and rehabilitative needs. The consumers are patients with complex needs. With increased awareness of healthcare, healthcare facilities and Consumer Protection Act, patients/clients are getting awareness about their rights. Nurses also have now the expanded role, with the result the legal responsibility is increased. Hence, it is important for nursing personnel working in hospital, community and educational field to develop understanding of Legal and Ethical issues of Nursing.

2 Origin and Development of Nursing

2.1 INTRODUCTION

The history of nursing spans from the history of human kind. For as long as there has been life, there has been the need to provide care and comfort to those suffering from illness and injury. From the dawn of civilization, evidence prevails to support the premise that nurturing has been essential to the preservation of life. Survival of the human race, therefore, is in inextricably intertwined with the development of nursing. Nursing has been called the oldest of the arts and the youngest of the profession. The word nurse evolved from the Latin word nutritious, which means nourishing.

The roots of medicine and nursing are intertwining and found in mythology, ancient eastern and western cultures and religion. Nursing is defined by various authors at various times. Anderson says "nursing is primarily assisting the individuals (sick or well) in the performances of those activities, contributing or its recovery (or to a peaceful death) that he would perform unaided, if he had the necessary strength, will or knowledge. The unique contribution of nursing is to help the individual to be independent or such assistance as soon as possible".

2.2 CONCEPT OF NURSING

The International Council of Nurses defines "Nursing is to assist the individual, sick or well in the performance of those activities contributing to health or to its recovery (or to peaceful death) that he would perform unaided if he had the necessary strength, will or knowledge. And to do this in such a way as to help in gain independence as rapidly as possible. Nursing, besides being a honorable profession, is one of the oldest arts and an essential modern occupation. Nursing is one of the greatest of humanitarian services and all people whether ill or well, rich or poor, literate or illiterate, young or old, at work or at play, in or out of hospital, are in some way or other, directly or indirectly closely associated with it.

Nursing has its own body of knowledge scientifically based and humanitarianism that promises expanded benefits to people and society. It assists the individual or family to achieve their potential for self-direction for health. Nursing is not only an applied science; it is also an art, which provides skillful care for the sick in appropriate relationship with the patient, family, physician and with others who have related responsibilities. It is concerned equally with the prevention of illness and the conservation of health. Skillful nursing care embraces the whole person, body, mind and soul, his physical, mental, social and spiritual well-being (holistic approach).

In its broadest sense, nursing covers not only the care of the sick, the aged, the helpless and the handicapped, but also cares for the promotion of health and prevention of illness.

2.3 ARTS OF NURSING

The arts of nursing had its birth in the earliest home where a mother cared for the well-being of the rest members of the family. It is this mother care that through the ages developed into a skilled art and a well-organized science. It will be interesting to know and understand the vast changes that nursing has passed through, in order to meet the needs of a changing civilization. A study of the development of nursing will throw light on some of the problems of the past, how they have been solved and how nursing has progressed rapidly despite various hindrances.

The paternal and maternal instinct in a human being is the main source of the nursing impulse, and is found in the hearts of people of all ages. A mother's care for her sick child always found expression in such acts to alleviate pain and help the child to get better. In a society, the noblest forms of humanitarianism are showing mercy, love and kindness to those in physical or mental distress. When this impulse is re-enforced by religious philosophies and beliefs, it inspires people to live a life of service and of self-sacrifice for the sake of others. Along with this spirit, special training and experience has made nursing an ideal and useful profession.

2.4 PRE-HISTORIC NURSING

Myths, songs and other findings of the archaeologists throw some light on prehistoric man's care for this sick. In the pre-historic era, it was believed that illness was caused by evil spirits within the body. In order to get rid of the evil spirit, the body had to be illtreated. This was done by starving, beating, and administering nauseous medicines, beating of drums, magic rites and ceremonies and by causing sudden fright. Sometimes, holes were made in the affected parts of the body to allow the evil spirit to escape.

Besides this, there were also many other ways of treating illness. Primitive man's skill in fighting disease has given us many medical and surgical treatments such as massage fomentations, trephining, bone setting, hot and cold baths, etc. The doctor cum nurse in such cases was the medicine man or the witch doctor or the priest physician.

2.5 NURSING IN EARLY CIVILIZATION

EGYPT: The Egyptians thought medicine to be of divine origin. One of the world's oldest medical records, dating back to 1600 B.C. comes from Egypt. Sources of medical history, description of diseases and their treatment, surgery and drugs used are found in the "Hieroglyphic writings" on papyrus from the temples of ancient Egypt and from the Pyramids. Temple took the places of hospitals and the doctor cum nurse was the priest. It is probable that high-ranking women who become the priestesses in the temples played the role of nurses.

Mothers and daughters nursed the sick at home. An outstanding priest physician was Imhotep. Because of his great love and kindness to his patients and of his success in healing, he was elevated to the rank of a deity. Embalming and bandaging of mummies led to the study of anatomy of the body and the study of various herbs and drugs in preservation of the same. The Egyptians recognized about 250 diseases and discovered suitable drugs and surgery for their treatment.

The sacred books were strictly followed by the priest physicians. He was taken to task, if he deviated from the teaching of these books and if his patient dies.

Even though Egypt had made much progress in medicine and nursing, it soon declined for no dissection was permitted and also no experiments in medicines were to be made. This together with the advent of the Romans led to its decline.

GREECE: Medicine was closely connected with religion in Greece as in India. According to Greek mythology, Apollo the Sun God was their **God of healing. Asclepius, the son of Apollo, was** the Greek, God of medicine. The Greeks prayed to Apollo and Asclepius, and the goddess of health, **Hygiea** the daughter of Apollo for magical cures for their illnesses. Temples, where people came to worship were also places for the treatment of the sick and the priest-physician was in charge of them. These temples were situated in a healthy location, in a cheerful and charming country-side with plenty of fresh air. In Greece, the emphasis was a positive health, in beauty and perfection - not sickness and misery. The young of Athens were taught to give their bodies exquisite care. It was in Greece that personal hygiene developed to a degree never previously or subsequently approached. Much emphasis was given to personal cleanliness, exercise and dietetics rather than to matters of environmental sanitation. **Hippocrates,** 100 BC known as **"Father of Scientific Medicine"** had a medical foundation to start with. He found that health and prevention of disease depends on certain laws of nature. He also established an **Ethical code of conduct** for all who practiced medicine. Parts of his code are being used by medical students today and it forms the base of the 'Nightingale's pledge'. He separated medicine from religion for the first time in the history. With the spreading of Greek's influence in other countries, the Greeks introduced establishments that may be considered as modern city hospitals. They also established scientific methods of diagnosis and systematic methods of recording.

ROME: The Romans are best known for advances in public health. Rome had proper sanitation, drainage and sewage system, public baths and a type of public dispensary. The Roman noble women cared for the sick. With the advent of Christianity, deacons and deaconesses performed the duties of nurses. **Galen,** a Greek physician who lived in Rome about 100 BC, performed numerous experiments on animals to learn about anatomy and disease.

HEBREWS: The writings of Hebrews in the Old Testament speak about laws and principles of sanitation in accordance with modern bacteriology. They mention about selection of food, sanitation, segregation of the sick, disinfection and midwifery.

CHINA: The Chinese were well-advanced in medicine and surgery. They had good knowledge of internal organs and knew about the circulation of the blood. They practiced dissection. They also practiced vaccination and physiotherapy. Liver for anemia, seaweed for thyroid were administered. The sick were prayed for in halls of healing. Intestinal infection was prevented by drinking of tea. Much importance was given to cleanliness and hygiene.

INDIA: In India, we had the **Ayurvedic system of medicine**, which can be traced back to about 3000 B.C. Ayurveda stressed on hygiene, prevention of sickness, inoculation against small pox, sanitation, lavatories, good ventilation, kitchen, construction of hospitals, cultivation of medicinal plants and suitable building for housing animals. **Atreya** was the first great physician and teacher of Ayurveda. He lived about 800 B.C. During 700–600 B.C **Sushruta** and **Charaka** started practice of surgery and medicine. **Sushruta Samhita** is written by the great surgeon Sushruta, who says "the physician, the patient, the drugs and the nurse are four feet of 'Padas' of the medicine, upon which the cure depends". He then explains how cash may be a true 'Pada' (Foot). The nurse is a pada when he is kindhearted, strong, trustworthy and mindful of the physician's orders.

The nurse is one who attends the patient; is cool headed and pleasant in his demeanour; does not speak ill of anybody; is strong and attentive to the requirements of the sick and strictly follows the instructions of the physicians.

The great physician **Charaka** has written the **Charaka Samhita** in which he explains details of the manner in which drugs should be prepared or compounded for administration. According to him, resourcefulness, devotedness to the patient waited upon, and purity of mind and body are the qualification of the attending nurse. The Charaka Samhita states that attendants on the sick should have good behavior and should be distinguish for purity and cleanliness of habits.

Nursing treatments prescribed are baths, enema to evacuate the bowels, emetics to produce vomiting, vaginal and urethral infusion (introducing a fluid under pressure), venesection (reducing of blood volume by opening the vein), gargles, massages, rubbing or pressing the limbs etc. A nurse is expected to assist the patient to walk or move about. She/he must know how to make clean beds. She should be skilled in compounding drugs and ever willing to do any work that her profession demands of her.

700–600 B.C - **Thiruvalluvar** in his songs speaks highly of medicine. He describes medical care as consisting of patients, doctors and nurses.

264 B.C - King Ashoka made a great stride in the care of the sick, both human beings and animals. He not only founded a large number of hospitals for the sick but also made provision for the education and training of women for that purpose.

Monastery Universities were founded and became famous for their medical schools. The ethical standards of conduct demanded from those who attended upon the sick were of an exceptionally high order. The nursing of patients seems to have been devoted primarily to men, a great deal of unrewarded work. The qualities expected of nursing attendants were good behavior, purity, cleverness, at kindness and skill.

2.6 EARLY CHRISTIAN ERA

Nursing in Pre-Christian times, religious beliefs had great bearing on the attitude towards the sick and the mode of caring for the sick and the suffering. Christianity believed that one should render services of love to humanity without any reward. It was equal to one's sincere love of God. This principle was absorbed in nursing and helped to improve the status of a nurse. Some of examples of such women are as follows:

Phoebe: She was the first deaconesses. She was intelligent and educated and the best nurse who could care for the sick in their homes. She can be compared to a modern public health nurse.

Fabiola: She was a young, beautiful and attractive woman. She was the daughter of a great Roman Noble. She converted her palace into a hospital and it was the first Christian hospital in Rome. She collected the poor and sick from the streets and cared for them herself, in her place.

Paula: She was a friend of Fabiola. She devoted herself for the services of the sick. She built a hospital for strangers, pilgrims, and travellers and for the sick. She constructed a monastery in Bethlehem. They gave good nursing care for the sick.

Marcella: She was a wealthy woman. Since, women of high rank had much freedom in Rome, she was able to lead a group of such women and induce them in works of charity.

During the middle Ages, monks and nuns devoted their life to the care and services of the poor and sick. The monasteries became the places of education, medical care and nursing. The following monks and the nuns devoted their life and services for the poor and the sick.

- St. Dominic (1170–1221),
- St. Francis of Assisi 1182–1226.
- St. Elizabeth of Hungary 1207–1231
- St. Catherine Sienna 1347–1380

The women who assisted in the work of clergy in the church were known as deaconesses. They were matured women, who did teaching, preaching and caring for the sick at the home. New thoughts and new ideas were introduced in the early Christian era. Even though many religious were fatalistic in their outlook on illness and looked upon it as a punishment or a necessary evil, Christianity introduced a new aspect on the subject, thus transforming nursing to a higher level and raising it to a professional standing.

This new aspect that of "altruism" was the highest motive given to mankind. It taught that one's sincere love for God and a desire to be like Him, would be the chief motive for one's selfless and sacrificial service to mankind without any hope of a reward. This inspired may godly men and women to step forward in the service of the sick, the suffering and the needy. They opened their homes to the sick and in need. Such homes were called "**Diakonia**". During the time of the persecution of the Christians, people turned to the Bishop of the Church for help. This necessitated the building of homes cum hospitals where the strangers, the orphans, the aged, the sick and the lepers were cared for.

These homes cum hospitals were known as **Xenodochia.**

One such outstanding hospital was founded at Casearia by St. Basil in 370 A.D.

The Christian church preserved records and from that time till today we have a continuous record of the history of nursing. Many rich and noble women launched out in groups and organizations in the service of the sick and the ailing and used their wealth for this cause. Monasteries came into being and became a heaven for those who needed help and care. Two notable names of people belonging to this era are worth mentioning. Celsius, a Greek, studied anatomy and knew how to do surgical operations for cataracts and hernias. Galen practiced dissection on animals and studied the anatomy and physiology of the heart and circulation, the respiratory and the nervous system. His writings together with his translations of Hippocrates were considered to be the chief medical authority by the Arabs.

2.7 MIDDLE AGES

Monks and nuns dedicated to the cause of human suffering worked as doctors and nurses. They were skilled in the use of home remedies. They got scientific knowledge in the care of the sick from the books in the monasteries. They did the groundwork for the development of universities. In the later middle ages, many social problems presented themselves with the disintegration of the protective units like monasteries, guilds and feudalism and resulting in redistribution of population. Late in the 12th and 13th centuries nursing become differentiated from medicine and surgery. Medicine went into a period of advancement while nursing declined. At such time may noteworthy men and women came out to serve the sick. During the medieval period, plague and pestilence were thought to be due to supernatural rather than natural causes. Religious expeditions like the crusades led to founding of secular as well as military hospitals.

Quarantine was instituted to check spreading of epidemics like plague. Social problems were solved to a great extent. The needs of abandoned children were met in hospital, leading to the founding of creches. People had an indifferent attitude towards sanitation and hygiene. The Dark Ages was marked by superstition, mysticism, persecution of free thinkers and religious wares. Use of talisman and incantations for healing the sick become quite common.

2.8 THE DAWN OF MODERN NURSING

From the late 1700s through 1853, the manner in which the sick were cared, remain essentially unchanged. In Europe, the dawn of nursing was underway.

The Deaconess Institute of Kaiserswerth, Germany was established in 1836 by Pastor Theodor Fliedner, to train the Deaconesses to care for the sick and the provision of social services. Graduates of the Kaiserswerth program spread their influence throughout the world.

Florence Nightingale: Everyone who had studied about Miss Florence Nightingale knows of her devotion to the services to the poor and the sick and is also aware of what she did for humanity and to raise the status of nursing profession. Florence Nightingale was born in a wealthy English family, on 12th May 1820. As she grew off, she became interested in people and in politics. She had great desire to become a nurse though her parents were not keen on her becoming one.

1. She was dissatisfied with the dealt routine lifestyle of the upper class women of their days. She had an active mind and an interest in her surroundings beyond household and socials events.
2. She had received a classical education equal to that of men of her day. This education provided her with an understanding of the circumstances of the world in which she lived.
3. She became aware of the inadequate care being provided in hospitals, when she accompanied her mother on visits to the ill. What Nightingale saw in the hospitals intrigued her and made her want to become more involved.

In 1846, in spite of the concerns of parents and friends Nightingale became to visit and care for the sick in her community.

In addition, she visited hospitals in England and throughout Europe.

Out of her experiences she recognized that nurses required knowledge, training and discipline, if they were to be effective. Nightingale learned about the school at Kaisersworth and in 1850, she was admitted to the training program. The three years of training she received were rigorous but helped her clarify what was lacking in the current training of English nurses. After her training, in 1853 she was appointed as Superintendent of the Institution for the Care of the Sick Gentlewomen in London.

She had an opportunity to give her best service to the wounded soldiers in the Crimean War in 1854. Florence Nightingale and her nurses attended thousands of wounded and dying soldiers. Every night Florence Nightingale walked about with a lamp in her hand to help the suffering soldiers. At this time, she helped them to write letters to their families and last messages for those who were dying. She was rightly known as "The Lady with the Lamp". Nightingale and a small band of untrained nurses went to the British hospitals at Scutari in Turkey. She found the patients were laid on the floor in bloody uniforms. Equipments and facilities were not present adequately. With great compassion, she set about the task of organizing and cleaning the hospital and provided care to the wounded soldiers.

Through her efforts and the help of others, Nightingale introduced numerous improvements in the military hospital. Her efforts were largely responsible for traumatic reductions (42 % to 2%) in the wartime death rate of British Soldiers.

She also founded the first training school for nurses (St. Thomas Hospital, London, 1860). Throughout the publication of countless articles and papers, she shared her ideas about nursing and nursing education. Miss Nightingale was the first to mention **Holism (**treating the whole patient) in nursing and the first who stated that a unique body of knowledge is required to practice professional nursing.

After the war, she worked to bring about better health conditions in the British army. Nightingale almost single-handedly tried to change health care in England. Nightingale was the founder of modern nursing education. She established the Army Medical School at the Fort Pitt. Despite her ill health she worked for the development of nursing services without taking sufficient rest.

Florence founded a training school for nurses in 1860 at St. Thomas Hospital London. The funds, which were raised by the British people for her service in the Crimean War, were used for this training school. She was very much interested in improving the conditions of the army in India also. She planned a complete public health program, which was practiced in all hospitals and in the fields of nursing. She died peacefully in her sleep at the age of 90 (13th May 1910) In recognition of her meritorious help to mankind she was offered the Order of Merit in 1907.She was the first lady recipient for such an honor.

CONCLUSION

Nursing has been called the oldest of the arts and the youngest of the profession. The word nurse evolved from the Latin word nutritious, which means nourishing. The roots of medicine and nursing are intertwining and found in mythology, ancient eastern and western cultures and religion.

Nursing is defined by various authors at various times. Hansderson says "nursing is primarily assisting the individuals (sick or well) in the performances of those activities, contributing or its recovery (or to a peaceful death) that he would perform unaided, if he had the necessary strength, will or knowledge. The unique contribution of nursing is to help the individual to be independent or such assistance as soon as possible. Nursing, besides being a honorable profession, is one of the oldest arts and an essential modern occupation. Nursing is one of the greatest of humanitarian services and all people whether ill or well, rich or poor, literate or illiterate, young or old, at work or at play, in or out of hospital, are in some way or other, directly or indirectly closely associated with it. Nursing has its own body of knowledge scientifically based and humanitarianism that promises expanded benefits to people and society. It assists the individual or family to achieve their potential for self-direction for health.

Section-2

Nursing as a Profession

3 Nursing as a Profession

3.1 INTRODUCTION

Knowledge of the professions history increases the nurses awareness and promotes an understanding of the social and intellectual origins of the discipline. From the earliest history nursing was a form of community services to protect and preserve the family. Historically men and women held the role of nurse. The Code points out very clearly the role of the nurse as a leader and an active participator in professional activities by setting up and carrying out desirable standards of nursing practice and nursing education.

3.2 QUALITIES OF PROFESSIONAL NURSE

For an efficient discharging of her/his duties and for a satisfactory fulfillment of all the aims and aspirations that her/his profession stands for, the following qualities in a nurse are inevitable.

1. **Love:** With all its other attendant qualities like mercy, kindness, gentleness, patience and understanding are a must in a successful nurse. All her service for the sick and disabled are sponsored by these qualities. Without these essential characteristics the nurse becomes only a mechanical aid.
2. **Willingness and self-sacrifice:** These two qualities are complimentary to each another. Because she is willing to serve under any trying situation, a nurse sacrifices her time, comfort and even material benefits. For example, Florence Nightingale at Scutari.

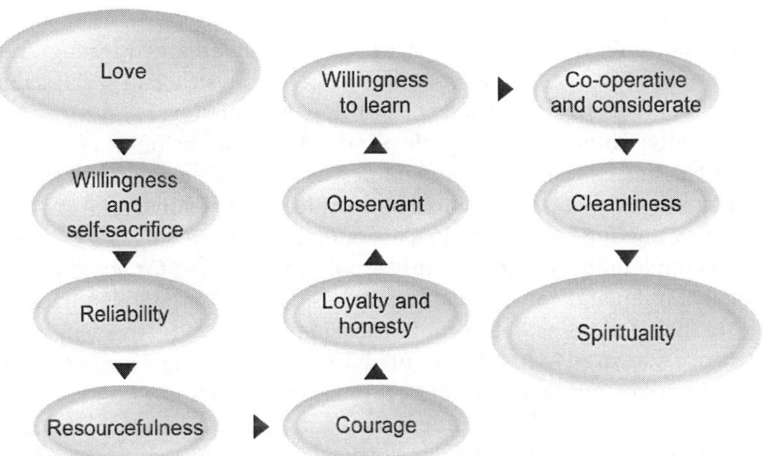

Fig. 3.1: Qualities of professional nurse

3. **Reliability:** A nurse is one who can be depended upon for a faithful discharging of her duties, the patients under her care, their families, doctors and members of the "health team" depend on her, for she is trust worthy and competent.
4. **Resourcefulness:** In critical circumstances, she uses her wisdom and knowledge and performs her duties to the best of her ability with whatever means that are at her disposal. She tackles situations with alacrity.
5. **Courage:** In times of confusion, calamity or catastrophe, the nurse manages her work with compassion and is ready to meet any problem with courage. She is cool and levelheaded and does not get agitated easily.
6. **Loyalty and honesty:** Her relationship with the patient, the doctor and her associates are marked by utmost loyalty and honesty.
7. **Observant:** A good nurse is always vigilant. She keeps a close and constant watch on the patients, their progress, their changes and reactions to treatment etc. and gives the doctor timely reports, A nurse should anticipate and meet the patients' needs.
8. **Willingness to learn:** A nurse must keep in touch with the latest discoveries and developments in medicine and treatment and must "maintain her knowledge and skill at a consistently high level".
9. **Cooperative and considerate:** A nurse learns to live in harmony with patients, doctors and other members of the health team and tries to help them in times of need.
10. **Cleanliness:** A nurse is always clean and neat personally and in her work. She must be tidy and demand high standards of cleanliness from those whom she is associated within her profession.
11. **Spirituality:** A nurse must learn to create a spiritual atmosphere for the patient and must try and help the patients to put their confidence and trust in a "Power" that is higher than any other power in the world.

3.3 NEW PERSPECTIVES OF NURSING PROFESSION

Historically, only medicine, law and the ministry were accepted as profession.

Criteria of a profession: Genevieve and Roy Bixler first wrote about the status of nursing as a profession in 1945. These criteria include the following.

1. **The services provided are vital to humanity and the welfare of the society:** Nursing is the service that is essential to the well-being of the people and to the society. Nursing promotes, maintains and restores the health of individuals, groups and communities. Assisting others to attain the highest level of wellness is the goal of nursing. Caring, meaning nurturing and helping others are the basic components of professional nursing.
2. **There is a special body of knowledge** that is continually enlarged through research. In the past, nursing was based on principles borrowed from the physical and social sciences and other disciplines. Today there is a unique body of knowledge to nursing.
3. **The services involve intellectual activities:** Individual responsibilities (accountability) are a strong feature. Nursing has developed and refined its own unique approach to practice. Nursing process is a cognitive activity that requires both critical and creative thinking and serves as the basis of providing nursing care. Individual accountability in nursing has become the hallmark of practice. Accountability is 'is being answerable to someone for something one has done I through legal opinion and court cases, society has demonstrated that nurses are individually responsible for their actions as well as for those of personnel under their supervision.
4. **Practitioners are educated in institution of higher learning**: There are basic nursing program, baccalaureate program, masters and Doctoral program in nursing.
5. **Practitioners are relatively independent and control their own policies and activities (Autonomy):** Autonomy or control over one's practice is another controversial area for nursing.

Although many nursing actions are independent, most nurses are employed in hospitals where authority resides in one's position.

6. **Practitioners are motivated by service (altruism)** and considered their work an important component of their lives. Nurses are dedicated to the ideal of service to others, which is known as altruism.
7. **There is a Code of Ethics to guide the decisions** and conduct of practitioners. The International Council of Nurses (ICN) has established Code of Nursing Ethics through which standards of practice are established, promoted and refined.
8. **There is an organization (Association)** that encourages and supports high standards of practice. Nursing has a number of professional associations that were formed to promote the improvement of the profession. Foremost among these, is the TNAI (The Trained Nurses Association of India). The purposes of TNAI are to foster high standards of nursing practice, promote professional and educational advancement of nurses and promote the welfare of the nurses.

3.4 CONCEPT OF PROFESSIONALISM IN NURSING

1. **The art of nursing:** Professional nursing practice is grounded in the art of nursing, described as taking a holistic, client-centered focus; being caring and ethical in interactions with patients, families and colleagues; having above-average interpersonal skills; and making sound judgments based on experience and knowledge, thus averting potential problems.
2. **Competence:** Professional practice demands competence in relation to knowledge and technical skills. This requires not only a broad base of knowledge, but also depth of knowledge in a chosen area of practice, a desire and ability to continue developing that knowledge base and to share it with others and critical thinking in decision-making.
3. **Attributes of practice:** Professional practice reflects a particular approach to one's work, with collaboration by far most salient characteristic. Professional nursing practice means working in partnership with other nurses and health professionals in providing client care, being highly organized in managing activities and time, having the ability to manage many complex tasks simultaneously, working autonomously as appropriate and having an open mind and nonjudgmental manner.
4. **Personal commitment:** In describing this element of professional practice, respondents referred to the importance of having confidence in one's abilities and taking responsibility for one's actions, including having a sound understanding of the boundaries and limitations of nursing practice. Having a balanced lifestyle and supporting the advancement of the profession were also considered important characteristics of a professional nurse.

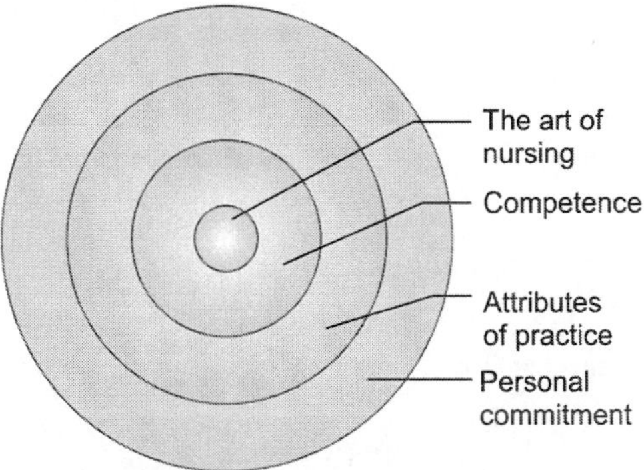

Fig. 3.2: Concept of professionalism in nursing

3.5 VALUES OF PROFESSIONAL NURSE

To be successful, nurses must be equipped with certain tools and abilities. These skills are developed over time as a nurse gains experience and confidence.

1. **Confidentiality and autonomy:** Nurses have to have an awareness of legislation on patient confidentiality and the policies of their own organization. Nurses should not breach confidentiality, unless the circumstances are exceptional. For instance, if the patient is threatening harm to himself or others. Nurses must not discuss patients' details outside of the care setting, and must take care of notes, paper and computer files. Nurses should make all efforts to promote the patient's rights to make her own decision whenever possible.
2. **Protection from harm:** The nurse's conduct must protect the patient from harm. He must not undertake something he thinks might cause harm to the patient even if he has been told or asked to do so by another person. The nurse is accountable for her own actions, and might be asked' to explain these in later proceedings. If the nurse sees anything she fears may endanger the patient, she must immediately report this to management.
3. **Professional development:** The nurse has a duty to keep up to date with all developments that may have an impact on his job. He must attend professional development and training activities. Part of his duty may involve training and mentoring new and junior staff. Nurses must meet training requirements and pay any fees needed to maintain licensing.
4. **Dedication:** Professional nursing is a difficult profession with many stressful scenarios. Nurses must work long shifts and deal with many vastly different issues on a daily basis. The combination of long work hours, constant care of patients, and the stress of seeing death can cause nurses to unravel. Thus, professional nurses need to be calm and level-headed, able to quickly handle a multitude of problems effectively. Nurses are responsible for patient quality of care and the execution of the health care plan. A dedication to the job is essential for a nurse to fulfill her nursing duties.
5. **Systems thinking:** A nurse is faced with a plenty of situations throughout each workday. Each patient has individual problems and requires a different approach. Nurses are expected to develop individualized decisions of care depending on the patient and the specific circumstances
6. **Caring:** Nurses are required to take care of the patient throughout the entire health care process. Their goal is to make the healing process and painless and comfortable as possible, without inflicting any unnecessary grief for the patient. In the case of imminent deal as of, nurses must console the patients and the families in order to ease the transition. According to the American Association of Critical Care Nurses, these duties of ca'-e include "vigilance, engagement, and responsiveness of caregivers, including family and healthcare personnel".

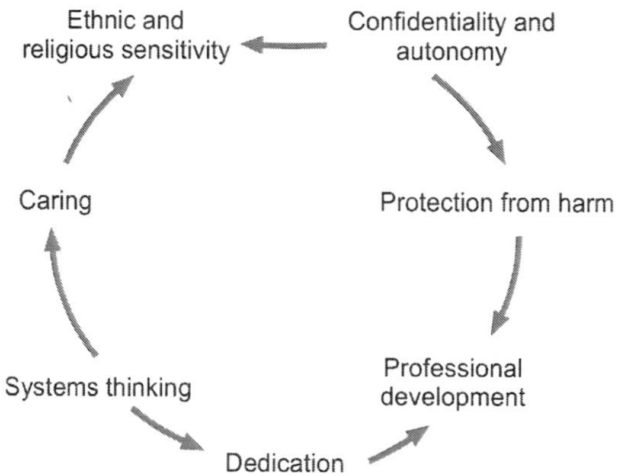

Fig. 3.3: Values of professional nurses

7. **Ethnic and religious sensitivity:** Nurses take care of patients from a variety of ethnic and religious backgrounds. Professional nurses must be sensitive to the specific requirements of various cultures and religions in order to facilitate the patient's health care. Nurses must demonstrate a desire to respect various practices while continuing to adhere to professional standards.

3.6 ROLE OF PROFESSIONAL NURSE

The professional nurse occupying a position of a professional nurse accepts responsibility and accountability in:

1. Provide quality nursing to the clients in their care, placing emphasis on the medical psychosocial, spiritual needs of the clients and be mindful of the needs of the relatives or attendants.
2. Cooperating with the nursing units and all other departments within the hospital.
3. Understanding all activities in relaxation to patient care and other assigned duties.
4. Actively participating in the nursing team.
5. Actively pursuing continuing self-education.
6. Actively providing appropriate health education to the individuals, families and groups and community at large in various settings.

3.7 FUNCTIONS AND RESPONSIBILITIES OF PROFESSIONAL NURSE

1. **Client care:** Providing safe and effective nursing care within a healthcare set up or community. It includes participating in the delivery of nursing care based on the best practice principles stated by statutory body, maintaining nursing standards, observing and participating in quality improvement programs, fostering congeniality between all members of the health care team, assisting with cost containment by utilizing resources effectively, participating in appropriate meetings, workshops or committees related to improving nursing care.

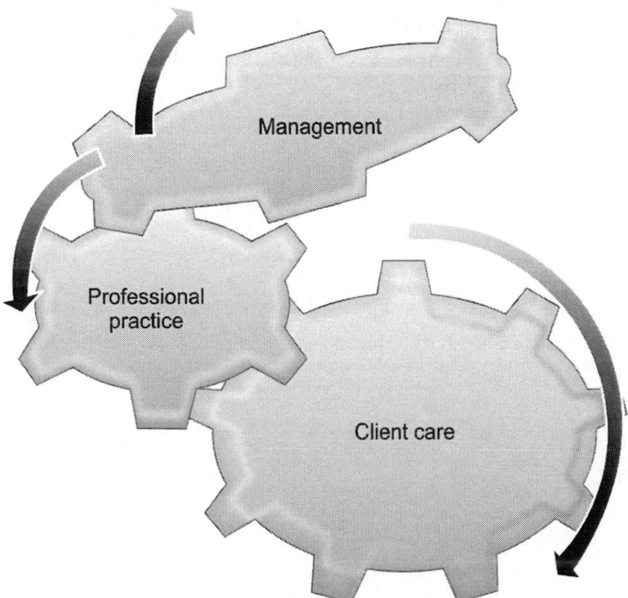

Fig. 3.4: Functions and responsibilities of professional nurse

2. **Professional practice:** In professional practice, the aspects included are maintaining confidentiality, taking reasonable care in health and safety of persons on the unit, being familiar with the resources to be used in case of any emergency or disaster, adhering to all infection control policies and safety rules, cooperating with management for health, safety and welfare provisions, actively seeking knowledge of the diagnosis and treatment given, actively participating with a zeal as a member of multidisciplinary team, complying with the professional code of ethics, demonstrating accountability and responsibility for the professional conduct, practicing with limits of own abilities and qualification, initiating and maintaining effective communication with others.
3. **Management:** There are three kinds of management roles, i.e. in planning and in organizing, in implementation and in evaluation.
    1. In planning, the management roles are to describe the planning process in the assigned clinical area, to assess client's needs, work environment and available resources, to set appropriate priorities for day's work, to anticipate and plan for potential problems or unpredictable events.
    2. In organizing, the management roles are to organize work activities, to delegate tasks and share responsibilities, to adhere to organizational policies and procedures, to describe instances of the incorporation of risk management concepts in the assigned clinical setting.
    3. In implementation, the management roles are to perform nursing procedures safely, accurately and scientific knowledge based, to describe the decision making process, to assure continuity of care, to communicate effectively with patients, families and other health personnel, to show sensitivity to the patients' needs, to bring change in the status of the organization as required.
    4. In evaluation, the management roles are to analyze the flow of communication in the unit and within the organization, to describe the nurse manager's role as evaluator of personnel performance, to assess patient care evaluation activities that are done in clinical setting.

CONCLUSION

Professional nursing practice is grounded in the art of nursing, described as taking a holistic, client-centered focus; being caring and ethical in interactions with patients, families and colleagues; having above-average interpersonal skills; and making sound judgments based on experience and knowledge, thus averting potential problems.

4 Expanded Role of the Nurse

4.1 INTRODUCTION

Contemporary nursing requires that the nurse possess knowledge and skills in a variety of areas. In the past, the principal role of nurses was to provide care and comfort as they carried out specific nursing functions, but changes in nursing have expanded the role to include increased emphasis on health promotion and illness prevention, as well as concern for the client as a whole. The contemporary nurse functions in the interrelated roles of care giver, clinical and ethical decision maker, protector and client advocate, case manager, rehabilitator, comforter, communicator, and teacher.

4.2 CARE GIVER

As care giver, the nurse helps the client regain health through the healing process. Healing is more than just curing a specific disease, although treatment skills that promote physical healing are important to care givers. The nurse addresses the holistic health care needs of the client, including measures to restore emotional, spiritual, and social well-being. The care giver helps the client and family set goals and meet those goals with a minimal cost of time and energy.

4.3 CLINICAL DECISION MAKER

To provide effective care, the nurse uses critical thinking skills throughout the nursing process. Before undertaking any nursing action, whether it is assessing the client's condition, giving care, or evaluating the results of care, the nurse plans the action by deciding the best approach for each client. The nurse makes these decisions alone or in collaboration with the client and family. In each of these situations, the nurse collaborates and consults with other health care professionals.

4.4 PROTECTOR AND CLIENT ADVOCATE

As protector, the nurse helps maintain a safe environment for the client and takes steps to prevent injury and protect the client from possible adverse effects of diagnostic or treatment measures. Confirming that a client does not have an allergy to a medication and providing immunization against disease in a community-based practice are examples of the nurse's protective role. In the role of client advocate, the nurse protects the client's human and legal rights and provides assistance in asserting those rights if the need arises. For example, the nurse may provide additional information for a client who is trying to decide whether to accept treatment. The nurse may also defend clients' rights in a general way by speaking out against policies or actions that might endanger client's well-being or conflict with their rights.

4.5 CASE MANAGER

As case manager, the nurse coordinates the activities of other members of the health care team, such as nutritionists and physical therapists, when managing a group of clients' care. In addition, nurses must also manage the own time and the resources of the practice settings. Differentiated practice models offer nurses opportunities to decisions about their career paths.

4.6 REHABILITATOR

Rehabilitation is the process by which individual's return to maximal levels of functioning after illness, other disabling events. Frequently, clients experience physical or emotional impairments that change their lives, and the nurse helps them adapt as fully as possible. Rehabilitative and restorative care activities range from teaching clients to walk with crutches to helping clients cope with lifestyle changes often associated with chronic illness.

4.7 COMFORTER

Comforter: The role of comforter, caring for the client as a person, is a traditional and historical one in nursing and has continued to be important as nurses have assumed new roles. Because nursing care must be directed to the whole person rather than simply the body, comfort and emotional support often help give the client strength to recover. While carrying out nursing activities, nurses can provide comfort by demonstrating care for the client as an individual with unique feelings and needs. As comforter, nurses should help the client reach therapeutic goals rather than encourage emotional or physical dependence.

4.8 COMMUNICATOR

The role of communicator is central to all oilier nursing roles. Nursing involves communication with clients and families, other nurses and health care professionals, resource persons, and the community. The quality of communication is a critical factor in meeting the needs of individuals, families, and communities.

4.9 TEACHER

As teacher, the nurse explains to clients concepts and facts about health, demonstrates procedures such as self-care activities, determines that the client fully understands, reinforces learning or client behavior, anti evaluates.

Progress in learning or client behavior, and evaluates progress in learning. Some teaching can be unplanned and informal, such as when a nurse responds to a question about a health issue in casual conversation. Other teaching activities may be planned and more formal, such as when the nurse teaches a client with diabetes to self-administer insulin injections. The nurse uses teaching methods that match the client's capabilities and needs and incorporates other resources, such as the family, in teaching plans.

4.10 CAREER ROLES

The proceeding roles and functions apply to all nurses in most practice settings.

Career roles, on the other hand, are specific employment positions. Because of increasing educational opportunities for nurses, the growth of nursing as a profession, and greater concern for job enrichment, the nursing profession offers expanded roles and different kinds of career opportunities. Examples of career roles include, nurse educators and advanced practice nurses, such as clinical nurse specialists, nurse practitioners, certified nurse midwives, anesthetists, administrators, and researchers. Additional no clinical roles include, risk managers, quality improvement nurses, and product consultants.

4.11 NURSE EDUCATOR

A nurse educator works primarily in schools of nursing, stall development departments (health care agencies, and client education departments. Nursing educators generally have a background in clinical nursing, which provides them with practical skills and theoretical knowledge. A faculty member in a school of nursing prepares students to function as nurses.

Nursing faculty members are responsible for teaching current nursing practice theory and necessary skills in laboratories or clinical settings. Nurse educators in nursing schools are usually required to have graduate degrees in nursing education. In addition, they generally have a specific clinical specialty and advanced clinical experience.

Nurse educators in staff development departments of health care institutions provide educational programs for nurses within their institution. These programs include orientation of new personnel, critical care nursing courses and instruction about new equipment or procedures. The primary focus of the nurse educator in an agency's department of client education is to teach or disabled clients and families to provide care in the home. In most of the care agencies, however, time budget dues not permit a separate client education department. Therefore, staff nurses usually incorporate education into a client's plan of care.

4.12 ADVANCED PRACTICE NURSE

The advanced practice nurse (APN) has a master's degree in nursing, advanced education in pharmacology and physical assessment, and certification and expertise in a specialized area of practice (American Nurse association, 1995). An APN usually works in primary, acute, restorative, or community health care agency. In addition, arm APN may specialize in the management of a disease such as cancer, diabetes, or cardiovascular or pulmonary disease or in a specific field such as pediatrics or gerontology.

4.13 CLINICAL NURSE SPECIALIST

Clinical nurse specialist: The clinical nurse specialist (CNS) has a master's degree in nursing and expertise in a specialized area of practice. A CNS may work in primary care, acute care, restorative care, and community-based settings. In addition, the CNS may specialize in specific diseases such as diabetes mellitus, cancer, or congestive heart failure or in a specific field such as pediatrics or gerontology. The CNS functions as an expert clinician, educator, case in manager, consultant, and researcher to plan or improve the quality of care provided to the client and family.

4.14 NURSE PRACTITIONER

The nurse practitioner provides health care to clients, usually in an outpatient, ambulatory care, or community-based setting and comprehensiveness of care. A significant percentage of primary care encounters extend beyond the boundaries of medicine and demand the expertise of the nurse. The nurse practitioner is able to establish a collaborative provider-client relationship. The major nurse practitioner categories are adult, family, pediatric, obstetrics- gynecology, and geriatric nurse practitioner. A nurse practitioner has the knowledge and skills necessary to detect and manage limited acute and chronic stable conditions. The nurse practitioner's educational preparation includes a practitioner program or a master's degree in nursing.

4.15 ADULT NURSE PRACTITIONER

Adult nurse practitioner (ANP) provides primary, ambulatory care to adults with a non-emergency acute or chronic illness, and in some settings tertiary care. ANPs are usually employed in ambulatory care centers or outpatient clinics and work in collaboration with a primary physician.

4.16 FAMILY NURSE PRACTITIONER

A family nurse practitioner (FNP) provides primary ambulatory care for families, usually in collaboration with a family care physician. The FNP meets the family's general health care needs, manages some illnesses by providing direct care, and guides or counsels the family as needed.

4.17 PEDIATRIC NURSE PRACTITIONER

A pediatric nurse practitioner (PNP) provides health care to infants and children. An obstetrics-gynecology nurse practitioner (OBGYN) provides primary ambulatory care to women seeking obstetrical or gynecological health care. The nurse practitioner who is also a certified nurse-midwife may independently deliver infants. GNP provides ambulatory or inpatient care to older adults. The GNP's activities include interventions for health maintenance, illness prevention, or health restoration.

4.18 CERTIFIED NURSE-MIDWIFE

Certified nurse-midwife (CNM): A CNM is an RN who is also educated in midwifery and is certified by the American College of Nurse-Midwives. The practice of nurse- midwifery involves providing independent care for women during normal pregnancy, labor, and delivery, as well as care for the newborn; it may include some gynecological services such as routine Papanicolaou (Pap) smears, family planning, and treatment for minor vaginal infections. A CNM practices with a health care agency that provides medical consultation, collaborative management and referral.

4.19 NURSE ANESTHETIST

A nurse anesthetist is an registered nurse (RN) who has received advanced training in an accredited program in anesthesiology. Nurse anesthetists provide surgical anesthesia under the guidance and supervision of an anesthesiologist, who is a physician with advanced knowledge of surgical anesthesia.

4.20 NURSE ADMINISTRATOR

Nurse administrator: A nurse administrator manages client care and the delivery of specific nursing services within a health care agency. This administrator may hold a middle-management position, such as head nurse or supervisor, or an upper-level management position, such as assistant or associate director or director of nursing services. Functions of administrators include, budgeting, staffing, strategic planning of programs and services, employee evaluation, and employee development. Middle-management position usually requires at least a baccalaureate degree in nursing, and upper-level positions generally require a master's degree.

4.21 NURSE RESEARCHER

The nurse researcher investigates problems to improve nursing care and to further define and expand the scope of nursing practice. The nurse researcher may be employed in an academic setting, hospital, or independent professional or community-service agency. The minimum educational requirement is now a doctoral degree, with at least a master's degree in nursing.

CONCLUSION

The nurses in India are also prepared and more privileged to face the changes and ready to accept the challenging roles and functions of the nurse as perceived in the globe because of the development in the education and training system. Contemporary nursing requires that the nurse possess knowledge and skills in a variety of areas. In the past the principal role of nurses was to provide care and comfort as they carried out specific nursing functions, but changes in nursing have expanded the role to include increased emphasis on health promotion and illness prevention, as well as concern for the client as a whole. The contemporary nurse functions in the interrelated roles of care giver, clinical and ethical decision maker, protector and client advocate, case manager, rehabilitator, comforter, communicator, and teacher.

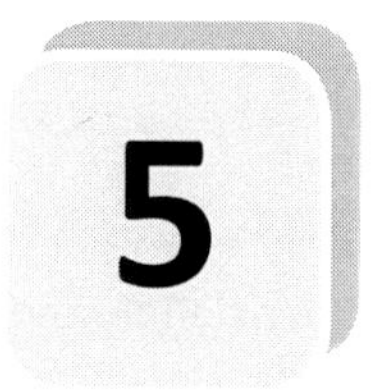

Career Opportunities in Nursing

5.1 INTRODUCTION

The goal of profession in nursing is to confirm and expand the present body of nursing knowledge, which in turn contribution to improved health care. Establishing a scientific base of nursing knowledge will provide nurses with most current principles of practice, e.g. if it could be demonstrated through research that one method of thermometer disinfections proved to be more effective than another, the better method could be adopted; a comparative study of the different methods of teaching family planning could aid in the selection of the best method for researching family planning; if a study of patient's comfort suggested that a relationship between high level of stress and visiting hours existed, visiting hours could be reduced and the effectiveness of reduced visiting hours could be further evaluated.

5.2 NURSING CAREER

Nursing shortages are often a symptom of wider health system or Nursing shortages are not just a problem for nursing stated Christine Hancock of Nurses. 'They are a health system problem, which undermines health social ailments, Nursing in many countries continues to be undervalued as 'Women's work,' and nurses are given only limited access to resources to make them effective in their jobs and careers. Health care is labor intensive and demands more nursing service. Policy makers in many countries have already recognized this fact and making necessary changes to attract the best nursing services in numbers and quality. Increases in demand are created due to these policies.

1. Be a serious student with proficiency in the health sciences.
2. Assume legal, moral and ethical accountability for your actions.
3. Use good judgment, and be loyal to patients and to the profession.
4. Demonstrate unbiased compassion for all by respecting all people regardless of age, race, social status, sexual orientation and religious beliefs.
5. Show highest degree of motivation to keep up with trends and research in the profession and to value life-long learning.
6. Learn to handle catastrophe and crisis, and everyday challenges, in a confident, efficient, and caring way.
7. Have good mental and physical health, plenty of stamina and endurance, a sense.

5.3 CAREER OPPORTUNITIES IN NURSING

1. **Nurse anesthetist:** Provides care to patients before, during and after surgery or delivery. Specific activities include physical assessment, preoperative teaching, and preparation, administration and maintenance of anesthesia. Responsible for constantly monitoring every function of the

patient's body while the patient is anesthetized. Provides care during the recovery period and as part of follow-up monitoring during the postoperative course.

2. **Nurse educator:** As the name suggests, the responsibilities include a verity of roles including teaching, research, and patient care. Central to effective teaching is the solid clinical skills developed from clinical practice. Nurse educator is responsible for lesson planning, instructing, evaluating learning, counseling, and assisting with solving learning problems. Serves as a primary resource for theory and knowledge development in the discipline of nursing.
3. **Staff nurse:** The entry-level nurse or nurse without any specialization is called staff nurse whose responsibilities include making nursing judgments based on scientific knowledge and relies on procedures and standardized care plans. The staff nurse has an incredibly complex job and advances to an intermediate level with experience and become more skilled in developing individual and innovative care plans to meet client needs.
4. **AIDS care nurse:** This is profession that takes care of a person who is certain to die within a specified time frame. AIDS care nurse responds to the physical, psychological, spiritual, and social concerns of patients with AIDS, cares for chronically ill and dying with numerous clinical manifestations.
5. **Ambulatory care nurse:** Provides for the health needs of individuals, families, and groups in diverse settings. Emphasis on helping patients stays well and independent in their home environment as long as possible.
6. **Cardiac rehabilitation nurse:** Meets the need for education and support of patients with coronary heart disease who are making lifestyle changes to prevent worsening of the disease. Monitors patients during physical workouts to prevent overexertion and or injury.
7. **Correction nurse:** Provides for the health care of inmates in correctional facilities such as juvenile offender homes, jails prisons and penitentiaries.
8. **Endoscopy nurse:** Provides essential care of patients undergoing procedures for screening, diagnosis and or treatment of gastrointestinal disorders and may specialize in endoscopy.
9. **Genetic nurse:** The genetic nurse care for people's genetic health-those with genetic problem-including screening, early detection, risk identification, treatment and testing.
10. **Infection control nurse:** Specializes in identifying, controlling and preventing outbreaks of infection in healthcare settings and the community in highly contagious situations. Activities include the collection and analysis of infection-control data; the planning, implementation and evaluation of infection prevention and control measures; the education of individuals about infection risk, prevention and control; the development and revision of infection control policies and procedures; the investigation of suspected outbreaks of infection and the provision of consultation on infection risk assessment, prevention and control strategies.
11. **Intravenous therapy nurse:** Initiates, monitors and terminates therapies including medications, antineoplastic agents, investigational drugs, blood products, and parenteral nutrition, performs venous and arterial punctures, maintain the intravascular side including tubing and dressings, monitor for infections, initiate emergency therapies, assess patients for adverse reactions and complications and document all patient-directed activities.
12. **Nephrology nurse:** Focuses on the prevention of disease and the care of patients with renal problems; works with patients in all stages of chronic renal failure, implementing treatment modalities including efforts to reserve renal function, hemodialysis, peritoneal dialysis, or transplant.
13. **Neuroscience nurse:** Care for individuals who have a dysfunction of the nervous system including alterations in consciousness and cognition, communication, mobility, rest and sleep, sensation and sexuality; plans and implements interventions to support bodily functions, promote healing, encourage adoption to persistent neurological difficulties and teaches patients and families about the illness.

14. **Occupational health nurse:** Occupational health nursing combines concepts of public health and nursing theory in an orientation toward primary prevention or keeping healthy workers healthy and includes managing workers' compensation records and counseling employees.
15. **Oncology nurse:** Cares for patients with the diagnosis of cancer in various settings; utilized an empathic and caring approach to patients whose diagnostics and treatment are often painful and life-threatening, administers chemotherapy, conducts patient teaching, and manages illness-treatment-related symptoms.
16. **Optholmic nurse:** Provides care to persons with disorders of the eyes including blindness or visual impairment; functions range from patient teaching to assistance in surgery.
17. **Perioperative nurse:** Provides for the surgical patient's needs by assessing, planning and implementing nursing care patient receive preoperatively, intraoperatively and postoperatively. Nursing activities performed by the preoperative nurse include patient assessment, creating and maintaining a sterile and safe environment.
18. **Orthopedic nurse:** Cares for the actual and potential health problem related to musculoskeletal function; relies on a holistic approach in their assessment of the impact of musculoskeletal conditions on self-care, patient management of the environment, available patient resources, and support systems.
19. **Prenatal nurse:** Cares for women, infants and their families from the onset of pregnancy through the first month of the newborn's life (prenatal period); monitors the pregnancy, assesses the progression of labor; monitors the status of mother and body, maintains a sense of clam and comfort during labor; fosters the new mother-infant relationship, teachers parenting skills, and assesses and supports the mother in her recovery from childbirth; evaluates the newborn's early adjustment to life.
20. **Psychiatric nurse:** Should possess the art of using one's self in therapeutic ways to assist patients to affect changes in self-understanding and behavior. Views individuals from a holistic perspective, taking into account both physical and mental health needs while focusing on human behavior.
21. **Plastic and reconstructive surgical nurse:** Cares for patients undergoing cosmetic and maxillofacial surgery, laser and microsurgery and nonsurgical treatments to correct aesthetic problems.
22. **Rehabilitation nurse:** The rehabilitation nurse cares for individuals who are experiencing temporary, progressive, or permanent illness or disabilities that are extensive enough to alter their normal functioning and interrupt their lifestyle.
23. **Respiratory nurse:** Promotes pulmonary health for individuals, families, and communities, and cares for persons with pulmonary dysfunction throughout the lifespan. Respiratory nursing may be preventive, acute or critical, or rehabilitative.
24. **Transplantation nurse:** Cares for recipient and living-donor patients throughout the transplantation process from and state disease to preoperative to intraoperative experience to aftercare and long-term follow up.
25. **Trauma nurse:** Trauma nursing involves responding quickly to a wide variety of single and multisystem trauma involving different patient needs, ages, cultures and severity of presenting symptoms. The trauma nurse must respond with decisiveness and clarity to unexpected events by assessing, intervening, and stabilizing patients about whom there is minimal information.
26. **Flight nurse:** Involves emergency and non-emergency air surface transport of ill and injured patients. This includes interfacility transport and emergency 'scene calls' for trauma and medical emergencies.
27. **Forensic nurse:** Forensic nursing combines clinical nursing practice with the law enforcement arena. It involves the investigation and treatment of victims of sexual assault, elder, child and spousal abuse, unexplained or accidental death, trauma and assault as well as perpetrators of these and any criminal activity.

28. **Holistic nurse:** Involves all aspects of wellness and healing of a holistic nature; holism being defined as the mind, body, spirit connection; that it, treating the whole person, not just a disease of symptom.
29. **Medical editor/author:** Involves all aspects of writing, editing and proofreading technical material for use in biomedical research, education and training, sales and marketing and other communication forms.
30. **Military nurse:** Provide all aspects of traditional nursing care and practice in both peace and wartime settings through various branches of the military service. Classifications include active duty, reserves, and civilian employment.
31. **Pediatric nurse:** Provides comprehensive care to children, adolescents and their families in various settings. Responds to the physical and psychosocial aspects of health and illness, concern for health promotion and disease prevention, management of physical and mental disabilities, and response to acute and chronic illness.
32. **Nursing informatics:** Involves all aspects of computerization as it relates to nursing and healthcare practice.
33. **Nurse anesthetist:** Perianesthesia nursing provides intensive care to patients as they awaken from anesthesia. The perianesthesia nurse prepares patients for the surgical experience, monitors and supports safe transition from anesthetized state to responsiveness, and readies patients for discharge from perianesthesia care unit.
34. **Career healing touch:** Nursing encompasses autonomous and collaborative care of individuals of all ages, families, groups and communities, sick or well and in all settings. Nursing includes the promotion of health, prevention of illness, and the care of ill, disabled and dying people. Advocacy, promotion of a safe environment, research participation in shaping health policy and inpatient and health system management, and education are also key nursing roles.
35. Nurse extends a caring hand; give a healing touch, a curing wish, and a mother's touch unconditionally to the person with a health condition of experiencing trauma. If personal and professional satisfaction and rewards are what you're looking for by caring the lives of others, nursing is for you. Nursing education makes intellectual demands on the student. Nursing career needs lot of stamina and patience.

CONCLUSION

Nurses work in all types of settings where there is a need for health care in communities, cities, and rural areas locally and globally, such as hospitals, community agencies, ambulatory care offices, home care settings, nursing homes, occupational settings, schools, public health clinics and government agencies. Nurses promote health, prevent disease and help patients cope with illness. They have a unique scope of practice and can practice independently, although they also collaborate with all members of the health care team to provide the care needed by each patient as an individual. Nurses are hands-on health professionals who provide focused and highly personalized care. The field has a wide range of career opportunities, ranging from entry-level practitioner to doctoral-level researcher. Nurses also serve as advocates for patients, families and communities. They develop and manage nursing care plans, instruct patients and their families in proper care and help individuals and groups take steps to improve or maintain their health.

Section-3

Ethical Issues

6 Nursing Ethics

6.1 INTRODUCTION

The word ethics is derived from the Greek word "Ethos" which means custom or guiding beliefs. Ethics are characteristics of a profession and are called as a "code". The ethics of nursing provides professional standards for nursing activities which protect the nurse and the patient. Ethics are the rules or principles that govern right contact. Ethics are designed to protect the rights of human being. Ethics are characteristics of a healthy profession. We have a set of ethics that is used by the nursing profession. It may be written or unwritten, but each profession has a set of ethics usually called a code. This code tells the members what kind of conduct is expected of them as they practice. It will state responsibilities of its members towards those whom they serve, their coworker, the profession and society as a whole. When a person becomes a member of a profession he/she accept the responsibility of living up to the code of ethics for that profession. It should be understood that a code of ethics is not a strict set of rules. It is a guide. Although, some behavior may be clearly correct or clearly wrong, other behaviors will depend upon the situation.

6.2 DEFINITION

1. Ethics is defined as rules for a correct behavior. Professional ethics for nursing will state the ideal way of a nurse behaving in all professional relationships (patient, patient's relatives, coworkers, members of other professions and the public).
2. Code of ethics defined what kind of conduct is expected of the members of a profession, it also used to guide professional behavior, help teachers plan education, prevent below standard practice, protect a nurse if falsely accused and guide direction for legal action.
3. Ethics is a system of understanding determinations and motivations based on individual conceptions of right or wrong. It is not determined by strict rules or rigid guidelines and although it is relatively stable, it can change over time.
4. Nursing ethics are the professional standard of conduct practiced by nurse practitioners related to or in accordance with approved moral behavior in rendering health care services.

6.3 IMPORTANCE OF ETHICS IN NURSING

1. Ethics used to guide professional behavior of the nurses.
2. It helps the teachers to know what must be taught in the education for the nurses.
3. It can be used to prevent a nurse from practicing if her/his conduct is poor and clearly below the standards set by the code.
4. It can used to protect a nurse who is falsely accused of doing something wrong.
5. It can also be used as a guide for direction when legal action must be taken in a law-suit.

6.4 HISTORY OF ETHICS IN NURSING

The primary body which creates ethical guidelines and monitors the field of nursing in the US is the American Nursing Association (Fowler, 2000). The present code of ethics for nurses was presented in 2001 and continues to be widely accepted as the correct set of ethical guidelines for the nursing field across the world. The code itself does not come out of thin air since more than a hundred years of perpetration started with the 'Nightingale Pledge' in 1893, which is similar to the Hippocratic Oath for doctors (Bett, 1960).

Nightingale Pledge

The pledge itself was little more than a paragraph and is reproduced below, but it must be noted that many of the ideals contained in the pledge continue to be seen in the present day code of ethics.

"I solemnly pledge myself before God and in the presence of this assembly, to pass my life in purity and to practice my profession faithfully. I will abstain from whatever is deleterious and mischievous, and will not take or knowingly administer any harmful drug. I will do all in my power to maintain and elevate the standard of my profession, and will hold in confidence all personal matters committed to my keeping and all family affairs coming to my knowledge in the practice of my calling. With loyalty will I endeavor to aid the physician, in his work, and devote myself to the welfare of those committed to my care (McDonald, 2006, Pg. 1)".

This pledge was used as the basis for developing a code of ethics by the American Nurses Association (ANA) which was founded in 1896. The association presented its first draft in 1926 and a tentative code in 1940, but it was only in 1950 that a code of ethics for nurses was first established. The code was revised and amended several times afterwards as the influence of time and society changed the scope of a nurse's duties and responsibilities (Rambur, 1998). Substantial revisions took place in 1968 when the code was condensed and later in 1985 with the additional of interpretive statements. The present code as it is seen today was created in 2001 (ANA, 2001).

It must be noted that whatever shape or form the code was presented in, the basic ideas behind the code of ethics have always remained the same. As discussed by the American Nursing Association (2001), these principles are:

Doing no harm, performing beneficial services, remaining loyal to the profession Honesty to oneself and the care receivers.

6.5 CURRENT ETHICAL GUIDELINES

The current code of ethics contains nine principles on which the entire structure is based. A brief description of those principles is given below, and an understanding of these principles is essential before their application and interpretation can be discussed. While some of the provisions are more or less self-explanatory, others require extensive explanations because the ethical questions associated with those provisions have no easy answers. The following summary of the provisions is a good starting point for ethics in nursing.

Provision 1: The first provision is possibly the simplest since, it asks nurses to treat all patients and professional associates with respect and compassion without any biases (ANA, 2001). The code seems to recognize that an individual can have several biases for or against people who are rich or poor, people who belong to a certain group, and individuals who have certain diseases, or even the personal characteristics of a patient/coworker. This does not stop a nurse from disliking someone for personal reasons but, in a professional capacity, the provision is very clear that there is no room for biases.

Provision 2: The second provision is the shortest of the nine since, it simply clarifies to all nurses that their main professional obligation is towards the patient. That patient can be one person or many persons in the shape of a family unit, or a group of people like a community (ANA, 2001).

While the provision is easy enough to understand, it is never easy to follow since very often a nurse could find that her behavior shows a greater commitment to her own person than anyone else (Rankin, 2000). This provision acts as a reminder that every ethical nurse will always keep the focus on the patient rather than any other individuals she comes across in a professional capacity.

Provision 3: The third provision also concerns itself with the patient, but here the focus is on the rights of the person who is being cared for. Ethically, a nurse should support and promote the rights of a patient as they are concerned with the privacy and confidentiality of the patient (ANA, 2001). At the same time, this provision demands that all nurses protect these rights and act with vigilance if they see the rights being tarnished in any way whatsoever. A breach of these rights can come from the nurse or those who are working with the nurse; therefore, the code also gives ethical guidelines on how a nurse is supposed to react to such issues. This idea is further explained in provision four of the code.

Provision 4: As is the case with other professions, whenever there is contact between two individuals certain responsibilities, duties and obligations are created based on ethical behavior (Lebacqz, 1985). This provision makes it clear that nurses are completely responsible and can be held accountable for their nursing practices (ANA, 2001). A nurse can certainly delegate certain duties to others but ethics demand that any such delegation should maintain the best ideals for patient care as a priority.

Provision 5: While several provisions ask the nurse to look outwards and focus on the patient or coworkers, provision five asks the nurse to look inwards because he owes the same responsibility to others as owed to himself (ANA, 2001). Ideally, a nurse should be able to spot problems with his own behavior and ethical lapses, if there are any, and personal integrity can be strongly supported by looking inwards (Curtin, 2000). The resulting practical benefit of this approach is increased self respect and an assurance that a nurse is experiencing continual growth in professional terms.

Provision 6: After looking inwards, the nurse can focus on the environment she is placed in to increase the value provided to patients as well as those who work in the same environment. Provision six asks nurses to work towards creating and keeping a work environment which is most conducive towards medical care (ANA, 2001). Undoubtedly, the environment has a great impact on how work is performed and how values are maintained in an office or hospital setting. Therefore, with individual and collective action, an ethical nurse should strive for improving his/her surroundings for the benefit of all concerned. At the same time, it must be remembered that the primary duty of all nurses has to be the medical care of the patients.

Provision 7: In an even larger sense, the environment of the profession can be improved if every nurse works ethically towards the improving the particular area she is focused on (ANA, 2001). For example, a nurse dealing with a patient can contribute by helping in research or by producing research material for other nurses. A nurse who works in administration can come up with better systems to manage a hospital. The methods for improvement are endless and it is an ethical obligation for all nurses to do whatever they can, whenever they can, to bring improvements to the field.

Provision 8: Of course such improvements in the local environment or the medical field may not be easy to do on your own. Therefore, provision eight recommends that it would be ethical, as well as a recommended procedure, to cooperate and collaborate with other nurses and health related professionals to bring about such changes (ANA, 2001). These efforts do not need to remain within the same state or even within the same country, since international collaboration is often required to understand how the profession can be developed further.

Provision 9: Finally, the ninth provision brings the focus back to the various bodies and groups who give ethical and other guidelines, and says that these organizations are ethically responsible for creating and maintaining the values for the nursing community (ANA, 2001). These groups also have the ethical responsibility to maintain and develop social policy and assist in the creation of local, as well as international laws, which deal with the medical fields.

Knowing all the provisions and the general flavor of the code of ethics is only the first step towards being an ethical nurse and a valued professional to the field (Walleck, 1989). The second and more important step is to understand how this code of ethics is actually beneficial for a nurse in his/her day to day work life. Additionally, the code provides significant benefits for patients under the care of the nurse; therefore it is doubly useful for all people who are influenced by the code.

6.6 NURSING ETHICS

The nursing ethics provide professional standards for nursing activities which protect the nurse and the patient. In 1973, the International Council for Nurses (INC) adopted code of ethics. The fundamental responsibility of the nurse is four fold: to promote health, to prevent illness, to restore health and to alleviate suffering. The need for nursing is universal. Inherent in nursing is respect for life dignity, and rights of men. It unrestricted by considerations of nationality, race, creed, color, age, sex, politics or social status.

Nurses render health services to the individual, the family and the community and coordinate their services with those of related groups.

Ethical involved in nursing: Ethical issues involved in various nursing branches in nursing, the branch/areas are:

1. Nursing research.
2. Nursing education.
3. Nursing administration.
4. Nursing management.
5. Intensive care unit.
6. Operation theater/surgical nursing.
7. Medical nursing.
8. Community health nursing.
9. Child health nursing.
10. Mental health nursing.
11. Maternity nursing.
12. Nursing procedures.

6.7 CODE OF ETHICS

The code of ethics will state what kind of conduct is expected from the members of a profession, what are the responsibilities of its members towards those whom they serve, their coworkers, the profession and the society as a whole. The nurse will adjust better if she understands what is a wrong/right behavior in different situations. The first such code of ethics, called the international code of nursing ethics, was adopted by the grand council of the international council of nurses at Sao Paulo, Brazil in 1953. It was later revised in Frankfurt, Germany in 1965 and then became known as International Council of Nurses (ICN) code of ethics. The most recent revision in 1973 took place in Mexico City, Mexico and resulted in the present code for nurses, revision of the code have resulted in clearer and broader standards which can be applied in any culture.

The International Code for Nurses adopted by the ICN (1973) is given in this unit. The code gives a general description of:

1. What the nurse does: the four-fold responsibility of promoting health, preventing illness, restoring health and alleviating suffering.
2. How nursing service should be given: unrestricted by nationality, race, creed, color, age, sex, politics or social status; coordinated with related groups.
3. To whom service is given: the individual, family and community.

The body of the code is made up of five sections.

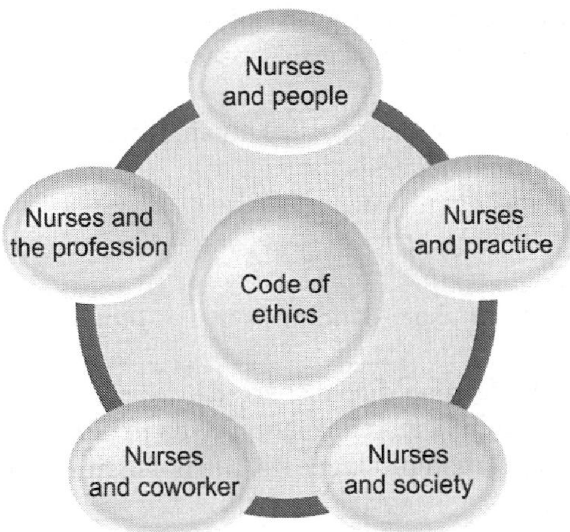

Fig. 6.1: Body of code

Nurses and people: The nurse's primary responsibility is to those people who require nursing care. The nurse holds in confidence personal information's and use judgment in sharing this information.
1. The nurse's primary responsibility is to those people who require nursing care.
2. The nurse, in providing care, promotes an environment in which the values, customs and spiritual beliefs of the individual are respected.
3. The nurse holds in confidence personal information and uses judgment in sharing this information.

Nurses and practice: The nurse maintains the highest standards of nursing care possible within the reality of a specific situation. The nurse when acting in a professional capacity should at all times maintain standards of personal conduct which credit upon the profession.
1. The nurse carries personal responsibility for nursing practice and for maintaining competence by continual learning.
2. The nurse maintains the highest standards of nursing care possible within the reality of a specific situation.
3. The nurse uses judgment in relation to individual competence when accepting and delegating responsibilities.
4. The nurse, when acting in a professional capacity, should at all times maintain standards of personal conduct which reflect credit on the profession.

Nurses and society: The nurse shares with other citizens the responsibility for initiating and supporting action to meet the health and social needs of the public.

Nurses and coworker: The nurse maintains a cooperative relationship with coworkers in nursing and other fields. The nurse takes appropriate action to safeguard the individual when his care is endangered by a coworker or any other person.
1. The nurse sustains a cooperative relationship with coworkers in nursing and other fields.
2. The nurse takes appropriate action to safeguard the individual when his care is endangered by a coworker or any other person.

Nurses and the profession: The nurse acting through the professional organization participates in establishing and maintaining equitable social and economic working conditions in nursing.
1. The nurse plays a major role in determining and implementing desirable standards of nursing practices and nursing education.
2. The nurse is active in developing a core of professional knowledge.
3. The nurse, acting through the professional organization, participates in establishing and maintaining equitable, social and economic working conditions in nursing.

The international code of nursing ethics is given below:

1. The fundamental responsibility of a nurse is to conserve life and to promote health. Every nurse is a teacher of health by example.
2. A nurse must be adequately prepared to practice nursing and be willing to continue to learn new ideas by reading, and attending meetings.
3. The nurse must learn to respect authority.
4. The nurse must carry out the doctor's orders accurately and sustain confidence in the doctor, and all members of the health team.
5. The nurse should report any unusual conditions or symptoms to the doctor or the in-charge nurse.
6. The religious beliefs of a patient should be respected.
7. The nurse should hold confidential all information given to her.
8. When a patient requires continued nursing care, the nurse must remain with the patient until adequate relief is available.
9. The nurse has the obligation to give conscientious service and, in return, is entitled to just remuneration.
10. A patient should always be called by his full name.
11. Punctuality is very important for every nurse.
12. Obedience is very important in observing rules and regulations.
13. Every nurse must have respect for authority and for rules and regulations.
14. Economy is important for all nurses to practice.

6.8 ETHICAL PRINCIPLES INVOLVED IN NURSING ETHICS

Ethical principles actually control professionalism nursing practice much more than to ethical theories. Principles encompass basic promises from which rules are developed. Principles are the moral norms that nursing, as a profession, both demands and strives to implement to every day clinical practice. Ethical principle that the nurse should consider when making decisions are as follows:

1. Respect for persons.
2. Respect for autonomy.
3. Respect for freedom.
4. Respect for beneficence (doing good).
5. Respect for nonmaleficence (avoiding harm to others).
6. Respect for veracity (truth telling).
7. Respect for justice (fair and equal treatment).
8. Respect for rights.
9. Respect for fidelity (fulfilling promises).
10. Confidentiality (protecting privileged information).

1. **Respect for persons:** Respect for persons not only applies to clinical situations, but also to all life's situations. It directs individuals to treat themselves and others with a respect inherent to man's humanness. It requires recognition on a sense that all mankind shared a common human destiny. The respect to persons needs to be simplified as it affects nursing practice.
2. **Autonomy:** Autonomy that individuals are able to act for themselves to the level of their capacity. It is the right of individual to govern their actions according to their own purpose and reason. Respect for autonomy requires that persons honor another's right to govern him or her. The legal doctrine of informed consent is the direct reflection of autonomy. So, it requires that health personnel obtain a patient's informed consent for treatment and for participation in research.

The followings are required for a patient to give informed consent for either:

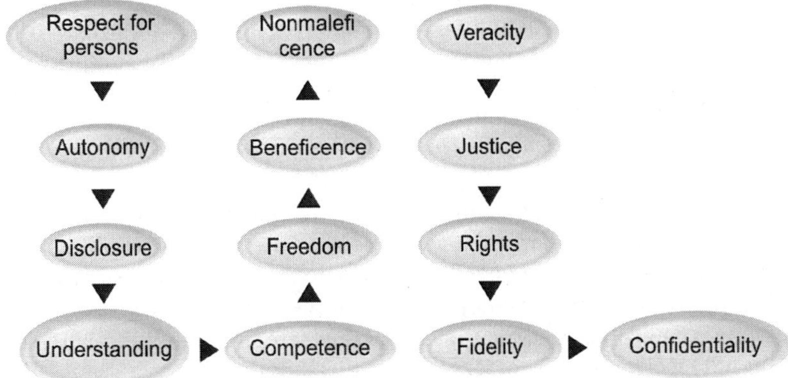

Fig. 6.2: Ethical principles involved in nursing ethics

3. **Disclosure:** Adequate presentation of relevant information about the proposed treatment or study.
4. **Understanding:** Adequate comprehension of the disclosed information.
   Voluntary agreement: Free assent, influenced by external controlling factors.
5. **Competence:** Adequate decision making capacity. There are three type of autonomy, i.e., freedom of action, freedom of choice and effective deliberation.
6. **Freedom:** The principle of individual freedom decrease that patients be exempt from control by others to select and pursue personal health goals. Nurses as a group believe that patient should have greater freedom of choice within the nation's health care system. This principle should be observed by staff nurses when planning patient care; by nurse manager when leading subordinates.
7. **Beneficence:** The beneficence principle states that the actions one takes should promote good. It dictates that a person is obliged to help others to advance their legitimate and important interests; it requires the balancing of harms and benefits. Benefits promote the client's welfare and health, whereas harms or risks detract from the client's health and welfare. In other words, providing benefits that enhance the others welfare, whereas balancing the benefits and harms of intervention made on the others behalf.
   Professional education provides awareness that most nursing interventions are capable of producing undesirable, as well as desirable, patient outcome. Therefore, the nurse is obliged to ascertain each care measure, likelihood of success, and balance the measures probable benefits and risks in order to select interventions that maximize patient's welfare.
8. **Nonmaleficence:** The corollary of beneficence, the principle of nonmaleficence states that one should do no harm. The nurse should interpret the term 'harm' to mean emotional and social as well as physical injury. Harm is thwarting, defeating, or setting back one person's interest through invasive action by another. Many nurses find it difficult to follow the principle when performing treatment and procedures that bring discomfort and pain to patients. When the principle of sanctity of human life guides healthcare decisions, the principle of nonmaleficence prohibits active and passive enthusive by caregivers of terminally ill patients. As nurse manager performing performance evaluation of subordinates should emphasize their good qualities and give positive direction for growth. Destroying the employees self-esteem and self-worth would be considered doing harm their principles.

9. **Veracity:** It concerns truth telling an incorporates the concept that individuals should always tell the truth. It requires professional caregivers to provide with accurate, reality-based information about their health status and care or treatment prospect. Truth telling is an ethical concern for nurse, because truth is the basis for mutual trust between patient and nurse, and trust is the basis for patient's hope of benefit from nursing services. Nurse managers use this principle when they give all the facts of a situation, truthfully and assist their employees to make decisions. However, truth telling may be difficult in a healthcare relationship. Some information that is transmitted from nurse to patient is depressing and/or frightening, e.g. bad news about personal health status.
10. **Justice:** It concerns the issue that persons should be treated equally and fairly. This principle of justice requires treating others fairly and giving persons their due. When there are resources to distribute in healthcare, nurses should allocate them in such a way that equal shares go to equal recipients. The following problems complicate the application of justice:
    1. Not everyone is equal in every way; sometimes there are situations in which it seems that one person should receive a greater or lesser share than another.
    2. Resources are limited. There is not always enough for each person to receive an equal share. Questions of justice relate to the fairness with which benefits and burdens are distributed among people. Experience in turn found various principles have to be proposed to guide fair distribution of society's good are as follows:
        a. Each person should receive an equal share.
        b. The amount given to each person should be proportional to his or her need.
        c. The amount given to each person should be proportional to the amount of his or her work effort,
        d. The amount given to each person should reflect the value of his or her work product.
        e. The amount given to each person should reflect his to her value to society.
        f. The amount given to each person should be determined by free market exchange. These principles usually arise in times of short supplies or when there is competition for resources of benefits.
11. **Rights:** Right is an entitlement to behave in certain way under circumstances, such as nurse's entitlement to freely express personal beliefs and preferences by voting in a political election. Another right is the prerogative to define another's behavior in selected situations, such as manager's prerogative to give assignments to subordinates. A right is also a claim to a specific good, service or prerequisite such as tea break time. Right is also used to mean agreement with justice, law and morality. So, right may be mental rights or legal rights related to respective profession.
    1. The patient has the right to every consideration of his privacy concerning his own medical care program.
    2. The patient has the right to expect that all communications and records pertaining to his care should be treated as confidential.
    3. The patient has the right to expect that within its capacity a hospital must make reasonable response to the request of a patient for services.
    4. The patient has the right to obtain information as to any relationship of his hospital to other healthcare and educational institutions in so far as his care is concerned and any professional relationships among individuals, by name, who are treating him.
    5. The patient has the right to be advised if the hospital proposes to engage in or perform human experimentation affecting his care or treatment and has the right to refuse to participate.
    6. The patient has the right to expect reasonable continuity of care.
    7. The patient has the right to examis and receive an explanation of his bill regardless of source of payment.
    8. The patient has the right to know what hospital rules and regulations apply to his conduct as a patient.

12. **Fidelity:** It is keeping one's promises or commitments. The principle of fidelity holds that a person should faithfully fulfill his duties and obligations. Fidelity is important in a nurse because a patient's hope for relief and recovery rests on evidence of caregiver's conscientiousness. Nurse managers abide by this principle when they follow through on any promise they have previously made to employees, such as promised leave, a certain shift to be worked or a promotion to perception within the unit.
13. **Confidentiality:** It is the duty to respect privileged information. The principle of confidentiality provides that caregivers should respect a patient need for privacy and use personal information about him or her only to improve care. Nurses should practice confidentiality to decrease patient vulnerability and share from widespread knowledge of personal information divulged during care.

6.9 STATEMENTS OF ETHICAL RESPONSIBILITY

1. Caring demands, the provision of helping services that is appropriate to the needs of the client and significant to others.
2. Caring recognizes the client's membership in a family and community, and provides for the participation of significant others in his or her care.
3. Caring acknowledges the reality of death in the life of every person, and demands that appropriate support provided to the dying person and family to enable that to prepare for, and to cope with death when it is inevitable.
4. Caring acknowledges that the human person has the capacity to fact up to health needs and problems in his or her own unique way, and directs nursing action in a manner that will assist the client to develop, maintain or gain personal autonomy, self-respect and self-determination.
5. Caring, as a response to a health need, requires the consent and the participation of the person who is experiencing the need.
6. Caring dictates that the client and significant others have the knowledge and information adequate for free and informed decisions concerning care requirements, alternative and preferences.
7. Caring demands that the needs of the client supersede those of the nurse.
8. Caring acknowledges the vulnerability of a client in certain situations and dictates restraint in actions which might compromise the client's rights and privileges.
9. Caring involving a relationship which is, in itself therapeutic, demands mutual respect and trust.
10. Caring acknowledges that information obtained in the course of the nursing relationship is privileged and that is requires the full protection of confidentiality unless such information provides evidence of serious impending harm to the client or to a third party, or is legally required by the courts.
11. Caring requires that the nurse represents the needs of the client and that the nurse takes appropriate measures when fulfillment of these needs is jeopardized by the actions of other persons.
12. Caring acknowledges the dignity of all persons in the practice of educational setting.
13. Caring acknowledges respects and draws upon the competencies of others.
14. Caring establishes the conditions for the harmonization of efforts of different helping professionals in providing required services to clients.
15. Caring seeks to establish and maintain a climate of respect for the honest dialogue needed for effective collaboration.
16. Caring establishes the legitimacy of respectful challenge and or confrontation when the service required by the client is compromised by in competency, incapacity or negligence or when the competencies of the nurses are not acknowledged or appropriately utilized.

17. Caring demands the provision of working conditions which enable nurses to carry out their legitimate and responsibilities.
18. Caring demands resourcefulness and restraint accountability for the use of time, resources, equipment, and funds, and requires accountability to appropriate individuals and/or bodies.
19. Caring requires that the nurse bring to the work situation in education, practice, administration or research, the knowledge, affective and technical skills required, and that competency in these areas be maintained and updated.
20. Caring commands fidelity, oneself, and guards the right and privilege of the nurse to act in keeping with an informed moral conscience.

6.10 MEANING AND RELATIONSHIP OF PROFESSIONAL ETHICS AND ETIQUETTES

Etiquettes mean good manners. We all learn certain standards of social etiquette in daily life. It means that we know how to behave with courtesy and respect as we relate with other people. For example, we learn when it is correct to remain seated or to rise in different kinds of social situations. We also learn how to make another person feel welcome comfortable and at ease, much of what we learn to do in these relationships depends upon the social customs of the community in which we live.

Professional etiquette means "good manners" in professional relationship just as we learn social etiquette, we must learn that etiquette is acceptable and expected of us in our professional relationships it is essential for successful working, relationships with those in authority nursing colleagues, members of other professions, patients and those in society.

To help us learn what professional etiquette is expected of us the following discussion is centered upon professional relationships and standards of behavior which have been developed and accepted by the nursing profession it must be remembered that these standards will vary according to the society in which they are practiced in all situations, however professional etiquette is based upon the same characteristic that is consideration and respect for others.

Nothing is more important than practicing these two things in everyday behavior. Developing good relationships in all area of life will help you to become a better person and will lead you to develop greater cooperation and understanding in your professional relationships and activities.

Professional etiquette: Etiquette means good manner, it tells how to behave with courtesy and respect as we relate with other people. Professional etiquette means good manner in professional relationship. It is essential for successful working relationship with those in authority, nursing colleagues, and members of other profession, patients and those in society. It must be remembered that these standards will vary according to the society in which they are practiced. Professional etiquette is based upon the characteristics, which are consideration and respect for others.

Employment etiquette: Professional success and reputation depend upon practicing good professional etiquette. Advertising in nursing journals and newspaper, direct contact with institutions and professional organizations and informal contacts with experienced nursing personnel's are the best sources of information about vacant positions. Application for a position may be sent through a letter or application with or without a resume, an application form supplied by an employer or by personal interview.

Resigning from a position: Resignation letter should be submitted in good business form, well in advance, of your planned departure, depending upon the circumstances. Early notification is helpful for staffing and planning by the administration under which you presently work. A resignation should never be written unless you are sure that you are leaving. The letter of resignation should be typed or printed clearly in approved business form on plain white paper. Your reasons for leaving should be expressed in a polite, honest and objective manner. You should also express appreciation for the experience you have had and express regret for the necessity of leaving. You should hand over charge to another responsible person before you quit the hospital. Proper notification is professional and important when submitting a resignation. A notice of one month is considered courteous except in emergency cases. Professional success and reputation depend upon practicing good professional etiquette.

6.11 PROFESSIONAL ETIQUETTES FOR NURSES

Etiquette is a code of good manners that a nurse should follow. The nurse is an important member of the health team that must work in cooperation and harmony for the care of the sick. For a smooth functioning and a good interpersonal relationship, you as a nurse should follow certain essential good manners.

1. The nurse should be courteous to all. Be gentle and polite in your talk.
2. The nurse should greet your seniors, coworkers, your patients etc. with appropriate words and according to the time of the day, e.g. good morning, good evening.
3. The nurse should address the seniors with proper title, e.g. sir, madam, sister, mister, miss, etc.
4. Stand up when people of higher rank enter your room.
5. Stand up when answering questions in the class room.
6. Open the door for the senior and stand aside for them to pass.
7. Excuse yourself when overtaking a senior person.
8. Stand aside and give way to senior when you cross them on the ways, e.g. in the corridors, on the staircases etc.
9. Maintain silence wherever and whenever necessary, e.g. class room, library, study room and dormitories.
10. Keep your dress neat and tidy (series arranged and the hair put up).
11. While on duty never use any form of jewellery that may interfere with work.
12. Obey seniors without arguing.
13. Help the seniors to carry a heavy load if you find them on the way.
14. Say “thank you” when some one is doing a favor for you, and also when someone corrects you.
15. Get prior permission from the sister in-charge before you take any article from any department.
16. Do not delay the answers to the questions. Give the answer immediately and appropriately.
17. Always be punctual.
18. Avoid thumb sucking and nail biting.
19. In an assembly, let the senior take the seat first.
20. Keep eye contact and sit face to face when listing to some one.
21. Say “Excuse me” even if you hurt others accidentally.
22. Never let others secret go out of you.
23. Always close the door after getting into a room or when you get out of the room, if so desired.
24. Knock at the door and wait for the answer before you enter into other’s room.
25. Do not cover the mouth while talking to others. Cover your mouth when you cough or sneeze.
26. Excuse yourself before you interfere with others engaged in talking or doing some work.
27. The nurse should not give and receive any gifts or present especially from the patients and their relatives.

CONCLUSION

Nursing ethics is a branch of applied ethics that concerns itself with activities in the field of nursing. Nursing ethics shares many principles with medical ethics, such as beneficence, nonmaleficence and respect for autonomy. It can be distinguished by its emphasis on relationships, human dignity and collaborative care. The need of nursing is universal. Inherent in nursing is respect for life, dignity, and rights of man; it is unrestricted by considerations of nationality, race, creed, color, age, sex, politics or social status. Nurses render health services to the individual, the family, and the community and coordinate their services with those of related groups.

7 Code of Ethics in Nursing

7.1 INTRODUCTION

Nursing has a code of ethics that defines the principles by which nurse provide care to their clients. In addition, nurses incorporate their own values and ethics into practice. The code of ethics for nurses with interpretive statements provides a guide for carrying out nursing responsibilities that provide quality nursing care and provides for the ethical obligations of the profession. Codes are effective in accomplishing their goals only to the extent that they are uphold by members of the profession.

7.2 DEFINITION

1. A code of ethics is a guide for an individual or group to follow in making decisions regarding ethical issues.
2. Code of ethics is a set of ethical principles that generally are accepted by members of a profession.
3. Ethical principles are moral norms that nursing as a profession, both demands and strives to implement in everyday clinical practice.

7.3 PURPOSES OF CODE OF ETHICS

A code of ethics is a formal statement of a group's ideals and values. Codes of ethics are usually higher than legal standards, and they can never be less than the legal standards of profession. Nursing code of ethics have the following purposes:

1. To inform the public about the minimum standards of the profession and to help them understand professional nursing conduct.
2. To provide a sign of the profession's commitment to the public it serves.
3. To outline the major ethical considerations of the profession.
4. To provide general guidelines for professional behavior.
5. To guide the profession in self-regulation.
6. To remind nurse of the special responsibility they assume when caring for clients.

7.4 FUNCTIONS OF CODE OF ETHICS

Nursing codes of ethics inform both nurses and society of the primary goals and values of the profession. These should compatible with the nurse's personal value system and moral code.

Table 7.1: Functions of ethics

S.N	Functions	Description
1	Responsibility	Indicating nursing acceptance of the responsibility and trust with which it has been invested by society.
2	Guidance	Providing guidance for conduct and relationships in carring out nursing responsibilities consistent with the ethical obligations of the profession and with the high-quality care.
3	Self-regulation	Proving a means for exercise of professional self-regulation.

7.5 INTERNATIONAL COUNCIL OF NURSING-CODE OF ETHICS

The fundamental responsibility of the nurse is fourfold-to promote health, to prevent illness, to restore health, and to alleviate suffering. The need of nursing is universal. Inherent in nursing is respect for life, dignity, and rights of humans. It is unrestricted by considerations of nationality, race, creed, age, sex, politics or social status.

Table 7.2: Code of ethics by ICN

S.N	ICN-Code	Description
1	Nurses and people	• The nurse primary responsibility is to those people who require nursing care. • The nurse in providing care, promotes an environment in which the values, customs and spiritual beliefs of the individual are respected. • The nurse holds in confidence personal information and use judgments in sharing this information.
2	Nurses and practice	• The nurse carries personal responsibility for nursing practice and for maintain competence by continual learning. • The nurse maintains the highest standards of nursing care possible with in the reality of a specific situation. • The nurse uses judgment in relation to individual competence when accepting and delegating responsibility. • The nurse when acting in a professional capacity, should at all times maintain standards of personal conduct that reflect credit on the profession.
3	Nurses and society	• The nurse shares with other citizen the responsibility for initiating and supporting action to meet the health and social needs of the public.
4	Nurses and coworker	• The nurse sustains a cooperative relationship with coworker in nursing and other fields. • The nurse takes appropriate action to safeguard the individual when his or her is endangered by a coworker or any other person.
5	Nurses and the profession	• The nurse plays the major role in determining and implementing desirable standards of nursing practice and nursing education. • The nurse is active in developing a core of professional knowledge. • The nurse, acting through the professional organization, participates in establishing and maintaining equitable social and economic working conditions.

7.6 AMERICAN NURSES ASSOCIATION CODE FOR NURSE

Founded in 1896 as the Nurses Associated Alumnae, the American Nurses Association is an organization that works to promote and protect the field of nursing. They are directly involved in establishing the standards of practice in the field, as well as promoting workplace rights and safe conditions for nurses. The organization has 54 constituent member associations. Multiple subsidiaries of the American Nurses Association exist that focus on more specific needs of nurses. The American Academy of Nursing works to improve nursing knowledge, while the American Nurses Foundation focuses on charitable work. At times, they come into conflict with other organizations, such as the American Diabetes Association, when they disagree on issues of health or safety.

A nursing code of ethics cannot remain a stagnant document. As new issues arise in nursing and healthcare practice, they must be addressed and possibly included in a formal statement. The American Nurses Association (ANA) Code for Nurses with Interpretive Statements was approved in 1985 and was still being used in mid-2001. A task force met in 1996 and began the process of reviewing and revising the code. A draft of the new code is anticipated to be approved and released in 2001. The new code is more comprehensive than the 1985 code. It is the responsibility of all professional nurses to be aware of the Code for Nurses and any changes that may be made in the future. It is also the responsibility of each individual nurse to practice ethical care on a daily basis.

Table 7.3: Code of ethics by ANA

S.N	Code	Description
1	Provide service	The nurse provides services with respect for human dignity and the uniqueness of the patient unrestricted by considerations and social or economic status, personal attributes, or the nature of health problems.
2	Confidentiality	The nurse safeguard the patient's right to privacy by judiciously protecting information of a confidential nature.
3	Safeguard the patient's right	The nurse acts to safeguard the patient and the public when health care and safety are affected by the incompetent, unethical, or illegal practice of any person.
4	Responsibility and accountability	The nurse assumes responsibility and accountability for individual nursing judgment and actions.
5	Competence	The nurse maintains competence in nursing
6	Informed judgment	The nurse exercise informed judgment and uses individual competence and qualifications as criteria in seeking consultation, accepting responsibilities and delegating nursing activities to others.
7	Contributes in developments	The nurse participates in activities that contribute to the ongoing development of the profession's body of knowledge.
8	Improvement of standards	The nurse participates in the profession's efforts to implement and improve standards of nursing.
9	Participates in professional efforts	The nurse participates in the profession's efforts to establish and maintain conditions of employment conductive to high quality nursing care.
10	Protect public	The nurse participates in the profession's efforts to protect the public for misinformation and misrepresentation and to maintain the integrity of nursing.
11	Practice environments	The nurse collaborates with members of the health professions and other citizens in promoting community and national efforts to meet the health needs of the public.

7.7 CANADIAN NURSES ASSOCIATION CODE OF ETHICS

The Canadian Nurses Association's *Code of Ethics for Registered Nurses* is a statement of the ethical values of nurses and of nurses' commitments to persons with health-care needs and persons receiving care. It is intended for nurses in all contexts and domains of nursing practice and at all levels of decision-making. It is developed by nurses for nurses and can assist nurses in practicing ethically and working through ethical challenges that arise in their practice with individuals, families, communities and public health systems. A value is something that is prized or held dear; something that is deeply cared about.

This code is organized around seven primary values that are central to ethical nursing practice:

Table 7.4: Code of ethics by CAN

S.N	Elements	Description
1	Health and well-being	Nurses values health and well-being and assist patients to achieve their optimal level of health in situations of normal health, illness or injury or in the process of dying.
2	Choice	Nurses respect and promote the autonomy of patients and help them to express their health needs and values and to obtain appropriate information and services.
3	Dignity	Nurses value and advocate the dignity and self-respect of human being.
4	Confidentiality	Nurses safeguard the trust of patients so that information learned in the context of a professional relationship is shared outside the health care team only with the patient's permission or as legally required.
5	Fairness	Nurses apply and promote principles of equity and fairness to assist patients in receiving unbiased treatment and a share of health services and resources proportionate to their needs.
6	Accountability	Nurses act in a manner consistent with their professional responsibilities and standards of practice.
7	Practice environments	Practice environments that are conducive to safe, competent and ethical care. Nurses advocate practice environments that have the organizational and human support system and the resources allocations necessary for safe, competent and ethical nursing care.

Each value is articulated by responsibility statements that clarify its application and provide more direct guidance. Where it is clear that an action or inaction would involve an ethical violation (i.e. the neglect of a moral obligation), the level of guidance is prescriptive. The statement is intended to tell the nurse and others what is ethically acceptable and what is not. Where the situation involves an ethical problem or dilemma, guidance is advisory. No ready-made answers can be offered and thoughtful consideration is required to increase the quality of decision-making.

Where the situation provokes feelings of guilt, concern, or distaste, it is a situation of ethical distress. In instances of ethical distress, the level of guidance is more limited but there remains a responsibility for the nurse to examine the situation in light of the provisions of the code. Decisions will be influenced by the particular circumstances of the situation. Ethical reflection and judgment are required to determine how a particular value or responsibility applies in a particular nursing context. There is room within the profession for disagreement among nurses about the relative weight of different ethical values and principles. More than one proposed intervention may be ethical and reflective of good practice.

Discussion is extremely helpful in the resolution of ethical issues. As appropriate, clients, colleagues in nursing and other disciplines, professional nurses' associations and other experts are included in discussions about ethical problems. In addition to this code, legislation, and the standards of practice, policies, and guidelines of professional nurses associations may also assist in problem-solving.

The values articulated in this code are grounded in the professional nursing relationship with clients and indicate what nurse's care about in that relationship. For example, to identify health and well-being as a value is to say that nurses care for and about the health and well-being of their clients. The nurse-client relationship presupposes a certain measure of trust on the part of the client. Care and trust complement one another in professional nursing relationships. Both hinge on the values identified in the code. By upholding these values in practice, nurses earn and maintain the trust of those in their care. For each of the values, the scope of responsibilities identified extends beyond individuals to include families, communities and society.

7.8 HEALTH AND WELL-BEING

Nurses value health and well-being and assist persons to achieve their optimum level of health in situations of normal health, illness, injury, or in the process of dying.

1. Nurses provide care directed first and foremost toward the health and well-being of the client.
2. Nurses recognize that health is more than the absence of disease or infirmity and assist clients to achieve the maximum level of health and well-being possible.
3. Nurses recognize that health status is influenced by a variety of factors. In ways that are consistent with their professional role and responsibilities, nurses are accountable for addressing institutional, social, and political factors influencing health and health care.
4. Nurses support and advocate a full continuum of health services including health promotion and disease prevention initiatives, as well as diagnostic, restorative, rehabilitative and palliative care services.
5. Nurses respect and value the knowledge and skills other health care providers bring to the health care team and actively seek to support and collaborate with others so that maximum benefits to clients can be realized.
6. Nurses foster well-being when life can no longer be sustained, by alleviating suffering and supporting a dignified and peaceful death.
7. Nurses provide the best care circumstances permit even when the need arises in an emergency outside an employment situation.
8. Nurses participate, to the best of their abilities, in research and other activities that contribute to the ongoing development of nursing knowledge. Nurses participating in research observe the nursing profession's guidelines, as well as other guidelines, for ethical research.

7.9 AUTONOMY

Nurses respect and promote the autonomy of clients and help them to express their health needs and values, and to obtain appropriate information and services.

1. Nurses seek to involve clients in health planning and health care decision-making.
2. Nurses provide the information and support required so that clients, to the best of their ability, are able to act on their own behalf in meeting their health and health care needs. Information given is complete, accurate, truthful, and understandable. When they are unable to provide the required information, nurses assist clients in obtaining it from other appropriate sources.
3. Nurses demonstrate sensitivity to the willingness/readiness of clients to receive information about their health condition and care options. Nurses respect the wishes of those who refuse, or are not ready, to receive information about their health condition.
4. Nurses practice within relevant legislation governing consent or choice. Nurses seek to ensure that nursing care is authorized by informed choice, and are guided by this ideal when participating in the consent process in cooperation with other members of the health team.
5. Nurses respect the informed decisions of competent persons to refuse treatment and to choose to live at risk. However, nurses are not obliged to comply with clients' wishes when doing so would require action contrary to the law. If the care requested is contrary to the nurse's moral beliefs, appropriate care is provided until alternative care arrangements are in place to meet the client's needs.
6. Nurses are sensitive to their position of relative power in professional relationships with clients and take care to foster self-determination on the part of their clients. Nurses are sufficiently clear about personal values to recognize and deal appropriately with potential value conflicts.

7. Nurses respect decisions and lawful directives, written or verbal, about present and future health care choices affirmed by a client prior to becoming incompetent.
8. Nurses seek to involve clients of diminished competence in decision-making to the extent that those clients are capable. Nurses continue to value autonomy when illness or other factors reduce the capacity for self-determination, such as by providing opportunities for clients to make choices about aspects of their lives for which they maintain the capacity to make decisions.
9. Nurses seek to obtain consent for nursing care from a substitute decision-maker when clients lack the capacity to make decisions about their care, did not make their wishes known prior to becoming incompetent, or for any reason it is unclear what the client would have wanted in a particular circumstance.

When prior wishes of an incompetent client are not known or are unclear, care decisions must be in the best interest of the client and based on what the client would want, as far as is known.

7.10 SELF-RESPECT OF HUMAN BEING

Nurses value and advocate the dignity and self-respect of human beings.

1. Nurses relate to all persons receiving care as persons worthy of respect and endeavour in all their actions to preserve and demonstrate respect for each individual.
2. Nurses exhibit sensitivity to the client's individual needs, values, and choices. Nursing care is designed to accommodate the biological, psychological, social, cultural, and spiritual needs of clients. Nurses do not exploit clients' vulnerabilities for their own interests or gain, whether this be sexual, emotional, social, political, or financial.
3. Nurses respect the privacy of clients when care is given.
4. Nurses treat human life as precious and worthy of respect. Respect includes seeking out and honouring clients' wishes regarding quality of life. Decision-making about life-sustaining treatment carefully balances these considerations.
5. Nurses intervene if others fail to respect the dignity of clients.
6. Nurses advocate the dignity of clients in the use of technology in the health care setting.
7. Nurses advocate health and social conditions that allow persons to live with dignity throughout their lives and in the process of dying. They do so in ways that are consistent with their professional role and responsibilities.

7.11 CONFIDENTIALITY

Nurses safeguard the trust of clients that information learned in the context of a professional relationship is shared outside the health care team only with the client's permission or as legally required.

1. Nurses observe practices that protect the confidentiality of each client's health and health care information.
2. Nurses intervene if other participants in the health care delivery system fail to respect client confidentiality.
3. Nurses disclose confidential information only as authorized by the client, unless there is substantial risk of serious harm to the client or other persons, or a legal obligation to disclose. Where disclosure is warranted, both the amount of information disclosed and the number of people informed is restricted to the minimum necessary.
4. Nurses, whenever possible, inform their clients about the boundaries of professional confidentiality at the onset of care, including the circumstances under which confidential information might be disclosed without consent. If feasible, when disclosure becomes necessary, nurses inform clients what information will be disclosed, to whom, and for what reasons.

5. Nurses advocate policies and safeguards to protect and preserve client confidentiality and intervene if the security of confidential information is jeopardized because of a weakness in the provisions of the system, e.g., inadequate safeguarding guidelines and procedures for the use of computer databases.

7.12 EQUITY OR FAIRNESS

Nurses apply and promote principles of equity and fairness to assist clients in receiving unbiased treatment and a share of health services and resources proportionate to their needs.

1. Nurses provide care in response to need regardless of such factors as race, ethnicity, and culture, spiritual beliefs, social or marital status, gender, sexual orientation, age, health status, lifestyle or the physical attributes of the client.
2. Nurses are justified in using reasonable means to protect against violence when they anticipate acts of violence toward themselves, others or property with good reason.
3. Nurses strive to be fair in making decisions about the allocation of services and goods that they provide, when the distribution of these is within their control.
4. Nurses put forward, and advocate, the interests of all persons in their care. This includes helping individuals and groups gain access to appropriate health care that is of their choosing.
5. Nurses promote appropriate and ethical care at the institutional/agency and community levels by participating, to the extent possible, in the development, implementation, and ongoing review of policies and procedures designed to make the best use of available resources and of current knowledge and research.
6. Nurses advocate, in ways that are consistent with their role and responsibilities, health policies and decision-making procedures that are fair and comprehensive, and that promote fairness and inclusiveness in health resource allocation.

7.13 ACCOUNTABILITY

Nurses act in a manner consistent with their professional responsibilities and standards of practice.

1. Nurses comply with the values and responsibilities in this code of ethics for registered nurses as well as with the professional standards and laws pertaining to their practice.
2. Nurses conduct themselves with honesty and integrity.
3. Nurses, whether they are engaged in clinical, administrative, research, or educational endeavors, have professional responsibilities and accountabilities toward safeguarding the quality of nursing care clients receive. These responsibilities vary but are all oriented to the expected outcome of safe, competent and ethical nursing practice.
4. Nurses, individually or in partnership with others, take preventive as well as corrective action to protect clients from unsafe, incompetent or unethical care.
5. Nurses base their practice on relevant knowledge, and acquire new skills and knowledge in their area of practice on a continuing basis, as necessary for the provision of safe, competent and ethical nursing care.
6. Nurses, whether engaged in clinical practice, administration, research or education, provide timely and accurate feedback to other nurses about their practice, so as to support safe and competent care and contribute to ongoing learning. By doing so, they also acknowledge excellence in practice.
7. Nurses practice within their own level of competence. They seek additional information or knowledge; seek the help, and/or supervision and help, of a competent practitioner; and/or request a different work assignment, when aspects of the care required are beyond their level of competence. In the meantime, nurses provide care within the level of their skill and experience.
8. Nurses give primary consideration to the welfare of clients and any possibility of harm in future care situations when they suspect unethical conduct or incompetent or unsafe care. When

nurses have reasonable grounds for concern about the behavior of colleagues in this regard, or about the safety of conditions in the care setting, they carefully review the situation and take steps, individually or in partnership with others, to resolve the problem.
9. Nurses support other nurses who act in good faith to protect clients from incompetent, unethical or unsafe care, and advocate work environments in which nurses are treated with respect when they intervene.
10. Nurses speaking on nursing and health-related matters in a public forum or a court provide accurate and relevant information.

7.14 PRACTICE ENVIRONMENTS

Practice Environments Conducive to Safe, Competent and Ethical Care

Nurses advocate practice environments that have the organizational and human support systems, and the resource allocations necessary for safe, competent and ethical nursing care.
1. Nurses collaborate with nursing colleagues and other members of the health team to advocate health care enof Athhvironments that are conducive to ethical practice and to the health and well-being of clients and others in the setting. They do this in ways that are consistent with their professional role and responsibilities.
2. Nurses share their nursing knowledge with other members of the health team for the benefit of clients. To the best of their abilities, nurses provide mentorship and guidance for the professional development of students of nursing and other nurses.
3. Nurses seeking professional employment accurately state their area(s) of competence and seek reasonable assurance that employment conditions will permit care consistent with the values and responsibilities of the code, as well as with their personal ethical beliefs.
4. Nurses practice ethically by striving for the best care achievable in the circumstances. They also make the effort, individually or in partnership with others, to improve practice environments by advocating on behalf of their clients as possible.
5. Nurses planning to participate in job action, or who practice in environments where job action occurs, take steps to safeguard the health and safety of clients during the course of the action.

7.15 APPLICATION OF CODE OF ETHICS IN SELECTED CIRCUMSTANCES

Some Suggestions for Application of the Code in Selected Circumstances

Steps to Address Incompetent, Unsafe and Unethical Care

1. Gather the facts about the situation and ascertain the risks.
2. Review relevant legislation and policies, guidelines and procedures for reporting incidents or suspected incompetent or unethical care and report, as required, any legally reportable offence.
3. Seek relevant information directly from the colleague, whose behavior or practice has raised concerns, when this is feasible.
4. Consult as appropriate with colleagues, other members of the team, professional nurses' associations, or others able to assist in resolving the problem.
5. Undertake to resolve the problem as directly as possible consistent with the good of all parties.
6. Advise the appropriate parties regarding unresolved concerns and, when feasible, inform the colleague in question of the reasons for your action.
7. Refuse to participate in efforts to deceive or mislead clients about the cause of alleged harm or injury resulting from unethical or incompetent conduct.

Nurse Managers, Professional Associations and Client Safety

1. Nurse managers seek to ensure that available resources and competencies of personnel are used efficiently.
2. Nurse managers intervene to minimize the present danger and to prevent future harm when client safety is threatened due to inadequate resources or for some other reason.
3. Professional nurses' associations support individual nurses and groups of nurses in promoting fairness and inclusiveness in health resource allocation. They do so in ways that are consistent with their role and functions.

Consideration in Student-Teacher-Client Relationships

1. Student-teacher and student-client encounters are essential elements of nursing education and are conducted in accordance with ethical nursing practices.
2. Clients are informed of the student status of the care giver and consent for care is obtained in compliance with accepted standards.
3. Students of nursing are treated with respect and honesty by nurses and are given appropriate guidance for the development of nursing competencies.
4. Students are acquainted with and comply with the provisions of the code.

Considerations in Taking Job Action

1. Job action by nurses is often directed toward securing conditions of employment that enable safe and ethical care of current and future clients. However, action directed toward such improvements could work to the detriment of clients in the short-term.
2. Individual nurses and groups of nurses safeguard clients in planning and implementing any job action.
3. Individuals and groups of nurses participating in job actions, or affected by job actions, share the ethical commitment to client safety. Their particular responsibilities may lead them to express this commitment in different but equally appropriate ways.
4. Clients whose safety requires ongoing or emergency nursing care are entitled to have those needs satisfied throughout any job action.
5. Members of the public are entitled to information about the steps taken to ensure the safety of clients during any job action.

7.16 PROFESSIONALISM AND CODE OF ETHICS

The International Council of Nurses (ICN) code of ethics is based on the idea that nurses respect human rights, including the patient's right to life and dignity. The code of ethics was adopted in 1953 and has served as a model for nurses worldwide ever since.

The ICN code: According to the ICN, a nurse's primary responsibility is to patients, and she should treat them with respect for their rights, values, customs and beliefs. Personal information she learns about them should remain confidential. In addition, she should continue her learning because she is personally responsible and accountable for good nursing practice, and she should take care of her own health so it doesn't interfere with her ability to care for others. She should cooperate with her coworkers but, if a patient's health or safety is threatened by others, she must take action to protect them.

The ANA code: Like the ICN, the American Nurses Association (ANA) believes that a nurse's first commitment is to her patient, and she should have compassion and respect for every individual no matter who they are, what kind of health problems they have, or what social and economic background they come from. A nurse also has a duty to establish, maintain, and improve health care environments and conditions of employment so that high quality health care can be provided. She should work to improve health care locally, nationally, and internationally, and she should also work through her professional associations to influence social policy concerning health care. Finally, she has a duty to maintain her own competence and to grow personally and professionally.

Types of ethical issues: Registered nurses (RN) responding to a 2006 survey reported 21 different ethical issues they faced while caring for their patients. These issues included the use of restraints, pain management, determining best interest of the patient, organ donation, life-sustaining treatment and end of life care, reporting errors, dealing with impaired nurses, conflicts of interest, justice for people with disabilities, the ethics of research and the use of information technology and confidentiality.

Nurse dissatisfaction: In a study investigating the relationship between ethics and the intent of nurses and social workers to leave their profession, researcher Connie Ulrich, PhD, RN discovered that 25 percent of practicing nurses and social workers wanted to leave the field. More than 52 percent of those who responded said they were frustrated with the ethical issues they faced. Hospital workers reported more ethical stress than caregivers who worked in other settings. Nearly 40 percent of hospital workers reported they had no organizational resources to help them with their ethical concerns, while another 25 percent said they had never received any ethical training.

Medical vs. nursing ethics: Since, the time of Florence Nightingale, nursing has subscribed to the ideal of caring for people. Medicine focuses on cures. Nursing is health-oriented while medicine is illness-oriented. Nursing emphasizes the preservation and restoration of health. Medicine emphasizes the treatment and prevention of disease. The word "nursing" reminds people of a mother who nurtures, teaches and cares for her young. Medicine, on the other hand, does not nurture. It combats illness and injury. Sympathy and support are primary virtues in nursing. Authority, courage, and risk-taking are the virtues of medicine. Although, both are concerned with healing, doctors and nurses have different points of views that shape their work ethics.

7.17 SAFE AND UNSAFE PRACTICE SITUATIONS

The goal of the RN is to provide safe, competent, ethical nursing care to the public. As changes in the health care system evolve, nurse administrators and staff nurses in all settings face the challenges of regionalization, reduced staff and budgets, caring for sicker patients, and changing roles and responsibilities of health care providers.

Addressing Unsafe Practice Issues

Unsafe practice situations are defined as particular circumstances in which the obligation of the RN to provide safe, competent, ethical care cannot be fulfilled. The unsafe practice situation could be a result of inadequate staffing, outdated policies and procedures, inappropriate or inadequate supplies and equipment, or inappropriate staff mix decisions. The following process can be used by registered nurses to address unsafe practice situations:

Step 1: Identify the Problem

1. What is the concern?
2. Why is it a concern?
3. What are the implications for patient outcomes and safety?
4. What evidence is there that a problem exists (e.g. incident reports)?
5. If it is a staffing concern, what are the needs for the skilled assessment, critical thinking, and critical judgment skills of the registered nurse in this situation?
6. Are other institutions or agencies concerned about this? Why?

Step 2: Assess the Environment

1. Who else is concerned about the problem (e.g. other professionals, the public)?
2. How could you work with others in addressing the problem?
3. What factors are impacting on the concern (e.g. economic, social, interpersonal, government or regional policy, administrative policy or philosophy, etc.)?

4. Who makes decisions? How are decisions made?
5. What resources do you have?
6. Who is the most appropriate person to take the concern to?
7. Are there committees in the institution or agency that should address problems of this nature? Are registered nurses on such committees?

Step 3: Document the Problem

1. State objective facts, dates, times, place, setting, people present.
2. Provide your professional opinion on the specific outcomes or consequences for the patient/ client. The AARN's Guidelines for Registered Nurses Part 3:
   Determining the Appropriate Category of Care Provider (September 1997) can be used as a framework for identification and documentation of the problem.
3. Document the problem when it occurs and keep a copy.
4. Document all conversations, meetings, and decisions made in relation to the problem.
5. Documentation is an essential step in the process of addressing unsafe practice situations.
6. The Canadian Nurses Protective Society (CNPS) can provide information as to the ethical and legal requirements for documentation, particularly when there are liability issues involved. If you are documenting anything which is hearsay or unsubstantiated speculation, note it as such in order that follow-up can occur with the original source.

Step 4: Plan Your Course of Action

1. Gather information and documentation to support your concern and course of action.
2. Brainstorm alternatives to address the problem.
3. Analyze the "pros" and "cons" of each alternative.
4. Develop a plan of action.
5. Work together and distribute the work involved in addressing the concern.

Step 5: Implement and Evaluate Your Plan

1. Decide the most appropriate level at which to address the problem—begin with your immediate supervisor and proceed as necessary.
2. Evaluate each part of the plan as you implement it.
3. Questions to ask:
   a. Is this approach effective - why or why not?
   b. Is more information needed?
   c. Are other resources needed?
   d. Do any of the steps of the action plan need to be repeated?

CONCLUSION

Code of ethics for nurses assumes various versions depending on the organization. For instance, the International Council for Nurses has embraced a code of ethics since 1953. It was in 2006, that it was revised as people and the demands of nursing have changed. This serves as a guide for right actions towards social values and needs. The code has been the basis of worldwide practice for ethical practice in nursing. The ICN Code of Ethics serves as the guiding light for professional nurses as they practice their skills whether on a hospital setting or community setting. This serves as a gauge whether nurses have given ethical care that encourages healing or preventing illness.

Nurses committed to high quality care based their practice of professional standards of ethical conduct. The study of professional ethical behavior begins in nursing school, continuous in formal and informal discussions with colleagues and peers and culminates when nurses try on and make their own the behaviors of role models who practice professional nursing consistent with high ethical standards. A professional code of ethics provides a framework for making ethical decisions and sets forth professional expectations.

8 Ethical Issues in Clinical Practice

8.1 INTRODUCTION

It is not possible in real life to separate "ethical behavior from all other behaviors". Almost everything we do can be judged as a moral action by some group of persons. It is because ethical behavior is important but not easily understood. From the time we were young we began to learn what was right and what was wrong. We learned this from our parents, relatives, friends, teachers and other authority figures. Much of what we learned was shaped by religious beliefs and the philosophy of life practiced in our home. By the time we become an adult we have a personal set of ethics to guide our behavior in daily life.

8.2 OBJECTIVES OF ETHICS IN CLINICAL PRACTICE

1. To recognize the ethical dimension of every healthcare encounter.
2. To understand the nature of values and how they impact on healthcare.
3. To identify the values that patients, families and members of the healthcare team bring to a specific healthcare decision.
4. To demonstrate moral reasoning skills in the process of choosing an appropriate course of action or resolving conflicting values.
5. To demonstrate the knowledge skills and attitudes for effective communication in eliciting and understanding the values of patients, negotiating an acceptable course of action and justifying that course of action.
6. To demonstrate knowledge of the professional ethical guidelines and legal framework within which healthcare decisions should be made.
7. To recognize their personal values and how these influence their decision-making.

8.3 ETHICAL PRINCIPLES RELATED TO CLINICAL PRACTICE

1. **Principles of autonomy:** It refers to a person's independence, e.g. It is the duty of the nurse to ask the clients wishes before a treatment and as a health care worker.
2. **Principles of beneficence:** It refers to taking positive actions to help medical orders but will act thoughtfully understand to help in meeting those needs.
3. **Principles of nonmaleficence:** It refers to avoidance of harm or hurt. In healthcare ethics, it is the duty of a nurse to practice not only the will to do well but also the equal commitment not to do any harm.
4. **Principle of justice:** It refers to fairness, e.g. For there were around 100 candidates waiting for liver transplants but only 50 organs were available such cases lottery system or randomization should not be practiced. It is the responsibility of nurse to maintain proper justice by providing organs to the first 50 who approached firstly.

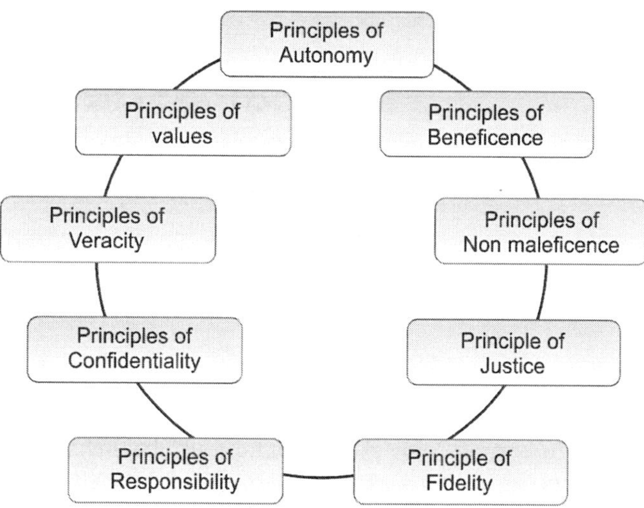

Fig. 8.1: Ethical principles

5. **Principle of fidelity:** It refers to the agreement to keep promises. For example, if a nurse assesses a client for pain and then offers a plan to manage the pain the standard of fidelity encourages nurse to monitor client response to plan.
6. **Principles of accountability:** Refers to the ability to answer for one's own acting. A nurse may know that a client who will be discharged soon remains confused, about how to administer insulin. The nurses sense of accountability guides actions that achieve this goal.
7. **Principles of responsibility:** The term responsibility refers to characteristics of reliability and dependability e.g., a nurse is responsible for assessing the clients' need for the drug, for giving it safely and correctly and for evaluating the response to it.
8. **Principles of confidentiality:** A nurse protects the privacy of a client without diminishing access to quality care.
9. **Principles of veracity:** In general, the term means accuracy or conformity to truth. It guides a nurse to practice truthfulness.
10. **Principles of values:** The work of nursing involves negotiation of values of a client, the physician, the employee or other groups. Understanding one's own values and assessing the value systems of other helps to facilitate decision making while ensuring respect for client autonomy.

8.4 ETHICAL ISSUES AND VALUE-BASED PRACTICE

Table 8.1: Value based practice

S.N	Areas	Description
1	Primary care management	1. Awareness of the range of values that may influence a patient's behavior or decision-making in relation to his or her illness. 2. How to integrate knowledge of patients' values with the relevant scientific evidence and clinical experience to achieve the best outcome for the patient. 3. Ability to recognize the ethical issues raised by public health programmes and develop appropriate approaches to their implementation. 4. Ability to recognize the needs and values and their impact on patient care.

Contd...

Contd...

2	Person centered care	1. Skills to achieve meaningful consent by a patient to a plan of management by seeing the patient as a unique person in a unique context. 2. Skills to balance conflicting duties to individual patients who are members of the same family. 3. Ability to apply the ethical guidance on consent and confidentiality to the particular context of primary care. 4. Ability to apply the law relating to making decisions for people who lack capacity to the particular context. 5. Awareness of the research evidence on patient values that are likely to influence a given healthcare situation. 6. Understanding the importance of continuity of care and long-term relationships with patients and their families in identifying and understanding the values that influence a patient's approach to health care. 7. Understanding of the relationship between the interests of patients and the interests of their careers.
3	Specific problem-solving approach	1. The skills to analyze the effect of different values on specific decisions by patients, families and health professionals. 2. Ability to draw on frameworks of moral reasoning to think through the issues and resolve conflicts of values.
4	Comprehensive approach	1. Understanding those patients' views and perspectives may change through the course of a chronic disease 2. Understanding that comorbidity or disease progression may affect decision-making capacity. 3. That they can recognize and respond to a patient entering a terminal stage of illness, and the values that are important in managing this. 4. Ability to identify potential ethical difficulties and develop proactive strategies to prevent or reduce the likelihood of conflict arising for themselves and for patients.
5	Community orientation	1. Understanding of the different conceptions of distributive justice that are used in resource allocation debates. 2. Recognition of the range of values that influence choices about healthcare provision. 3. Awareness of the obligation to use public resources in a prudent manner to benefit the whole community. 4. Ability to give morally relevant reasons for decisions that balance individual patient needs with the needs of the wider community.
6	Holistic approach	1. Understanding of the complexity of values that influence patients' attitude to their illness and their health care. 2. Ability to identify and involve appropriate resources and skills in other disciplines and other agencies to respond to the patient's individual needs and concerns 3. Understanding that respect for patient autonomy is in essence a holistic approach. To enable a patient to make choices about how he or she wishes to live his or her life, a General Practitioner must explore what is important to the patient overall and not restrict information-sharing to clinical data.
7	Contextual aspects	1. Understanding of the local community and culture. 2. How the values and beliefs prevalent in the local culture impact on patient care. 3. Understanding of how the social context of primary care frames the identification and resolution of ethical issues by general practitioners. 4. The ability to apply the results of research appropriately to the needs of individual patients and their families.

8.5 NURSING PRACTICE STANDARDS

The establishment of Nursing Practice Standards is essential for a self-regulating profession. Nursing Practice Standards represent acceptable requirements for determining the quality of nursing care, a patient/client receives. The AARN's Nursing Practice Standards have been developed to:

1. Guide and direct nursing practice.
2. Promote professional nursing practice.
3. Facilitate evaluation of nursing practice.
4. Enable the patient/client to judge the adequacy of nursing care.
5. Provide guidelines to nurse researchers in identifying and exploring relationships between nursing practice and patient care outcomes.
6. Provide guidelines for nurse administrators to support and facilitate safe, competent, and ethical nursing practice within their agencies.
7. Provide guidelines for nurse educators in setting objectives of educational programs.
8. Provide a framework for developing specialty nursing standards.
9. Facilitate articulation of the role of nursing within the health care team.

I. **Professional responsibility:** The registered nurse (RN) is personally responsible and accountable for ensuring that her/his nursing practice and conduct meet the standards of the profession and legislative requirements.
    1. The RN is accountable at all times for his/her own actions.
    2. The RN follows current legislation, standards, and policies relevant to the profession or practice setting.
    3. The RN questions policies and procedures inconsistent with therapeutic patient/client outcomes, best practices, and safety standards.
    4. The RN supports the continuing competence process.
    5. The RN participates in quality improvement activities.
    6. The RN has a professional responsibility to practice competently.
    7. The RN demonstrates competence by regularly evaluating his/her practice and taking necessary steps to improve personal competence.
    8. The RN is responsible for ensuring her/his own fitness to practice.

II. **Knowledge-based practice:** The registered nurse continually strives to acquire knowledge and skills to provide competent, evidence-based nursing practice.

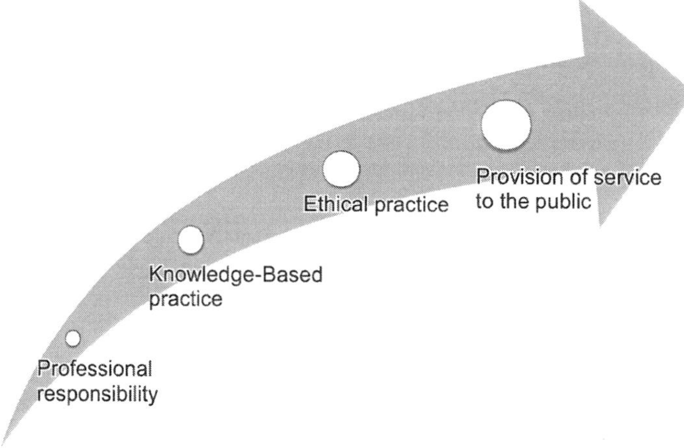

Fig. 8.2: Standards of nursing practice

1. The RN supports decisions with evidence-based rationale.
2. The RN accesses appropriate information and resources that enhance patient care and achievement of desired patient outcomes.
3. The RN demonstrates critical thinking in collecting and interpreting data, planning, implementing, and evaluating all aspects of nursing care.
4. The RN exercises reasonable judgment in practice.
5. The RN practices within own level of competence.
6. The RN documents timely, accurate reports of data collection, interpretation, planning, implementing, and evaluating care.
7. The RN sets justifiable priorities when giving care.
8. The RN supports, facilitates, or participates in research relevant to nursing.

III. **Ethical practice:** The registered nurse complies with the Canadian Nurses Association's Code of Ethics for Registered Nurses (1997).
1. The RN practices with honesty, integrity, and respect.
2. The RN reports unskilled practice or professional misconduct to appropriate person, agency, or professional body.
3. The RN acts as an advocate to protect and promote a client's right to autonomy, respect, privacy, dignity, and access to information.
4. The RN assumes responsibility for ensuring that her/his relationships with clients are therapeutic and professional.
5. The RN advocates for practice environments that have the organizational and human support systems, and the resource allocations necessary for safe, competent, and ethical nursing care.

IV. **Provision of service to the public:** The registered nurse provides nursing service in collaboration with the client, significant others, and other health professionals.
1. The RN collaborates with the client/significant others and other members of the healthcare team regarding activities of care planning, implementation, and evaluation.
2. The RN uses communication and team building skills to enhance client care.
3. The RN is accountable for her/his delegation of care to other health team members.
4. The RN explains nursing care to clients and others.

8.6 ETHICO-LEGAL ISSUES IN CLINICAL PRACTICE

In nursing practice it means the way in which you are obligated to obey the law in professional activities. Disobedience of the law results in punishment. Legal responsibility is stated and enforced by law.

Guides for Legal Responsibilities

1. Central and State government act are binding by law.
2. International code of nurses.
3. Institutional rules and regulations.
4. Standing orders and precedent or an example of what court decision has been made in similar case.
5. Central Government services conduct rules.
6. State Nursing Council's conduct rules and disciplinary actions.

There are certain determinants of legal framework for nursing practice in India.

1. **Registration:** Licensing is a mandatory procedure for practice of nursing. Registration aims at protecting patients by providing qualified nurses. The nurse is responsible to obtain registration in the respective State Nursing Registration Council. Employers should recruit only registered nurses as per the State Nursing Home Act.

2. **Legal Liability/Act of Negligence Criminal (IPC):** Under Section 304 of Indian Penal Code (IPC) (e.g. wrong medication leading to death of patient), it is important that nurse is careful while administering medications and follows all the seven "R's" every time (i.e. right patient, right medicine, right dose, right time, right route, right reason, right documentation). Civil Tort in Civil Court (Negligence, e.g. not giving railing bed to unconscious patient causing fall of patient).
3. **Medicolegal Case (MLC):** A medicolegal case (MLC) is a patient who is admitted to the hospital with some unnatural pathology and has to be taken care of in concurrence with the police and/or court.

   Types of clients, which are categorized as MLC in a hospital, are:
   1. Road traffic accident (RTA)
   2. Injuries inflicted during brawls/fights, shooting, bomb blasts etc.
   3. Suicide
   4. Homicide
   5. Bums
   6. Poisoning
   7. Rape victim
   8. Assault

   Nurse role in a medicolegal case:
   1. Obtain complete history from patient or significant other (s).
   2. Inform the police officer/constable on duty in the hospital and the Chief Medical Officer (CMO).
   3. When it is made a MLC, then record it on the patient's case sheet with red ink right hand top corner.
   4. Do not give any statement about patient's condition to police, magistrate or media. Only a doctor is to give information.
   5. When a patient has to be discharged, inform the police officer/ constable on duty in hospital and/or the CMO, after clearance from others, then only discharge.
   6. If an MLC patient absconds inform the CMO and the treating doctor, immediately.
   7. No MLC patient can go LAMA.
   8. Document the care given to the patients timely, accurately and duly sign the nurse's notes.
   9. Records and all documents pertaining to patient and his care, during his stay in the hospital, must be kept safely, should be handed over to the authorized person as designated by the hospital authority.
   10. In case of death of an MLC, the body is not to be handed over to the relatives. It needs to be accurately labeled and sent to the mortuary. CMO and/or police officer should be informed simultaneously. Appropriate authority must be informed.
4. **Consent**
   1. Consent is a written acceptance from the patient.
   2. "Every adult of sound mind has a right to determine what shall be done with his body".
   3. Consent has to be valid, must be a free and informed consent:
      a. The patient must be able to understand the choices he or she is required to make.
      b. Consent must be free and voluntary.
      c. The procedure for which consent is sought must have been explained to the patient. It may be negligent to withhold important information.
      d. Consent must not be procured by deceit.
   4. Less than 12 years cannot give consent for general physical examination. It should/must come from parent/guardian.
   5. 12–18 years can give consent for general physical examination only.
   6. More than 18 years must come from patient himself/herself except in certain circumstances:

Consent-should come from parent/guardian/significant others in case of patients who are not in a capacity to decide for themselves such as: patient with dementia/delirious patient/ mentally challenged/deaf and mute/patients with mental disorders/unconscious/gravely ill etc.

5. **Correct identity**
    1. A nurse/midwife is responsible to make sure that all babies born in hospital are correctly labeled at birth and handed over to right parent.
    2. Unknown/unconscious patients must be labeled as soon as their identity is known.
    3. Patients who have to undergo surgery should be appropriately identified and labeled.
    4. Site of operation to be correctly marked particularly where symmetrical sides or organs are there.

    Operation theatre (O.T): Scrub nurse has to see that all instruments/swabs are returned. She has to say 'OKAY' before closure by the surgeon.
6. **Left against Medical Advice (LAMA):** Inform medical officer in-charge. Signatures of both patients and witness to be taken as per institutional policy.
7. **Patient's property:** Inform patient on admission that hospital does not take responsibility of his belonging. If patient is unconscious/or otherwise required, then a list of items must be made, counter checked by two staff nurses and kept under safe custody.
8. **Dying declaration:** Doctor or nurse should not involve himself or herself in dying declaration, in case where police records the dying declaration. Dying declaration is to be recorded by the magistrate.

    But if condition of patient becomes serious then Medical Officer can record it along with two nurses as witnesses. Dying declaration can be recorded by nursing staff with two nurses as witnesses when Medical Officer is not present. Then, the declaration is to be sent immediately under sealed cover to the Magistrate.
9. **Wills:** For this doctor has to be present or he can record if requested.
10. **Examination of rape case:** Female attendant/female nurse must be present during the examination.
11. **Artificial Human Insemination**
    1. Written consent should be obtained from both donor and recipient.
    2. Donor and recipient must have the same blood group.
    3. Donor and recipient's identity should be kept confidential.
    4. All related documents should be kept confidential and safe.
12. **Poison Case**
    1. Do not give either verbal or written opinion.
    2. Do not allow taking photos unless appropriate authority grants special permission.
    3. Do not give information to public or press.
    4. Preserve all evidence of poisoning.
    5. Collect and preserve all excreta, vomits and aspirates, seal them immediately and send to forensic laboratory at the earliest.
13. **Consumer Protection Act (1986):** Consumer Protection Act (CPA) was passed by the Parliament in 1986 to provide for better protection of the interest of consumers and focuses on consumer justice through the establishment of consumer councils and other authorities for the settlement of consumer's disputes and matters connected therewith. The scope of the Act is wide enough to include a vast variety of services.

    Under this act, consumer can complain in redressal forum. It enables the consumer! Patient to make a complaint to a redressal forum in respect of defective services provided.

    Rights of a Consumer/Patient are:
    1. Right of safety
    2. Right to be informed

3. Right to choose
4. Right to be heard
5. Right to seek redressal
6. Right to consumer education.

Nurses role to prevent legal complications:

1. Review nursing practice periodically. Update knowledge and improve skills by attending short-term courses, in-service education and continuing education programmers.
2. Should have complete knowledge of all rules and regulation of hospital and know their job descriptions (duties and responsibilities).
3. Follow nursing practice standards/Protocols.
4. Be a keen observer.
5. Written instructions must be displayed in all nursing units for necessary guidance and protection of the staff regarding issues related to patient care.
6. All hospitals must have rules and code of practice laid down to ensure the safety and well-being of patients and nurses.
7. Maintain records and reports of the unit properly.
8. Follow 7 R's - right patient, right drug, right dose, right time, right route, right reason and right documentation.
9. Check the treatment order and use professional judgment before implementing.
10. Do not attempt anything beyond the level of competence and scope of nursing practice. If there is any doubt in mind, seek advice from professional colleagues.
11. Do not exceed the limits of nursing procedure laid down by statutory bodies.

8.7 SOURCES OF ETHICS IN NURSING

The individualistic ethic and the aggregate ethic of nursing are contained in:

1. Professional statements on standards.
2. Social policies.
3. Clinical and other research.
4. Code of ethics.
5. Government policies and the type of govt.

There are differing interpretations of the professional ethic in many of those professional statements. There are differing interpretations of the individualistic ethic and the aggregate ethic of nursing practice.

8.8 THEORETICAL FOUNDATIONS OF NURSING PRACTICE

Theoretical foundations for the ethic of promoting individual good and ethic of promoting aggregate good can be derived from theories of distributive justice:

1. Egalitarian theory.
2. Utilitarian theory.

a. Egalitarian theory of justice requires the equality of net welfare for individuals.
b. Utilitarian theory of justice claims that justice is served by promoting aggregate goods at the least cost.

In Egalitarian theory, the distribution of good in the community means taking the needs of all citizens into account equally amount of good or health resources for all individual to seek health services and do not limit the liberty of seeking basic health services.

Aggregate good enters the egalitarian system of through the acknowledgment that it is impossible to provide for an equal amount of good health resources for all individuals as resource are limited. Aggregate good reduces the obligation to provide for individual good.

Where as in utilitarian system of justice, resources among citizens are distributed by deciding how expenditure or the use of resources will achieve the greatest net total of good and serve the largest number of people.

8.9 IMPLICATIONS FOR NURSING PRACTICE

1. Potential over riding of individual liberties and values for the common good.
2. Role of aggregate good in policy decisions have long-term effects: It is often uncertain how short-term effects on aggregate good are stressing in long-term effects, the individual as well as aggregate interests in health may be sacrificed for perceived future. This can have a devastating effect on role and functioning of nurses.
3. Planned distribution of nursing resources: Prioritizing of health interests and the various ways to carry out these priorities may create conflicts of interest among health providers. Hence, there is a need for coordination, with available resources of other health care providers is essential.

8.10 STRATEGIES OF NURSING PRACTICE

There are several strategies that may appeal in distribution of nursing resources on ethical manner.

1. Focus nursing services on those who have the most reasonable chance of benefiting from nursing services, e.g. Maternal and child health (MCH) services. It is cost effective and greatest net benefit is there.
2. Provide basic nursing service on first come, first served basis. This cost more and overlap services. It is not an efficient means of distributing nursing resources.
3. Focus nursing care services on those who are able to pay for services. This has limited relevance to identified needs of individuals and aggregate groups.
4. Categorize clients according to health needs and decide who should receive first priority — this approach has a decided utilitarian twist to it and limits the access of some groups to nursing services. It is not in accordance with the moral ethics of nursing.

8.11 ACCOUNTABILITY IN NURSING PRACTICE

Nurses are responsible for how they promote, protect and meet the health needs of clients, individuals as well as aggregate groups.

1. No nurse should be expected to provide nursing care services to individual clients or population at physical risk to oneself or when client's need for health goods infringe on the nurse's personal life or responsibilities to other clients.
2. The obligation to promote individual good at expense of aggregate good is limited by consideration of disruptive justice and impossibility of meeting every individual health care needs.
3. The obligation to promote good is like wise limited by consideration of individual rights, especially the right of all members of society to be able to secure an adequate level of care without excessive burden.

8.12 ETHICAL TENSION IN NURSING PRACTICE

The professional nurse experience ethical conflict in many aspects of health care delivery. The fundamental conflict today is tension between the obligation to benefit the individual client and the obligation to benefit society.

The nurse must decide whether her primary obligation to promote individual good or to promote aggregate good. Recent concerns about the equitable distribution of health care resources, cost containment in health care, and the availability of innovative health care, have added new substance to this tension, in nursing practice.

The individual ethic:

1. International Council of Nurses Code for nurses claims that the nurse renders "health services to the individual family and the community".
2. Canadian Nurses Association: "Nurse is obliged to treat clients with respect for their individual needs and values.
3. American Nurses Association believes that "Nurses are morally accountable for how they provide health care services according to "the uniqueness of the client".
4. Canadian Public Health Association: "The nurse assists the individual, family and community to assume responsibility for sound health practices". Regardless of the source, the individualistic focus of nursing practice is a fundamentally important component of ethical nursing practice. Nurse is expected to provide services for the benefit of the individual patient and is expected to promote individual good in matters of health.

The aggregate ethic:

1. International Council of Nurse's: "Nurse shares with other citizens and responsibility for initiating and supporting action to meet the health and social needs of the public".
2. Canadian Nurses Association: "The public is owed the same duties—as are clients within the employment setting.
3. American Nurses Association: "Nurses must also recognize the situation in which individual rights to self determination in health care may temporarily be altered for common good. It also claims the main responsibility of nursing is good.
4. American Nurses Association (ANA's): A social policy statement: "Nursing is owned by society and must be perceived as serving interest of larger whole of which it is part".
5. American Public Health Association: "In providing the health of entire community or as planning for a community as a whole rather than individual".

The ethical focus of science of nursing and science of public health is different. This is a conflict in the synthesis of two. Nurse may have to decide, whether to honor the obligation to promote individual good or to honor important for all nurses to understand how choices between the two ethics can be justified according to the requirements for normal accountability in nursing practice.

CONCLUSION

In conclusion, in meeting moral accountability requirements in nursing practice, nurses are not merely answerable for how they have promoted, protected and or met the health needs of the clients, individual as well as groups, they are also accountable for determining justifiable reasons for limiting the provision of good in specific situations.

Every nurse should act as per the legal guidelines for nursing practice while caring for patients since negligence may cause a great distress to nurse, the patient and others, as well as to reputation of the institution. "Every individual is ordinarily liable for their own negligence". Therefore, nurses have a responsibility of seeing that no harm comes to their patients and also to themselves. "Ignorance of law is no excuse for negligence".

9 Ethical Dilemma

9.1 INTRODUCTION

A dilemma is defined as situations requiring a choice between two equally desirable or undesirable alternatives. In ethical dilemma, each alternative course of action can be justified by two ways in which a person views the course of action based on his or her value system. Issues in healthcare delivery practices present different alternatives based on whether the issue or course of action is viewed by the patient, the healthcare agency, the legal system or the nurse. Increasingly, staff nurses and nurse managers face difficult decisions caused by tensions between technological capabilities, budgetary structures, and quality of life concerns.

9.2 DEFINITION

"Situations arising when equally compelling ethical reasons both for and against a particular course of action are recognized and a decision must be made". (CNA code) Decision making; and it requires a systematic framework for addressing the complex and often controversial moral questions. The Ethical Model for Ethical Decision Making (McGonagall, 2000) provides a systematic framework to examine ethical dilemmas focusing on the following steps:

E : Examine the ethical dilemma.
T : Thoroughly comprehend the possible alternatives available.
H : Hypothesize ethical arguments.
I : Investigate, compare, and evaluate the arguments for each alternative.
C : Choose the alternative you would recommend.
A : Act on your chosen alternative.
L : Look at the ethical dilemma and examine the outcomes while reflecting on the ethical decision.

We will use this each step of this model to examine a case involving the dilemma of balancing the protection of privacy while protecting patients from harm.

9.3 MEANING OF ETHICAL DILEMMA

Ethical problems can cause distress and confusion for both clients and care givers. Controversy is the very nature of ethical problem and few people like conflict to overcome controversy and determined a course of action. Ethical issues are processed carefully and deliberately, wherever an ethical dilemma is resolved-in a committee setting, at the bed side or in a family a nurse should apply a careful, critical processing of the dilemma. It requires deliberate, systematic thinking, the nurse gathers information through assessment planning intervention and evaluation she distinguishes the problems and solves deliberately.

9.4 TYPES OF ETHICAL DILEMMA IN NURSING

An ethical dilemma in nursing occurs when a nurse is in a situation that involves a conflict between two contradictory principles or values. In an ethical dilemma, moral principles do not easily determine the correct course of action.

There are many ethical issues in nursing that suggest two or more equally compelling courses of action that appear to be morally right. The nurse trying to make an ethical decision may recognize that one specific course of action will uphold some ethical principles but not all of them. Ethical dilemmas in nursing are commonly discussed during the course of nursing education. The goal is to not only inform students of the issue, but also to provide them with guidelines for handling these dilemmas.

Table 9.1: Ethical dilemma types

S.N	Types	Description
1	Patient's rights	A patient's rights and dignity must always be respected, and a variety of ethical dilemmas arise from this nursing principle. Although, a nurse may want to administer life-saving drugs to a dying patient, she is unable to do so if the patient refuses treatment.
2	Family's rights	Ethical dilemmas in nursing may also involve patient families. For example, although a mother and father may wish to be in the operating room with their dying child, hospital regulations may not allow this.
3	Internal dilemmas	Some nurses have may face ethical dilemmas that stem from their own culture or religion. Although, a nurse's own culture or religion may not believe in organ transplantation, blood transfusions or in vitro fertilization, she is still responsible for providing these treatments to his patients when necessary.

9.5 PROCESS OF AN ETHICAL DILEMMA

Step 1: Is this an ethical dilemma? If a review of scientific data does not resolve the question, the question is perplexing, and the answer will have profound relevance for several areas of human concern, then an ethical dilemma may exist.

Step 2: Gather all of the information relevant to the case. To be sure it is a true dilemma, it will be important to review all pertinent information. Occasionally, an overlooked fact may provide quick resolution. At this point, client, family, institution, and social perspectives are important sources of relevant information.

Step 3: Examine and determine your own values on the issues. Values clarification provides a foundation for clarity and for confidence during discussions that will be necessary for resolution of a dilemma.

Step 4: Verbalize the problem. A clear simple statement of the dilemma may not always be easy, but it is essential for the next step to take place.

Step 5: Consider possible courses of action to respect all sides of an issue, it is helpful to list potential actions, especially when the list will reflect opinions that conflict.

Step 6: Negotiate the outcome. Sometimes courses of action that seem unlikely at the beginning of the process take on new possibility as they are put to rational and respectful consideration. Negotiation requires a confidence in one's own point of view and a deep respect for the opinions of others.

Step 7: Evaluate the action.

9.6 ETHICAL DILEMMA IN NURSING

Nurses in all clinical and functional specialities face the following ethical dilemmas:

1. Need to ration patient care to conserve scarce resources.

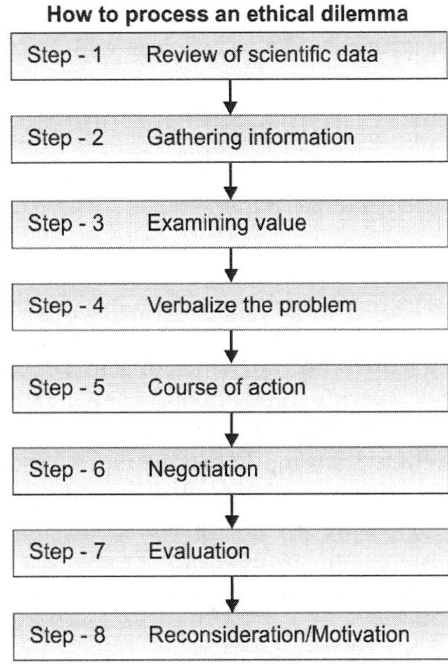

Fig. 9.1: Steps of ethical dilemma process

2. Need to make treatment and care decisions for terminally ill patients.
3. Need to obtain patients informed consent for care and treatment orders and measures such as:
   a. Do not resuscitate order.
   b. Withholding/withdrawing nutrition and fluids.
   c. Starting/discontinuing life support system.
4. Response to patient request for assisted suicide.
5. Need to balance the patients need for confidentiality and privacy against society's needs for protection from unreasonable risk.
6. Need to protect autonomy rights of children and incompetent adults concerning consent for research participation.
7. Need to protect justice rights of patients who participate in random trials of experimental treatment.

Usually, the dilemma occurs when opposing views are seen for the solution of an issue and a decision must be made. There is no set of procedures or easy answers for how an ethical dilemma should be resolved. Ethical decision making is needed in all steps of the nursing process and all phases of the nursing management process. Ethical reasoning is similar to the nursing process in that it requires critical thinking skills. A nurse can best resolve ethical dilemma, by systematically considering all options for solving the dilemma. A ethical dilemma occurs as a result of conflict between moral principles that support different courses of action.

9.7 ETHICAL DECISION-MAKING

Nurses decisions are increasingly constrained by ethical issues. Ethical decision making involves reflection on the following:

1. Who should make the choice?
2. Possible options or courses of action.
3. Available options.

4. Consequences, both good and bad, of all possible options.
5. Rules, obligations and values that should direct choices, and
6. Desired outcomes.

When making decisions, nurses need to combine all of these elements using an orderly, systematic, and objective method. There are various models for ethical decision making. Perhaps the easiest ethical decision making model to remember and to implement in practice is the "moral model" developed by Thirona and Halloraw as follows:

M-Massage the dilemma: Identify and define the issues in the dilemma. Consider the opinions of all major players in the dilemma as well as their value system. This includes patient's family members, nurses, doctors, priest and any other interdisciplinary healthcare team member.

O-Outline the options: Examine all options including those less realistic and conflicting; this stage is designed only for considering options and not for making final decision.

R-Resolve the dilemma: Review the issues and options, applying the basic principles of ethics to each option. Decide the best option based upon the views of all those concerned in the dilemma.

A-Act by applying chosen action: This step is usually the most difficult as it requires actual implementation. While the previous steps had only allowed for dialogue or discussion.

L-Look back and evaluate: The entire process including the implementation. No process is complete without a thorough evaluation. Ensure that those involved are able to follow through on the final option. If not, a second decision may be required and process must start again at the initial step.

Another exchange of traditional model of ethical decision making are as follows:

1. Identify the problem.
2. Gather data to analyze the causes and consequence of the problem.
3. Explore the optional solutions to the problem.
4. Evaluate the optional solution.
5. Select the appropriate solution from all the options.
6. Implement the selected solution.
7. Evaluate the result.

9.8 GUIDELINES FOR MAKING ETHICAL DECISION

A nurse may be caring for a client who is faced with a problem having many ethical ramifications. The client may ask for assistance in resolving the dilemma. Nurses can clarify their own ethical position as well as help families to make their decision by using these guidelines:

1. **Establish a complete data base:** Find out all the information about the situation, including data about those involved; their physical, psychological, financial and support resources; the proposed action and the reason behind it; and the possible results of the reason behind it; and the proposed action.
2. **Identify the ethical conflicts created by the problems:** Determine what the ethical problems are for the clients, the family, the health care agency and the various health professionals involved in care.
3. **Outline various courses of action:** Present alternative solutions to the problem and discuss with healthcare providers.
4. **Determine possible outcomes of the suggested actions:** Determine the consequences of the various courses of action as well as the proposed action.
5. **Determine who "owns" the problem and who should make the decision:** The following factors must be considered: who will be affected by the decision, for whom is the decision being made for, whose moral principles or legal responsibilities are being affected and what degree of constancy is needed from those involved.

6. **Define the obligations of the nurse:** In situations requiring ethical decision-making, nurses must determine their obligations both to the client and to themselves.
7. **Formulation of nursing ethical committee:** Nursing Ethical Committees are a means for nurses to develop their base of power when dealing with ethical situations. They provide a forum for nurses to verbalize viewpoints without infringing on the views of others. It can be consist of Chief Nursing Officer, Assistant Chief Nursing Officer, Departmental In-charges, Clinical Nurses, Psychologist, Psychiatric Nurse, Dean or Medical Superintendent and Concerning Medical officers of Units.

Role of Ethical Committee

1. Identification, exploration and resolution of ethical issues in nursing practice.
2. Education of nurses in bioethics and nursing ethics.
3. Preparation of nurses for participation interdisciplinary decision-making.
4. Service as a resource group.
5. Review of nursing ethics material.
6. Review of departmental policies related to ethics.
7. Involvement in nursing ethics research.
8. Preparation of nurses to serve on information, education and communication.

9.9 NURSING ISSUES RELATED TO ETHICAL DILEMMA

Nurses adhere to certain ethical principles when caring for patients. These principles include beneficence which is doing no harm to the patient, maleficence which is doing harm to a patient for positive outcome, justice in allocating care based on need not status and patient autonomy which is respecting the patient's right to make health decisions. Conflict with these principles results in an ethical dilemma.

Table 9.2: Ethical dilemmas in nursing

S.N	Issues	Description
1	Unsafe patient to nurse ratio	The nurse has an ethical duty to keep her patients safe. An ethical dilemma happens when a nurse finds herself in a situation where she has too many patients and cannot provide adequate care for all of them on her own.
2	Inappropriate medication orders	Giving wrong medication dosages or medication for the wrong illness is unsafe for patients and may lead to death. Nurses can find themselves in an ethical dilemma when they have to challenge a medication order written by a physician.
3	Unresponsive physicians	Nurses often have to call on physicians in situations beyond their scope of practice such as medical emergencies. The nurse finds herself in an ethical dilemma if the physician does not respond and her patient's condition goes from bad to worse.
4	Inappropriate tasks	Nurses float from department to department in the course of their career. When a nurse finds herself in an unfamiliar department and is asked to provide care she is inadequately trained for, she may have to refuse to provide care to avoid making the patient unsafe.
5	Life-threatening patient decisions	Patients sometimes make decisions that are unsafe, such as refusing treatment for a baby, medication or life saving procedures. The nurse finds herself in an ethical dilemma because not giving the needed treatment goes against beneficence and giving it ignores patient autonomy.

9.10 PROFESSIONAL RESPONSIBILITY IN ETHICAL DILEMMA

Professional responsibilities, tradition, and personal conscience along with legal, philosophical, and religious convictions dictate nursing interventions. Inevitably, these factors embrace life-sustaining therapies; however, in view of complications, prognosis, pain and suffering, and their own views of quality of life, some patients express wishes inconsistent with life-sustaining measures. In other situations, the healthcare provider as well as the patient may view heroic efforts as more debilitating than resortative.

1. Resolving the conflict while preserving the patient's best interests requires a confrontation with the status of "do-not resuscitate" policies within the nurse's institution, informed consent, refusal, and competency as the necessary underpinnings for the development of an ethical and legal posture within the profession, with which to approach significant decisions regarding life-sustaining therapies.
2. Literally, every hour of every day nurses are immediately and directly involved with resolving ethical dilemmas based upon judgments and interpretations of oral or written orders, patient and family wishes, professional training, and an infinite number of other factors.
3. When clear policies or orders are lacking, the nurse is left with the burden of making a life or death decision. It is imperative that professional nurses assess the administrative, legal, and ethical ramifications of their actions in terms of ethical codes of practice, patients' rights, institutional and personal liability, civil and criminal laws, and private conscience.
4. An understanding of these issues, passive and active euthanasia, state and national trends, and uniform legislation can assist in resolutions of the no-code dilemma.
5. Nursing as a profession must strive to develop sound and consistent guidelines and rationale for the scope of practice in ethical dilemmas.

9.11 NURSES ROLE IN ETHICAL DILEMMA

Nurses usually receive little or no formal training in ethics and law, and so are unqualified to deal with these issues when they encounter them in the clinical setting (Ramsey, 2000).

1. Ethical and legal issues stemming from such medical issues as organ donation, end-of-life care, euthanasia, physician-assisted suicide, genetic engineering, and managing patient confidentiality in the age of electronic data management are all part of the modern practice of nursing, and there are ethical, legal, and regulatory mandates that require a knowledge of these subjects in healthcare professionals so they can participate in ethical decision-making.
2. Many nurses feel powerless and this often leads to inaction in nurses faced with these decisions, and so they withdraw from the issue and nothing changes.
3. Nurses need to become proactive in ethical and legal issues relating to the care of their patients, and need to spearhead a move to form ethics committees, or to participate in those already in place in their healthcare organizations. This knowledge is vital to nurses, and they need guidance on how to deal with their inadequacies in this area of nursing.
4. Nurses are increasingly realizing that they can offer relevant information and participate in decision-making involving ethical issues. However, inter-professional communications are frequently inadequate, and do not permit exchange of opinions. The consequences are often frustrating and upsetting for nurses whose care is affected by others' policies.
5. Nurses should practice nursing in an ethical way at all times. At times, though, they may face ethical problems.
6. Nurses may be asked to administer improper medications or treatments, to perform duties outside the scope of their practice, to share information that should be kept confidential, to ignore patients' rights or to do something else improper or unethical.

7. Sometimes nurses can clearly see what to do but other times there are gray areas and nurses find themselves facing ethical questions and must determine the proper course of action.

9.12 CHECKLIST FOR ETHICAL DECISION-MAKING

A sound ethical decision-making process may incorporate the following abilities:

1. The ability to identify all related issues pertaining to the incident/issue/dilemma.
2. The ability to sort morally relevant issues from morally irrelevant issues in any given situation.
3. The ability to unpack the elements of morally relevant information.
4. The ability and willingness to research issues and reflect upon them.
5. The ability and willingness to seek advice.
6. The ability to form a well-reasoned, unbiased, and morally defensible conclusion in any given situation.
7. The ability to justify this position and act upon it.
8. The ability to challenge one's own moral framework in light of recalcitrant experiences.
9. Being in possession of a consistent moral framework.

CONCLUSION

Ethics offer moral principles, roles or standards that govern the conduct of members of a group. Since, the beginning of the human civilization ethical codes of conduct approach human behavior from a philosophical standpoint' by stressing objectively defined, but essentially idealistic, standards (or laws) of right and wrong, good/evil, and virtue/vice such as those applicable to the practices of lawyers and doctors.

Ethical dilemmas are everywhere and aesthetic medicine is no exception. Many would argue that they might even be more prevalent in this area. As this specialty area continues to grow, daily ethical reflection becomes necessary. As enhancement procedures are elective and based on patient choice, the ethical principle of autonomy becomes a dilemma for the provider. It becomes more of an ethical responsibility not to succumb to patient desires alone. It becomes apparent that it is necessary to develop frameworks that resolve such dilemmas in this specialty area As a new doctor of nursing practice, nurse practitioners will aspire to a higher level of ethical practice and lead efforts to formulate frameworks to achieve resolution of such dilemmas so that this higher level of ethical practice may be accomplished by each and every provider.

Section-4

Legal Issues

10 Legal Issues in Nursing

10.1 INTRODUCTION

Knowledge of legal aspects in nursing is absolutely essential for each nurse to safeguard self and clients from legal complications. Consumers are becoming increasingly aware of their legal rights in the healthcare. It is essential therefore, a nurse should know her legal rights and professional boundaries and their consequences of nonconformity. The law constitutes body of principles recognized or enforced by public and regular tribunals have the administration of justice. The law is the body of principles recognized and applied by the state and the administrations of justice. Law is that portion of the established thought and habit which has gained district and formal recognition and the shape of uniform rules backed by the authority and power of the government.

10.2 TYPES OF LAWS

1. **Civil law** includes rules and regulations that specify the required course of action to be followed by an individual in business and social relationships with others. It is concerned with relationships among people and the protection of a person's rights.
2. **Criminal law** defines offences that affect public welfare and security and impose penalties. It includes rules forbidding conduct that is injurious to public order and specifying punishments to be administered to individual who exhibits injurious conduct.

10.3 COMMON LEGAL ISSUES

1. Wrong medications, wrong dosage, wrong route of administration and wrong concentration.
2. Mistaken identity—prepare the wrong patient for an operation, to exchange babies in the labor room. To exchange dead bodies in the mortuary.
3. Failure to communicate.
4. Maintenance of record.
5. Giving explanation and getting the concerned.
6. Bums and false.
7. Counting sponges and instruments during surgery.
8. Loss or damage to patient's property and fame.
9. Euthanasia or mercy killing—taking positive step to kill a person in order to end his suffering is a murder.

10.4 LEGAL RESPONSIBILITIES OF A NURSE

1. **Responsibility of appointing and assigning:** The nurse administrators have responsibility for staffing and supervising nursing units to ensure safe, effective patient care. Therefore, they have

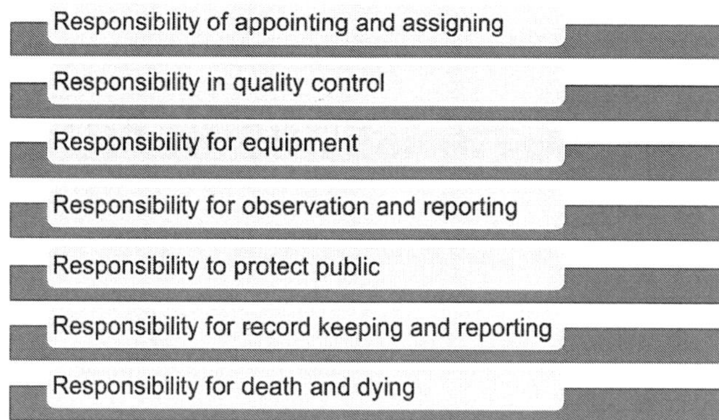

Fig. 10.1: Legal responsibilities of nurse

the authority to temporarily reassign a nursing employee to compensate for emergency staff shortages.

2. **Responsibility in quality control:** A nurse manager's legal responsibility for quality control of nursing service imposes a duty to observe report and correct the incompetence of any patient care provider.
3. **Responsibility for equipment:** To protect the patients and employees from injury, a nurse manager must ensure that all patient care equipments are fully functional and that defective equipment is promptly repaired or replaced.
4. **Responsibility for observation and reporting:** Consequently nurses have a legal duty to observe patients frequently and report findings that have diagnostic or treatment value for the patient's physician and other members of the patient's treatment team.
5. **Responsibility to protect public:** The nurse has a legal duty to protect the public from injury by dangerous patients. The manager must ensure that nursing personnel follow the procedures to alert community members to the presence of a potentially dangerous patient in their midst.
6. **Responsibility for record keeping and reporting:** Nurses have legal responsibility for accurately reporting and recording patient's conditions, treatments and response to care. The medical record is an information source document that should be used to plan care, evaluate care, allocate costs, educate personnel, research care measure, and substantiate legal claim.
7. **Responsibility for death and dying:** Nurses must be aware of legal definition of death because they must document all events that, when the patient is in their care.

10.5 LEGAL PERSPECTIVES IN NURSING

1. **Nurse Practice Act:** Each state has what is called a Nurse Practice Act. The Guidelines and laws outlined in the act pertain to all nurses who are licensed in that particular state. Nurse limitation is one of those laws. Each nurse has a limitation on what she is allowed and trained to do. She must follow the chain of command, especially with the care of a patient. If she does not have the authority or knowledge to give a prescription, analyze a lab report, or advise the patient on treatment, she may not legally do so. Any wrong information or practice he commits is punishable by the law and the patient or family may file a suit against her and the health agency or hospital she works for.
2. **Patients Advocate:** A nurse has a legal obligation to act as the patients advocate in case of emergency. The nurse is to act as the liaison between the patient and the healthcare provider, such as a physician. The nurse will monitor the patient, ensuring that if any complications or abnormalities arise, a physician notified immediately. The nurse is legally obligated to keep the

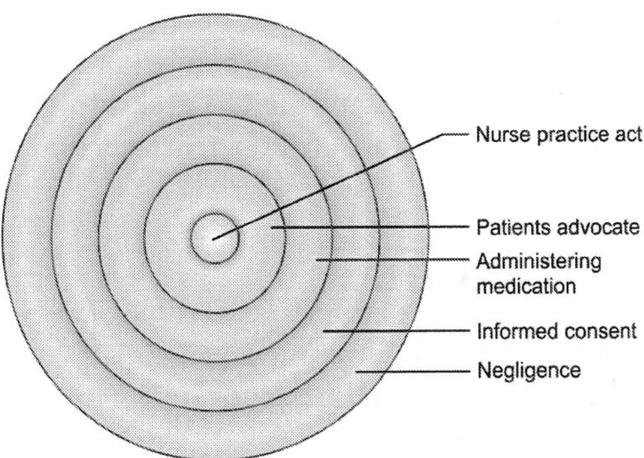

Fig. 10.2: Legal respectives in nursing

personal data and information of the patient confidential not doing so is a violation of the code of ethics for nurses.

3. **Administering medication:** Nurses are responsible for administering the correct doses and medications to patients. If the nurse gives a fatal dosage amount, she may face legal malpractice suits. It is also the responsibility to research the patient's records, or ask the patient and family members if there are any allergies or complications that may pose a risk if a certain medication is administered.
4. **Informed consent:** When a nurse is administering treatment, she must explain what the effects and outcomes could be, and any other important information. It is the responsibility of the nurse to confirm that the patient or family member who will sign the informed consent form is coherent, and understands all the negatives and aspects of the treatment. The nurse, patient, or patient family member will sign the informed consent form in front of a witness, a physician or another nurse. Not having this legal document signed and in front of a witness could be a legal issue for the nurse if complications arise during treatment.
5. **Negligence:** It is the responsibility of the nurse to monitor the patient. If a patient calls for a nurse to come and assist him in going to the restroom for example, the nurse is to assist, or if she is busy with another patient, have another nurse assist the patient. Ignoring the patient or responding after a a lengthy delay could be considered negligence, and if the patient is hurt from trying to move himself, the nurse could face legal suits. Also, it could be considered negligence if a physician orders the nurse to administer a prescription, and the nurse did not do so.

10.6 LEGAL ISSUES RELATED TO NURSING REGISTRATION

A registered nurse (RN) is a nurse who has graduated from a college's nursing program or from a school of nursing and has passed a national licensing exam. A RN helps individuals, families, and groups to achieve health and prevent disease. They care for the sick and injured in hospitals and other healthcare facilities, physicians' offices private homes, public health agencies, schools, camps, and industry. Some RN are employed in private practice. A RNs scope of practice is determined by each state's Nurse Practice Act. It outlines what is legal practice for RNs and what tasks they may or may not perform. Nurse Practice Acts also dictate the scope of practice for nurse practitioners (NPs). An example is prescriptive authority for NPs. In some states, NPs can practice completely autonomously and prescribe any category of medications. In other states, NPs cannot prescribe controlled substances and may only practice with the collaboration of a physician.

Civil law penalties for registered nurses: Registered nurses have penalties that are inflicted on them for transgressions such as medical malpractice and breach of confidentiality. These civil law penalties can cause them to be suspended or banned from the nursing practice.

License revocation or suspension procedure: According to Tennessee law, the reasons for a Tennessee registered nurses license being denied, suspended or revoked are: fraudulent activity with respect to certification, established' I guilt before a court of law, medical negligence or malpractice, mental dysfunction, unprofessional conduct, drug use and complicity in a crime with another.

10.7 PATIENTS BILL OF RIGHTS

In 1973, the American Hospital Association adopted Patient's Bill of Rights as national policy statement and distributed it to its members in the healthcare organizations throughout the nation. There are twelve rights summarized below:

1. The patient has a right to a considerate and respectful care.
2. The patient has a right to obtain complete and concerned information concerning the diagnosis, treatment and prognosis from his physician for the patient's expected understanding.
3. The patient has a right to receive the necessary information from his physician regarding the treatment and the procedures involved in it.
4. The patient has a right to refuse the treatment to the extent permitted by the law and to be informed about the medical consequences of his action.
5. The patient has a right to privacy concerning his own medical care program.
6. The patient has a right to expect all communications and records pertaining to his care should be treated as confidential.
7. The patient has a right to expect within the capacity a hospital must make reasonable response to the request made by the patient for services.
8. The patient has a right to obtain information as to any relationship of his hospital to other healthcare institution a care is concerned.
9. The patient has a right to be advised if the hospital proposes to engage him in or perform human experimentation affecting his treatment.
10. The patient has a right to expect reasonable continuity of care.
11. The patient has a right to examine and receive an explanation of his hospital bills regardless of the source of payment.
12. The patient has a right to know what hospital rules and regulations apply to his conduct as a patient.

10.8 STANDARDS FOR BREACH SANCTIONS

Important Practice Standards for Breach Sanctions

The disparity in organizational response to employee malfeasance has a far-reaching impact on the healthcare industry. Consequences include the following:

1. **Confusing message:** An inconsistent organizational response to a breach sends a confusing message to both staff and the public. Healthcare workers moving from one organization to another find differing tolerance levels for enforcing the same directives.
2. **Poor compliance:** Staff in organizations with less stringent enforcement may weigh the level of risk to themselves against the potential advantages. Inequity in sanction application encourages poor compliance by individuals who know they will escape any serious consequence for breaching privacy and security policies.
3. **Erosion of public trust:** Public trust is eroded when significant variation is blatantly apparent in how healthcare organizations respond to a privacy or security breach both within and across entities and systems. The public must feel assured their personal health information

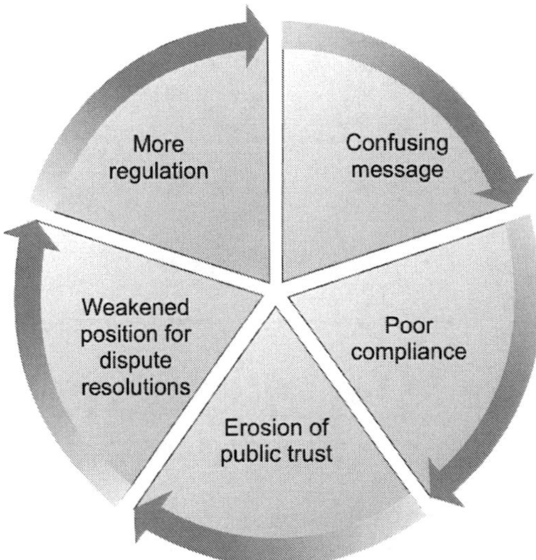

Fig. 10.3: Standards for breach situation

has sufficient protections across the healthcare spectrum, particularly in this era of health information exchange.

4. **Weakened position for dispute resolutions:** Inequitable application of sanctions can affect the outcome of personnel actions at arbitration and grievance proceedings. Unequal penalties for similar offenses undermine the organization's ability to prevail in dispute resolutions.
5. **More regulation:** Poor and inconsistent implementation of privacy and security safeguards invites further state and federal intervention. Such laws place an additional administrative and financial burden on facilities. If the industry does not self-correct, then it leaves open the door to state and federal government intervention.
6. **Questionable research:** The validity of research may be called into question when privacy or security breaches are not handled consistently and expeditiously patients.

10.9 LEGAL SAFEGUARDING OF NURSE

1. **Licensure:** All nurses who are in nursing practice have to possess a valid licensure, issued by the respective State Nursing Council/Indian Nursing Council.
2. **Good Samaritan laws:** In response to health professionals, fear of malpractice claims, most states enacted. Good Samaritan Laws that exempt doctors and nurses from liability when they render help during emergency. These laws limit liability and offer legal immunity for people helping in an emergency.
3. **Good rapport:** Developing good rapport with the client is very important to prevent malpractice. The ability to develop good rapport with client is dependent on the nurse having good interpersonal communication skills, e.g. listening.
4. **Standards of care:** All professional practicing in the medical field are held to certain standards when administering care. It is always better to follow standards of care to avoid malpractice and do not attempt anything beyond the level of competence.
5. **Standing orders:** Although, a nurse may not legally diagnose illness or prescribe treatment, she or he may after assessing patients condition apply standing orders or treatment guideline that have been established by the physician or doctor as appropriate for certain problems and conditions.

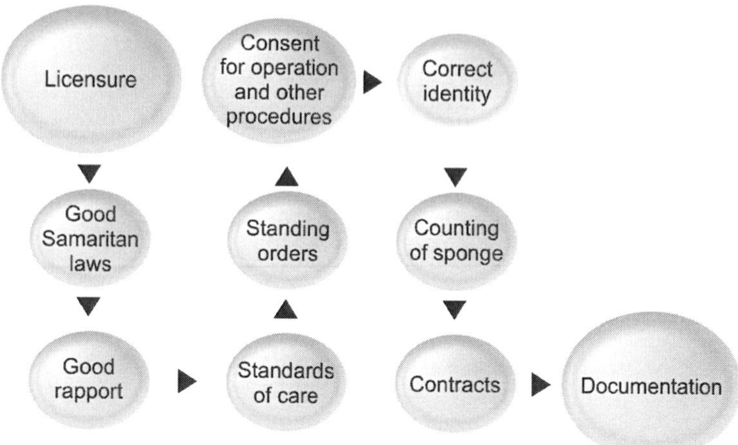

Fig. 10.4: Legal safeguarding of nurse

6. **Consent for operation and other procedures:** A patient coming in to hospital still retains his rights as a citizen and his entry only denotes his willingness to undergo an investigation or a course of treatment. Any investigation or treatment of a serious nature, or an operation in which an anesthetic is used, requires the written consent of the patient.
7. **Correct identity:** The nurse or the midwife has the great responsibility to make sure that all babies born in the hospital are correctly labeled at birth and to ensure that at no time they are placed in the wrong cot or given to the wrong mother.
8. **Counting of sponge instrument and needles:** Nurses advocate that sponge, instrument and needle counts be performed for all surgical procedures taking place in operation theatre. When an instrument left in a patient's body the nurse will probably be liable for any patient injury caused by the presence of foreign body.
9. **Contracts:** A contract is a written or oral agreement between two people in which goods or services are exchanged.
10. **Documentation:** Documentation is by far the best once a lawsuit field. The medical record is a legal document admissible in court as evidence.

CONCLUSION

Legal responsibility in nursing (service) practice is the way in which the nurses are obligated to obey the law in professional activities. The law is the final authority for regulating activities of all citizens including professional practitioner. Disobedience of the law results in punishment. It is always better that all nurses should understand the legal responsibility. When assuming a position to take care of a client, as a professional, nurse needs to update with the fast changing and advancing professional knowledge to provide safe nursing to their consumer on the basis of their needs. And nursing professionals should be aware of their limitations and shall be familiar with the law of nursing practice. Nurses should not give any room for any tort, i.e. negligence or malpractice in their practice. Torts may be unintentional, e.g. negligence and intentional torts are willful acts that violate another's right, e.g. invasion of privacy, and fraud.

11 Patients' Bill of Rights

11.1 INTRODUCTION

Patients' rights are among the most important of the issues involved in biomedical ethics influencing almost every aspect of the professional's ethical considerations. The American Hospital Association (AHA) has recognized the importance of patients rights and published a patients Bill of Rights. Patient awareness of individual rights and needs and availability of the various imaging techniques provides both opportunities and complications for the imaging professional. Nurses are not all levels of healthcare, but they are primary functionaries and the largest component of health manpower. Nurses while rendering care in a politically oriented health under the consumer protection act are increasingly facing ethical issues. Nursing ethics are the professional standard of conduct practiced by nurse practitioners related to or in accordance with approved moral behavior in rendering healthcare services.

11.2 GOALS OF PATIENTS' BILL OF RIGHTS

The Patients' Bill of Rights was created to try to reach three major goals:

1. To help patients feel more confident in the US healthcare system; the Bill of Rights: Assures that the healthcare system is fair and it works to meet patients needs, Gives patients a way to address any problems they may have encourages patients to take an active role in staying or getting healthy.
2. To stress the importance of a strong relationship between patients and their healthcare providers.
3. To stress the key role patients play in staying healthy by laying out rights and responsibilities for all patients and healthcare providers.

This Bill of Rights also applies to the insurance plans offered to federal employees. Many other health insurance plans and facilities have also adopted these values. Even Medicare and Medicaid stand by many of them.

11.3 AREAS OF PATIENTS' BILL OF RIGHTS

Table 11.1: The 8 key areas of the Patients' Bill of Rights

S.N	Areas	Description
1.	Information for patients	The patient has the right to accurate and easily-understood information about your health plan, health care professionals, and health care facilities. If you speak another language, have a physical or mental disability, or just don't understand something, help should be given so you can make informed health care decisions.
2.	Choice of providers and plans	You have the right to choose healthcare providers who can give you high-quality healthcare when you need it.

Contd...

Contd...

3.	Access to emergency services	If you have severe pain, an injury, or sudden illness that makes you believes that your health is in danger, you have the right to be screened and stabilized using emergency services. You should be able to use these services whenever and wherever you need them, without needing to wait for authorization and without any financial penalty.
4.	Taking part in treatment decisions	You have the right to know your treatment options and take part in decisions about your care. Parents, guardians, family members, or others that you choose can speak for you if you cannot make your own decisions.
5.	Respect and nondiscrimination	You have a right to considerate, respectful care from your doctors, health plan representatives, and other health care providers that does not discriminate against you.
6.	Confidentiality (privacy) of health information	You have the right to talk privately with healthcare providers and to have your healthcare information protected. You also have the right to read and copy your own medical record. You have the right to ask that your doctor change your record if it is not correct, relevant, or complete.
7.	Complaints and appeals	You have the right to a fair, fast, and objective review of any complaint you have against your health plan, doctors, hospitals or other healthcare personnel. This includes complaints about waiting times, operating hours, the actions of health care personnel, and the adequacy of healthcare facilities.
8.	Consumer responsibilities	In a healthcare system that protects consumer or patients rights, patients should expect to take on some responsibilities to get well and/or stay well (for instance, exercising and not using tobacco). Patients are expected to do things like treat health care workers and other patients with respect, try to pay their medical bills, and follow the rules and benefits of their health plan coverage. Having patients involved in their care increases the chance of the best possible outcomes and helps support a high quality, cost-conscious healthcare system.

11.4 PATIENTS' BILL OF RIGHTS

1. Understand and use these rights. If for any reason you do not understand or you need help, the hospital must provide assistance, including an interpreter.
2. Receive treatment without discrimination as to race, color, religion, sex, national origin, disability, sexual orientation, source of payment, or age.
3. Receive considerate and respectful care in a clean and safe environment free of unnecessary restraints.
4. Receive emergency care if you need it.
5. Be informed of the name and position of the doctor who will be in-charge of your care in the hospital.
6. Know the names, positions and functions of any hospital staff involved in your care and refuse their treatment, examination or observation.
7. A no smoking room.
8. Receive complete information about your diagnosis, treatment and prognosis.
9. Receive all the information that you need to give informed consent for any proposed procedure or treatment. This information shall include the possible risks and benefits of the procedure or treatment.
10. Receive all the information you need to give informed consent for an order not to resuscitate. You also have the right to designate an individual to give this consent for you if you are too ill to do so. If you would like additional information, please ask for a copy of the pamphlet "Deciding About Health Care — A Guide for Patients and Families".

11. Refuse treatment and be told what effect this may have on your health.
12. Refuse to take part in research. In deciding whether or not to participate, you have the right to a full explanation.
13. Privacy while in the hospital and confidentiality of all information and records regarding your care.
14. Participate in all decisions about your treatment and discharge from the hospital. The hospital must provide you with a written discharge plan and written description of how you can appeal your discharge.
15. Review your medical record without charge. Obtain a copy of your medical record for which the hospital can charge a reasonable fee. You cannot be denied a copy solely because you cannot afford to pay.
16. Receive an itemized bill and explanation of all charges.
17. Complain without fear of reprisals about the care and services you are receiving and to have the hospital responds to you and if you request it, a written response.
18. Authorize those family members and other adults who will be given priority to visit consistent with your ability to receive visitors.
19. Make known your wishes in regard to anatomical gifts. You may document your wishes in your health care proxy or on a donor card, available from the hospital.

11.5 WHO-DECLARATION OF PATIENTS' RIGHTS

Formalized in 1948, the Universal Declaration of Human Rights recognizes "the inherent dignity" and the "equal and unalienable rights of all members of the human family". And it is on the basis of this concept of the person, and the fundamental dignity and equality of all human beings, that the notion of patient rights was developed. In other words, what is owed to the patient as a human being, by physicians and by the state, took shape in large part thanks to this understanding of the basic rights of the person.

Patients rights vary in different countries and in different jurisdictions, often depending upon prevailing cultural and social norms. Different models of the patient-physician relationship—which can also represent the citizen-state relationship—have been developed, and these have informed the particular rights to which patients are entitled. In North America and Europe, for instance, there are at least four models which depict this relationship: the paternalistic model, the informative model, the interpretive model, and the deliberative model. Each of these suggests different professional obligations of the physician toward the patient. For instance, in the paternalistic model, the best interests of the patient as judged by the clinical expert are valued above the provision of comprehensive medical information and decision-making power to the patient. The informative model, by contrast, sees the patient as a consumer who is in the best position to judge what is in her own interest, and thus views the doctor as chiefly a provider of information. There continues to be enormous debate about how best to conceive of this relationship, but there is also growing international consensus that all patients have a fundamental right to privacy, to the confidentiality of their medical information, to consent to or to refuse treatment, and to be informed about relevant risk to them of medical procedures.

The Universal Declaration of Human Rights has been instrumental in enshrining the notion of human dignity in international law, providing a legal and moral grounding for improved standards of care on the basis of our basic responsibilities towards each other as members of the "human family", and giving important guidance on critical social, legal and ethical issues. But there remains a great deal of work to be done to clarify the relationship between human rights and right to health, including patient rights. Recognizing this challenge, the United Nations Commission on Human Rights (UNHCR) has designated a Special Rapporteur to provide it with a report that examines and clarifies the broader relationship between human rights and the right to health. This report has great importance for the World Health Organization (WHO), whose mission is to ensure "health for all". Grounding this mission in a fundamental human right to health would be an important milestone, and a great step forward realizing this goal.

11.6 CANCER PATIENTS BILL OF RIGHTS

1. All private, health insurers and all managed care plans shall cover in full all cancer screening and early detection protocols pursuant to the best evidence of appropriate screening protocols.
2. Every person diagnosed with a suspicious tissue growth, which has a reasonable, medical probability of being malignant shall have a right to immediate referral to a specialist, board-certified in cancer diagnosis and treatment.
3. Every patient with a confirmed diagnosis of cancer shall have a right to treatment by a multi-disciplinary team of oncology specialists, including but not limited to, medical oncologists, surgical oncologists, radiology oncologists, plastic surgeons, rehabilitation specialists, and counseling.
4. Every cancer patient, whether in treatment or after treatment, shall have the right to use a medical specialist as his/her primary care physician with full insurance coverage for same and without penalty within a managed care plan.
   Every competent, adult cancer patient shall participate in the formation of his/her treatment and rehabilitation plan and his/her pain management protocol.
5. Every hospital or research center rendering care to cancer patients shall respect such patients? Advance directives for discontinuation of care. If such hospital or research center for policy or religious reasons cannot respect advance directives, the patient or the patients designated representative shall be so informed as soon as possible.
6. Medical treatment facilities shall make every effort to acquaint each cancer patient with a recovering cancer patient who shall serve as the in patients personal counselor and advocate.
7. Cancer diagnostic testing and cancer treatment side effects shall be minimized to the extent practical under current standards of treatment.
8. Cancer patients have the right to continuity of care, including post-discharge aftercare.
9. Cancer patients shall receive from the primary, cancer treatment provider continuous and lifelong monitoring of health and emotional well-being with particular emphasis on vigilance for cancer recurrence and for long-term after effects of cancer treatment.
10. Cancer patients have the right to lifelong, continuing education on all aspects of cancer prevention, diagnostic tests, and treatment protocols.
11. Cancer patients have a right to participate in unapproved alternative or complimentary cancer treatments and to have their healthcare plan or health insurance provider pay for such treatments with certain noted restrictions. A competent, adult cancer patient may participate in alternative, unapproved treatments if he/she has received from his/her primary healthcare provider a written statement of such treatments known or probable risks and a written statement disclosing any readily available, known failures of such treatment.
12. Cancer patients shall participate in their own pain management and shall have the right to have their pain complaints believed, the right to aggressive pain management, and the right to know what limitations on pain management is the policy of the primary healthcare provider.
13. At the end of life, every competent adult or his/her legal representative shall have the right to request all available, pain management protocols, including opiates which might hasten death. No lawfully licensed physician shall be sanctioned for prescribing aggressive pain management even if death by sedation is a possible contraindication. No physician shall participate directly in physician-assisted suicide which shall be defined as deliberate administration of pain medication at a deliberately lethal dose with the intent of hastening a patients death.

14. Cancer survivors have a right to gainful employment commensurate with their talents and abilities, without regard to their history of cancer diagnosis.
15. Cancer survivors have a right to be included in employers group healthcare plans without prejudice against pre-existing cancer diagnosis.
16. Cancer survivors have a right to private health insurance at reasonable cost without prejudice against pre-existing cancer diagnosis if such patients have been in remission for at least two years.

CONCLUSION

A patient is a person with unique problem. A patient is a person who is suffering and needs help. It is necessary to recognize his /her needs. These rights are equal to those of anyone else in health. The patient has the right to obtain complete current information concerning his diagnosis, treatment and prognosis. In terms the patient can be reasonably, expected to understand. Nurses are accountable for judgments made and actions taken in the course of nursing practice.

12 Informed Consent

12.1 INTRODUCTION

Informed consent is a person's agreement to allow something to happen based on full disclosure of facts needed to make an intelligent decision. Nurses need to ensure that the patient/competent and responsible adult relative of the patient signs the consent form of the hospital.

12.2 PURPOSE OF INFORMED CONSENT

1. To ensure that the patient understands the nature of treatment including the potential complications.
2. To indicate that the patients decision was made without pressure.
3. To protect the patient against unauthorized procedures.
4. To protect the hospital staff and the hospital against legal action by a patient who claims that an unauthorized procedure was performed.

12.3 REQUIREMENTS OF INFORMED CONSENT

Table 12.1: Informed consent requirements

S.N	Requirements	Description
1	Disclosure	Adequate presentation of relevant information about the proposed treatment or study.
2	Understanding	Adequate comprehension of the disclosed information.
3	Voluntary agreement	Free assent, influenced by external controlling factors.
4	Competence	Adequate decision-making capacity. There are three types of autonomy, i.e., freedom of action, freedom of choice and effective delibration.
5	Freedom	The principle of individual freedom decrease that patients be exempt from control by others to select and peruse personal health goals.

12.4 KEY ELEMENTS OF INFORMED CONSENT

1. The consent must be given voluntarily by a mentally competent adult. The patient should not be coerced into giving consent.
2. Patient must understand exactly what he/she consenting to. If a patient speaks a foreign language or is deaf, an interpreter must explain the consent.

3. The consent should include risk to the procedure, alternative treatment available, and prognosis if the treatment is refused.
4. The consent is usually written, to provide a record of the transaction.
5. Consent to treatment a minor is usually given by the parent or the legal guardian; but nowadays, children who are at least seven years old are included in the decision-making process.

12.5 INFORMED CONSENT IN CLINICAL RESEARCH

1. Investigators should ensure that they obtain approval for the written consent form to be used in the study from the ethics committee prior to the trial starting.
2. Consent forms and information sheets should be revised when important new information becomes available that may be relevant to participant's consent. Revised consent forms should first be approved by the ethics committee before being used.
3. Neither the investigator nor the trial staff should coerce or unduly influence an individual to participate or to continue in a trial.
4. The investigator or the person designated by the investigator should fully inform the participant or the participants's legal representative of all the pertinent aspects of the trial including the written information provided to participants.
5. The language used in the oral and written information about the trial should be non-technical as practical and should be understandable to the participants and the participant's legal representative (where applicable).
6. Before consent is obtained, the investigator should provide participants with ample time and opportunity to inquire about details of the trial and decide whether or not to participate.
7. Prior to participant's recruitment to the trial, the written informed consent form should be signed and dated by the participant or by the participant's legal representative.
8. If a participant is unable to read, or the representative unable to read, an impartial witness should be present during the entire consent discussion and oral consent may be given. The witness confirms that the study information was understood and that informed consent was given freely.
9. Both the informed consent discussion and the written information sheet should include explanations about what the trial involves, the purpose of the trial, the trial treatment and whether randomization occurs as well as details.

12.6 INCAPACITY CRITERIA TO CONSENT

Table 12.2: Incapacity criteria to consent

S.N		Description
1	Neonates	1. Neonates cannot think like adults. It is therefore impossible for them to be able to make decisions, to understand information, to process information rationally or to desire reasonable outcomes. 2. As decisions have to be made about them, the best candidates for this role are the parents, on the assumption that above all people they will have the best interests of their child at heart. However, in some cases parents do not make decisions in the best interests of their children. 3. In those cases, it is possible for the state to step in and remove the decision-making role from them. This is done by making the child a ward of the court.

Contd...

Contd...

2	Children	1. It might appear that children cannot think like adults. Whilst this is certainly true of very young children, as children develop they show marked differences from each other. 2. The United Nations Convention on the Rights of the Child (UNROC) asserts that children have the right to say what they think should happen when adults make decisions that affect them and to have their opinions taken into account (Article 12), have the right to get and share information (Article 13), have the right to think and believe what they want and practice their religion as long as they do not stop other people enjoying their rights (Article 14), and have the right to privacy (Article 16). 3. Research activities involving children are carried out to learn more about the nature of pediatric development, disease and potential treatments. 4. An important safeguard required to minimize loss of respect for autonomy is the general rule that where the research can be carried out by employing adults then children should not be used.
3	Confused elderly patients	1. Various forms of neurological deterioration including Alzheimer's disease rob people of the powers to make decisions. 2. Relatives or true friends who knew them when well should be asked to help to build a picture of the patient's life, the preferences, the values and the wishes in which one can locate the decision that should be made. 3. A hypothetical consent is a consent which would likely be in accord with the feelings of the patient when well.
4	Patients with learning difficulties	1. It is important not to confuse intellectual impairment with mental illness. Patients with learning difficulties represent a wide range of intellectual ability and no simple standard of capacity can be assumed between them. 2. In each case an assessment according to the criteria outlined above is called for in combination with an awareness of the nature of the decision to be made. Only in extremely serious cases will a person with this problem be unable to make a decision about anything. 3. In those cases where either the impairment is so severe that the decision is too onerous or complex to be grasped by the person, a best interest judgment on their behalf should be made.
5	Mentally ill patients	1. As with intellectual impairment so with mental illness, one cannot assume that all persons possess equal capacity or otherwise. 2. On the one extreme, demented people cannot make coherent choices. 3. On the other hand when not in florid state a person with schizophrenia might be quite clear about how he feels about matters of life and how he would wish to address them.
6	Unconscious patients	1. Such documents as Advance Directives or Living Wills might be valuable guides but have inherent weaknesses that should be taken into account. 2. They might be old and out of date, they express hypothetical wishes, and there is always the need to know under what circumstances the documents were produced. The documents should be in accordance.

12.7 ELEMENTS OF INFORMED CONSENT IN RESEARCH

Table 12.3: Elements of informed consent in research

S.N	Elements	Description
1	Researchers role	1. The researcher must identify himself/herself and present qualifications to conduct study. 2. Nurse researcher in clinical practice must take extra precautions to inform client that they are acting in their capacity as researcher and not as nurse. 3. Potential subjects may not be able to differentiate the roles of nurse as caregiver and investigator.

Contd...

Contd...

2	Subject selection process is described	1. The subjects should be told how they were chosen to participate in the study. 2. If they must meet certain criteria to be eligible, these criteria should be presented early in the request for their participation.
3	Purpose of the study is described	1. The purpose or objects of the study should clearly present. 2. The material should be in the preferred language of the potential subject and at the subjects reading level for all printed material. 3. The researcher should be honest and open in presenting the purpose of the study.
4	Study procedures are discussed	1. All the subjects of the study should be fully explained. 2. This includes telling the potential subjects when the study will take place and where. 3. The researcher must stress the subjects' time involved and all activities that the subjects must perform. 4. This aspect of informed consent is particularly important in experimental studies where people will participate in or receive some type of treatment. 5. It is necessary to withhold information about a study from potential subjects, they must be informed of this before the study, and a debriefing session must be held afterwards. 6. This debriefing session will be used to ensure the participants understanding of the reasons and the justification for procedures used in the study.
5	Potential risks are discussed	Subject must be told of any possible discomforts, either physical or psychological, that might occur as a result of participation.
6	Potential benefits are described	In describing benefits to potential subjects, the investigator should describe both those applicable to the people involved in the study as well as how the results could benefit others.
7	Compensation if any discussed	1. Monetary compensation or any other type of compensation is involved in a research study, the possibility exists that biased results may be obtained. 2. Subjects may try to perform in a manner that will fulfill the researcher's expectations. Hence in nursing research, the researcher should avoid monetary compensations. 3. Subject compensations should come from those items listed under potential benefits. 4. The researcher should cover the cost of such items as laboratory tests and travel expenses for subjects.
8	Alternative procedures, if any, are disclosed	1. Potential subjects are informed of any alternative procedures that may be followed, such as you may fill out the questionnaire here or take it home. 2. Subjects more importantly, must be given an explanation of alternative procedures or treatment that may be received by others. 3. for example, a control group of subjects in an experimental study must be made aware that other subjects will be receiving some type of treatment. If the subjects have a choice of groups, this option is presented to them.
9	Anonymity or confidentiality is assured	1. Anonymity occurs when no one, including the researcher, can link subjects with the data they provide. 2. If the subjects can be liked to data, the researcher has the obligation to address confidentiality. 3. Confidentiality involves protection to the subjects identify by the researcher. 4. In many research studies, it is not possible to maintain anonymity. The researcher will usually come face to face with subjects in experimental study. 5. To maintain confidentiality, data are frequently coded and subject's names and code number are kept in a separate location that is only accessible to the researchers or members of the research team. 6. Any list that links subject names with data should be destroyed at the conclusion of the study.

Contd...

Contd...

10	Right to refuse to participate or to withdraw from study without penalty is assured.	1. All participation in nursing research studies must be voluntary. Even if a random sampling procedure is adopted also provide opportunity to decide if they wish to participate. 2. There must be no penalty involved for non-participation. Student's grades in a course should not be influenced by research participation.
11	Offer to answer all questions is made	1. Potential subjects must always be given the opportunity to ask questions that they have about the study. 2. It is almost impossible for the researcher to include every aspect of the study in a verbal or written explanation. Subjects frequently have questions about the study, and an opportunity should be presented for these questions during the verbal explanation of the study.
12	Means of obtaining study results is presented	1. Research subjects should always be given the opportunity to maintain the study results. 2. This does not mean that a copy must be sent to all participants. In fact, many participants are not interested in the results.
13	Documentation of informed consent	1. The researcher must document that informed consent was obtained. 2. If self-report questionnaires are used, a statement should be included on the questionnaire, in capital letters, similar to the following. Return of this questionnaire will indicate your consent to participate in this study. 3. In other type of research studies, consent is obtained in written form, stating that the study has willingly given permission and is aware of the risk and benefits. 4. Oral permission can be obtained, but must be witnessed by a third person. If the subject is a minor or is not able to give informed consent because of mental or physical disabilities, the consent of a legally authorized representatives, such as a child's parent, must be obtained.
14	The nurse researchers as a patient advocate	1. The nurse researcher has the responsibility to protect the privacy and dignity of the people involved in the research and to protects them from harm. 2. Even if study subjects willingly and knowingly agree to participate in a study involving undue physical risks, psychological risks, or both, the researcher has an obligation to refrain for conducting such research. 3. The nurse researcher must assume responsibility for study conditions and avoid undue physical or psychological risk to the subjects.

CONCLUSION

When a nurse is administering treatment, she must explain what the effects and outcomes could be, and any other important information. It is the responsibility of the nurse to confirm that the patient or family member who will sign the informed consent form is coherent, and understands all the negatives and aspects of the treatment. The nurse, patient, or patient family member will sign the informed consent form in front of a witness, a physician or another nurse. Not having this legal document signed and in front of a witness could be a legal issue for the nurse if complications arise during treatment.

13 Negligence and Malpractice in Nursing

13.1 INTRODUCTION

Negligence is described as lack of proper care and attention, carelessness. Negligence is the failure to meet an ordinary standard of care, resulting in injury to the patient or plaintiff.

13.2 DEFINITION

The basic and legal definition of negligence means breach of duty or injury. Standards of care in nursing generally mean those practices that "reasonably prudent nurses would use." So, a good nurse knows and understands ethics in the medical field.

13.3 COMMON SOURCES OF NEGLIGENCE

1. Medication errors that results in injury to the patient.
2. In intravenous infusion therapy error resulting in infiltration of phlebitis.
3. Burns to patients caused by equipment bathing or spills of hot liquids and food.
4. Falls resulting in injury to the patients.
5. Failure to uses aseptic techniques where required.
6. Failure to give a report or giving incomplete report to an oncoming shift.
7. Infection due to lack of aseptic techniques.
8. Error in sponge, instrument in surgical cases.
9. Error in patient identification.
10. Failure to adequate monitoring the patient.
11. Failure to meet the standard of care.

13.4 BREACH OF DUTY

Examples of breach of duty, which may be considered negligent under certain circumstances, may include doing something which a reasonably prudent person would not do, or the failure to do something which a reasonably prudent person would do, under circumstances similar to those shown by the evidence.

1. **Injury:** For an injury to be considered caused by negligence, records must show that the nurse failed to perform her duties with the patient in question. In such cases, the failure of duty must then be proven as directly related to the injury of the patient. For example, if a nurse fails to give medications as directed then the patient's condition worsens or he dies, the nurse may be found negligent.
2. **Performance failures:** Inadequate nursing skills or attention to tasks may result in a suit of negligence against a nurse who chronically fails to provide approved standards of care. Such

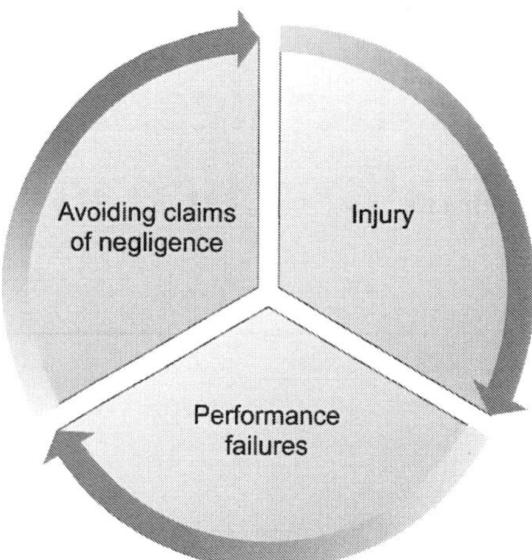

Fig. 13.1: Breach of duty

incidents include, but are not limited to, habitual medication errors, failure to follow protocol or orders and improper use of equipment.

3. **Avoiding claims of negligence:** A good nurse is well-informed regarding health and safety laws, as well as board regulations and customs of nursing. He is diligent in preventing injuries and falls, knowing his duties and is familiar with medications and dosage ranges for all patients under his care. A good nurse will avoids negligence when she practices good communication with patients and physicians and works within legal guidelines.

13.5 NEGLIGENCE IN NURSING PRACTICE

Negligence occurs when a nurse performs an act that is deemed below a competence level that is expected of someone in their position. Consequences to the nurse can range from suspension or firing to malpractice suits and loss of license. Neglect can be intentional or unintentional and can occur for many different reasons.

1. **Charting:** Failing to record vital information on the patient's chart can be considered negligent, especially if it results in further damage.
2. **Doctor's orders:** Failing to follow a doctor's orders can be grounds for malpractice if it results in damage to the patient.
3. **Confirming patient identity:** Before giving a patient medication or performing a medical procedure, the nurse must be sure that the right patient.
4. **Intentional neglect:** Many cases of neglect result from poor planning and other unintentional errors in judgment, but sometimes a nurse knows she is doing something wrong and chooses to do it anyway.

13.6 MALPRACTICE IN NURSING PRACTICE

Malpractice is one type of negligence and includes professional misconduct, breach of a duty or standard of care, illegal or immoral conduct or failure to excise reasonable skill, all of which lead to harm. Malpractice also professional misconduct performed in professional practice, any unreasonable lack of skill in professional duties or illegal or immoral conduct that results in injury or death to the client or consumer.

Common malpractices issues are:

1. Leaving foreign objects inside the client's body during surgery.
2. Failure to observe and report a change in the patient's condition.
3. Failure to get informed consent from the patient.
4. Medication error, giving wrong medication to the patient or wrong dosage.
5. Failure to follow physicians order.
6. Delaying patients care or failure to monitor the patient.
7. Incorrectly performing a procedure or trying to perform a procedure without training.
8. Documentation error.
9. Failure to provide patients education.

Avoiding nursing malpractice: Nursing is a highly respected and rewarding career, but it can also be very stressful and demanding. Even so, nurses make every effort to meet and exceed standards of care. The nurse should keep abreast of standards of care and standards of practice. Always follow facility policies and procedures to the letter. Above all, document, be sure to note the date and time on nurses' notes, and record all patient assessments and nursing interventions.

13.7 STANDARDS OF NURSING PRACTICE

Nurses are judged against specific standards of care. Simply put, standards of care delineate what nurses should do in the performance of their role. Standards of practice are more specific and outline how the care is to be delivered. For example, a standard of practice for a critical care nurse might be: Vital signs will be monitored continuously and recorded on the patient's medical record every fifteen minutes for the first 24 hours following admission. Standards of care are outlined within the state's Nursing Practice Act, facility departmental policy/procedure manuals, and within the specific area of practice.

CONCLUSION

Negligence is the responsibility of the nurse to monitor the patient. If a patient calls for a nurse to come and assist him in going to the restroom. For example, the nurse is to assist, or if the is busy with another patient, have another nurse assist the patient. Ignoring the patient or responding after a lengthy delay could be considered negligence, and if the patient is hurt from trying to move himself, the nurse could face legal suits. Also, it could be considered negligence if a physician orders the nurse to administer a prescription, and the nurse did not do so. Malpractice is a term used for negligence. Malpractice specifically refers to negligence by a professional person with a license. You can be sued for malpractice once you have your LPN license. If you are a nursing assistant right now, you may be negligent, but it wouldn't be malpractice because you are not licensed.

14 Public Health Legislations

14.1 INTRODUCTION

Law has had important contributions to several public health achievements but, despite this, the conceptual framework for its effective application has not been fully explicated. Medicine has moved beyond treating disease to promoting health, which entails policy interventions and regulations at different levels to bring about behavioral changes in individuals. The chief objective of public health laws at national level is proper regulation and management of health services. By logical utilization of health laws and acts, it is possible to improve national health status, through them, along with qualitative changes in health indices; the health objectives can also be achieved.

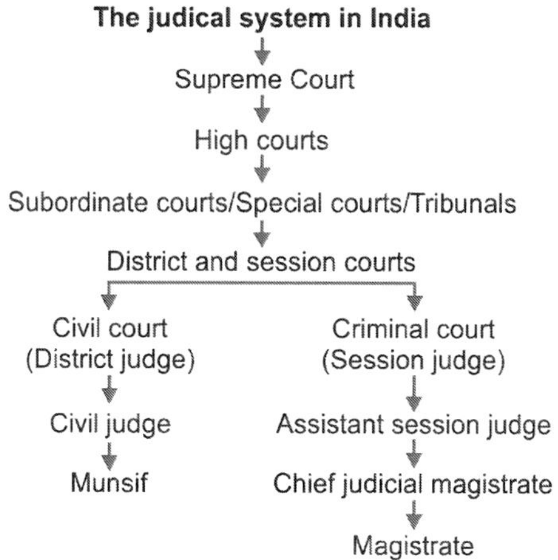

14.2 DEFINITION

Public health law focuses on legal issues in public health practice and on the public health effects of legal practice. Public health law typically has three major areas of practice: police power, disease and injury prevention, and the law of populations. Law is an important public health tool that plays a critical role in reducing illness and premature death. Public health law examines the authority of the government at various jurisdictional levels to improve the health of the general population within societal limits and norms.

14.3 SCOPE OF PUBLIC HEALTH LAW

The reach of public health law is as broad as public health itself and both have expanded to meet the needs of society. The scope of the right to health and its correlation with the right to healthcare was first outlined in the Universal Declaration of Human Rights in 1948, wherein while the right to health was conceived as an individual's civil right, states were bound to provide minimum conditions to enable individuals to enjoy this right and provide primary health services in an equal and fair manner. It is important to note that while the right to health is considered an inherent human right, the right to healthcare is its progressive realization through declared constitutional and legal rights, in particular, through public health law. Public health law could be defined as the study of the legal powers and duties of the State, to ensure conditions for people to be healthy with collaboration from multiple stakeholders (e.g. healthcare professionals, business, community, media and academe). Unlike at the turn of the century, today the field of public health has expanded from areas of communicable diseases and environmental sanitation to address enlarged health concerns, for instance, chronic diseases and mental health as well as provide services to create a healthy environment.

14.4 GOOD SAMARITAN LAW

This legislation applies to physicians, surgeons, registered professional nurses, licensed practical nurses, and licensed mobile emergency medical technicians in situations when aid is given in an emergency or accident and occurs outside of a health care setting. When any of the above health care providers render, in good faith, emergency care or assistance at the scene of an emergency or accident, no liability may be imposed for any civil damages arising from acts or omissions in rendering such emergency care. There is no protection, however, for gross negligence or willful or wanton acts or omissions. Thus, it should be noted that this legislation is only applicable if the care is rendered without compensation. This law further protects the rendering of emergency care or assistance to any minor involved in any accident, injured in competitive sports, or affected by any other emergency at the scene of an accident without first obtaining the consent of a parent or guardian. Again, there is no protection from civil liability for gross negligence or willful or wanton acts or omissions.

14.5 IMPORTANCE OF PUBLIC HEALTH LAWS

There is need for public health law to realize the urgency of regulating the modifiable patterns of behavior among people to strengthen the capacity of the community against public health risks involving, in particular, use of tobacco, diet and exercise. However, it is important to highlight that such legislations might have limitations and the level of effectiveness and enforcement can affect a law's effectiveness in achieving the intended public health goals. Laws should, therefore, not be used in isolation but as one of several tools for the attainment of public health goals. The importance of public health laws are described below:

1. Strengthen the nation's health infrastructure.
2. Following the international health laws (with suitable changes according to national needs).
3. Encouragement of unified group activity for health.
4. Identification of government's limitations in the area of health.
5. Making necessary financial provision for health.
6. Maintaining the federal form of the nation so that in a concurrent area like health there is no difference of opinion between center and states.
7. Proper exploitation and utilization of national resources.
8. Better coordination between health planning and finance departments.
9. Maintaining economic discipline in the area of health.
10. Protection of environmental health.
11. Protection of food and maintaining nutritional level.
12. Protecting citizens from drug addiction, alcoholism and other unhealthy and dangerous habits.

13. Protection to consumers of health services.
14. Protection from environmental pollution and other health risks.
15. Following codes of ethics in health and medical services, education, training and research.

In addition to these, through health laws, protection from violence and accidents, better control over private health services, etc. are also possible.

14.6 NEED OF PUBLIC HEALTH LEGISLATIONS

The *Public Health Act* is a product of extensive stakeholder consultations. Significant changes to the new Act include:

1. The modernization of powers and duties of public health officials for communicable disease prevention and control, environmental health hazard response, chronic disease and hazard prevention, and public health emergency response, e.g. updated inspection powers, powers to issue orders, quarantine and isolation provisions.
2. Improved health monitoring abilities such as being able to require the reporting of indicators of hazardous environmental exposures, e.g. blood levels of lead and mercury.
3. The ability of health officers to order groups of people to take prevention measures to control a health hazard. Previous to this new provision, each individual affected by a health hazard had to be issued a separate and unique order. After the SARS outbreak, public health officials identified the need for more effective management strategies to cope with groups of potentially infected people.
4. Ability to require public health planning.
5. New powers to regulate operations, activities or conditions that could pose a health hazard or a threat to long-term population health.
6. Provisions that ensure administrative fairness.
7. Strengthened relationships with and clarification of responsibilities of local governments regarding public health, and
8. Modernization of enforcement, sentencing, and penalty provisions.

The new *Public Health Act* reflects and supports many of key public health objectives raised by the Conversation on health, such as more proactive measures to promote health and prevent disease and injury. The Conversation noted a strong desire for better environmental protection, better availability of immunizations, and a need to strengthen the public health system's ability to address infectious disease outbreaks. Issues raised in the Conversation on Health addressed by the *Public Health Act* are:

1. **Health protection and environmental health issues:** The *Public Health Act* will allow development of mandatory reporting provisions in addition to those currently in place for communicable diseases to ensure that necessary information is collected for public health interventions and monitoring the health of the public. These provisions will allow for monitoring of body levels of pollutants (e.g. lead, mercury) and contribute to preventing the potential negative health effects associated exposure to environmental contaminants and poisonings.
2. **The Act provides health officials the authority and tools** to prevent and control the spread of disease and other health hazards by allowing for preventive interventions (e.g. vaccination, ordering examinations and quarantine). The Act strengthens the inspection and enforcement powers of health officials which enables them to monitor and ensure compliance with the Act, enter places, engage the assistance of peace officers, and obtain warrants and court orders. During a public health emergency, such as a pandemic flu outbreak, public health officials have additional authority to respond immediately to protect the public from significant harm.
3. **Health Promotion:** The *Public Health Act* allows the minister to require development of public health plans. The purposes of public health plans could include: promoting and protecting the health and well-being of British Columbians, identifying the needs of specific populations

(i.e. aboriginals, new immigrants), addressing mental health and substance use issues, and preventing and mitigating the adverse affects of diseases, disorders, disabilities, and injuries.

14.7 PUBLIC HEALTH LEGISLATIONS

Besides the committees which are appointed from time to time, the Union Ministry of Health and Family Welfare pilots draft legislation in the legislature. These laws assist in the formulation and execution of National health policy. These laws also empower health authorities to implement health policies. The first health legislation dates back to the year 1825 when the Quarantime Act was passed. Since, the first Lok Sabha, the following laws related to health have been enacted which are classified as:

I. Laws related to drugs, food adulteration and cosmetics:

1. Drugs and Magic Remedies Act, 1934, 1963 (Objectionable advertisement), 1964.
2. Prevention of Food Adulteration Act, 1934, 1964 (Amendment) 1971.
3. Drugs Act, 1953.
4. Opium laws 1957.
5. Poisonous Act, 1938.
6. Drugs Act, (Amendment) 1962.
7. Drugs and Cosmetics Act, 1964, 1972 (Amendment).
8. Medicinal and Toilet Preparation (Amendment) Act 1961.

II. Medical education:

1. Dentists (Amendment) Act, 1955, 1972.
2. Indian Medical Council Act, (Amendment) 1936,1938, 1964.
3. Indian Nursing Council Act, 1957.
4. Pharmacy Act, 1959.
5. Indian Medicine Central Council Act, 1970.
6. All India Institute of Medical Sciences Act, 1936.
7. PGIMER Chandigarh Act, 1956.
8. Homeopathy Central Council Act, 1975.

III. Maternity:

1. Maternity Benefit Act, 1972.
2. MTP Act, 1971.

IV. Miscellaneous:

1. Registration of Births and Deaths Act, 1969.
2. St. John Ambulance Association Act, 1956.
3. Indian Red Cross Society Act, 1956.
4. Countess of Dufferin Fund Act, 1957.

Public health laws provide the working tools to health administrators for safeguarding the communities from health hazards and for promoting health. Such legislation would help in the demarcation of the functions at various levels. Union, state and local would bring about uniformity in procedure and action. Nowadays, the health laws in India are scattered in piece-meal enactments. Some of them have become outmoded while others need change in contents because of the environmental changes. The present campus of legislation is inadequate. Regulations are taking in many vital subjects. There is a model of Public Health Act, 1955. But most of the states have not come forward to adopt this legislation. There is an urgent need to enact and approve this legislation as it would provide guidance to the policy makers, planners and health administrators.

1. **Medical Termination of Pregnancy Act (1971):** In this Act, unless the context otherwise requires, (a)"guardian" means a person having the care of the person of a minor or a lunatic; (b)"lunatic" has the meaning assigned to it in section 3 of the Indian Lunatic Act, 1912 (4 of 1912); (c)"minor" means a person who, under the provisions of the Indian Majority Act,

1875 (9 of 1875), is to be deemed not to have attained his majority; (d)"registered medical practitioner" means a medical practitioner who possesses any recognized medical qualification as defined in clause; (h) of section 2 of the Indian Medical Council Act, 1956, (102 of 1956), whose name has been entered in a State Medical Register and who has such experience or training in gynecology and obstetrics as may be prescribed by rules made under this act.

2. **Prenatal Diagnostic Techniques (Regulation and Prevention of Misuse) Act, 1994:** An Act to provide for the regulation of the use of prenatal diagnostic techniques for the purpose of detecting genetic or metabolic disorders or chromosomal abnormalities or certain congenital malformations or sex linked disorders and for the prevention of the misuse of such techniques for the purpose of prenatal sex determination leading to female foeticide; and, for matters connected there with or incidental thereto. (1) This Act may be called the Prenatal Diagnostic Techniques (Regulation and Prevention of Misuse) Act, 1994. (2) It shall extend to the whole of India except the State of Jammu and Kashmir. (3) It shall come into force on such date as the Central Government may, by notification in the Official Gazette, appoint.
3. **Food Safety and Standards (Contaminants, toxins and Residues) Regulations, 2011:** "Crop contaminant" means any substance not intentionally added to food, but which gets added to articles of food in the process of their production (including operations carried out in crop husbandry, animal husbandry and veterinary medicine), manufacture, processing, preparation, treatment, packing, packaging transport or holding of articles of such food as a result of environmental contamination.
4. **In the Hindu Marriage Act, 1955** (hereafter in this Chapter referred to as the Hindu Marriage Act), in section 13B, in sub-section (*2*), for the words, brackets and figure "On the motion of both the parties made not earlier than six months after the date of the presentation of the petition referred to in sub-section (*1*) and not later than eighteen months after the said date, if the petition is not withdrawn in the meantime", the words, brackets and figure "Upon receipt of a petition under sub-section (*1*)" shall be substituted.
5. **Women the right to protection against sexual harassment and towards that end for the prevention and redressal of sexual harassment of women (2010):** Whereas Sexual harassment infringes the fundamental right of a woman to gender equality under Articles 14 and 15 of the Constitution of India and her right to life and live with dignity under Article 21 of the Constitution which includes a right to a safe environment free from sexual harassment. And whereas the right to protection from sexual harassment and the right to work with dignity are recognized as universal human rights by international conventions and instruments such as Convention on the Elimination of all Forms of Discrimination against Women (CEDAW), which has been ratified by the Government of India. And Whereas the Supreme Court in Vishakha *vs* State of Rajashthan [1997 (7) SCC 323] has formulated guidelines to address sexual harassment until a suitable legislation is enacted in this respect.
6. **Child abuse or neglect:** Covered entities may disclose protected health information to report known or suspected child abuse or neglect, if the report is made to a public health authority or other appropriate government authority that is authorized by law to receive such reports. For instance, the social services department of a local government might have legal authority to receive reports of child abuse or neglect, in which case, the privacy rule would permit a covered entity to report such cases to that authority without obtaining individual authorization.

14.8 HEALTH MANAGEMENT SYSTEM (HMS) ACT

In addition to law of similar there are four other cardinal laws or principles. These are:

1. **The law of direction of cure:** The direction of cure states that during curative process the symptoms disappear in the reverse order of its' appearance- from above downwards, from more important organs to less important organs/from center to periphery etc.

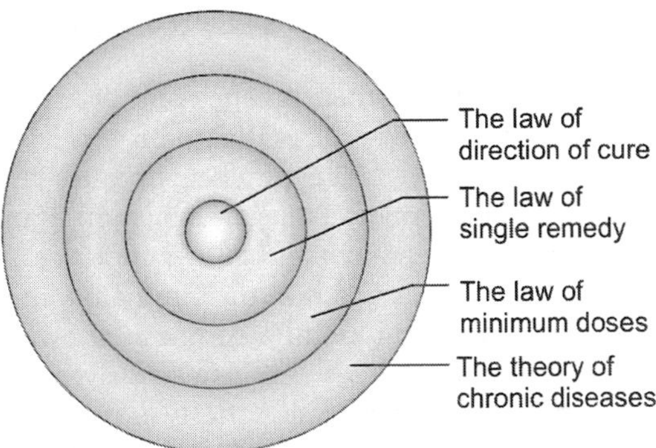

Fig. 14.1: Cardial laws

2. **The law of single remedy:** Homeopathy generally uses only a single medicine which has a true similarity of symptoms with that of the remedy. This process of selecting the correct remedy is done on the basis of individualization. The intensive process of individualization distinguishes this system from other system in its approach to the holistic concepts in therapeutics. The physician adopts a detailed case study by exploring the physical, psychological, biomedical constitution of the individual.
3. **The law of minimum doses:** The doses applied are the minimum possible, just sufficient to correct the diseased state.
4. **The theory of chronic diseases:** The theory of chronic diseases states that most of the diseases are due to three chronic latent affinities known as Psora, Syphilis and Sycosis in the human being which normally remain dormant but express their presence when conducive environment for disease such as irregular living, constant exposure to unhealthy situations, emotional stress, atmospheric influences etc., overpower the immune system/health. The modern concept of the host, and agent environment reaction (triad) in the causation of diseases is well-documented by Hahnemann in his Masterpiece Organaon of Medicine. Homeopathy attaches significance to the nomenclature of disease to the extent of choosing the auxiliary mode of treatment, prevention, and clinical management, prognosis etc., not in selection of the remedy. The concept is that the physical, mental and spiritual expression of the sick forms the totality of the disease.

Thus, Homeopathy is highly individualizing process. The physician's interest is to alleviate the present symptoms and also long-term well-being. The physician requires long duration to interview the patient to probe deeply into the most subtle and unique response of the patient's defence mechanism to varying stress.

14.9 LAW AND NURSING/MEDICAL PROFESSION

Doctors, nurses and other paramedical staff working in the field of public health are responsible and accountable to both, their profession and national law. Here some aspects of judiciary in India are being described in brief. The community/public health nurse may be a witness or a defendant in legal proceedings. Common legal proceedings are civil lawsuits, criminal prosecutions, professional discipline hearings, inquests, and labor arbitrations. Less common are public inquiries and human rights tribunals.

Legislative and legal control for nursing practice has been established to clarify the boundaries of nursing practice and to protect patients. The leader/manager uses established legal guidelines to role model nursing practice that meets accepted standard of care. Important leadership roles in law and legislation are those of vision, risk taking and energy. The leader who is active in professional organizations and groups define what nursing is and what it should be in the future.

This is an internalized responsibility that must be adopted by many nurses if the profession is to be recognized.

Managers are responsible for seeing that their practice and practice of their subordinates are in accord with current legal guidelines. This requires that managers have a working knowledge of current laws and legal doctrines that effect nursing practice. Because laws are not static, this is an active and ongoing function. The managers have a legal obligation to uphold the laws, rules and regulations, affecting the organization, the patient and nursing practice.

Managers have a responsibility to be fair and non-discriminatory in dealing with all members of the work force, including those whose culture differs from their own. The effective leader goes beyond merely preventing discrimintory charges and instead strives to develop sensitivity to the needs of a culturally diverse staff. Caring, respect and honesty as part of nurse patient relationships are emphasized if these functions and roles are truly integrated. The risks of patient harm and nursing liability are greatly reduced.

14.10 LEGAL RESPONSIBILITIES IN NURSING

Legal responsibility in nursing (service) practice is the way in which the nurses are obligated to obey the law in professional activities. The law is the final authority for regulating activities of all citizens including professional practitioner. Disobedience of the law results in punishment.

It is always better that all nurses should understand the legal responsibility. When assuming a position to take care of a client, as a professional, nurse needs to update with the fast changing and advancing professional knowledge to provide safe nursing to their consumer on the basis of their needs. And nursing professionals should be aware of their limitations and shall be familiar with the law of nursing practice. Nurses should not give any room for any tort, i.e. negligence or malpractice in their practice. Torts may be unintentional, e.g. negligence and intentional torts are willful acts that violate another's right, e.g. invasion of privacy and fraud.

Some of the Guidelines for Nurses for their Safe Practice

1. Document all unusual accidents.
2. Report all unusual incidents.
3. Follow policies and procedures as established by your employing agency.
4. Keep current year license.
5. Perform procedures.
6. Protect patient from injuring themselves.
7. Don't remove side rails.
8. Don't allow patients to leave the hospital without an order which is signed.
9. Don't witness patients will.
10. Don't accept money or gifts from patients.
11. Don't take medications that belong to patient.

Legal Responsibilities of Nurse

1. Responsibility of appointing and assigning.
2. Responsibility in quality control.
3. Responsibility for equipment.
4. Responsibility for observation and reporting.
5. Responsibility to protect public.
6. Responsibility for record keeping and reporting.

CONCLUSION

Public health laws provide the working tools to health administrators for safeguarding the communities from health hazards and for promoting health. Such legislation would help in the demarcation of the functions at various levels. Union, state and local would bring about uniformity in procedure and action. Nowadays the health laws in India are scattered in piece-meal enactments. Some of them have become outmoded while others need change in contents because of the environmental changes. The present campus of legislation is inadequate. Regulations are taking in many vital subjects. There is a model of public health act, 1955. But most of the states have not come forward to adopt this legislation. There is an urgent need to enact and approve this legislation as it would provide guidance to the policy makers, planners and health administrators.

15 Consumer Protection Act

15.1 INTRODUCTION

Consumer Protection Act (CPA) was passed by the Parliament in the year 1986. This Act considers patients as consumers, i.e. buyers of services and doctor as the provider of these services on payment. During last few years, due to increased availability of sophisticated investigative and therapeutic technology, modern practice of medicine is dehumanized. This fact is partly responsible for loss of mutual trust.

15.2 CONSUMER PROTECTION ACT

Consumer Protection Act (CPA) was passed by the Parliament in 1986 to provide for better protection of the interest of consumers and focuses on consumer justice through the establishment of consumer councils and other authorities for the settlement of consumers disputes and matters connected therewith. The scope of the Act is wide enough to include a vast variety of services. Under this Act consumer can complain in redressal forum. It enables the consumer or patient to make a complaint to a redressal forum in respect of defective services provided.

Rights of a Consumer/Patient are:

1. Right of safety.
2. Right to be informed.
3. Right to choose.
4. Right to be heard.
5. Right to seek redressal.
6. Right to consumer education.

15.3 IMPORTANT FEATURES OF CONSUMER PROTECTION ACT

Important features of this act are following:

1. Services rendered by a doctor, hospital or any other health care organization for carrying out consultation, diagnosis, investigations and treatment fall within the purview of this act.
   The services rendered may be free, on payment, in charitable hospital or in profit making paying hospital.
2. If the charges are reimbursible or there is third party payment, e.g. employer, insurance company etc., and then also the act is applicable.
3. If the services rendered are totally free, then the act is not applicable.
4. The act is applicable to the patients who are treated free in paying hospitals.
5. The act is applicable to all the patients free and paying in the free hospitals having paying beds, paying section or payment required for any service.
6. Consumer does not have to pay court fees or process fees.

7. Prescribed time limit for settling the dispute is three months. If expert examination is required, longer time is permitted.

15.4 AUTHORITIES INVOLVED IN CONSUMER PROTECTION ACT

The act permits examination by the following bodies:

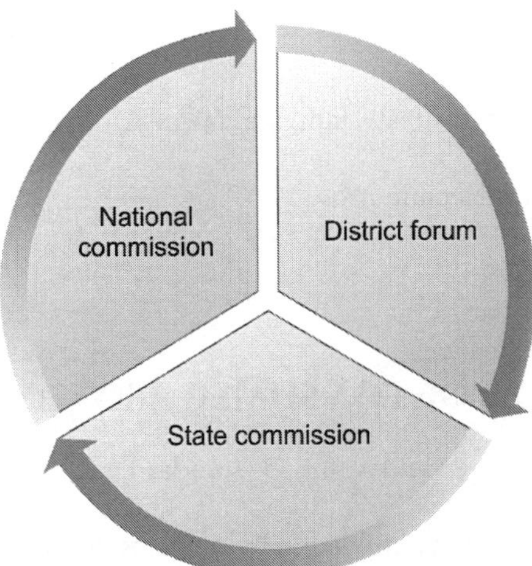

Fig. 15.1: Authorities involved In CPA

1. **District forum: The forum consists of three persons.** a. District judge as president, b. Two persons having knowledge of any of the following i. Law, ii. economics, iii. Commerce, iv. Accounting, v. Administration, vi. Industry.
   They should be having ability and integrity. At least one person should be a woman. Compensation not exceeding ₹ 5 lakhs is the limit of this body. Complaints demanding higher compensation are outside its purview. If the complaint is not satisfied with the decision he/she can appeal to state commission within 30 days.
2. **State commission: Consists of 3 members.**
   a. Sitting or past judge of high court as president.
   b. Two persons as described in the composition of district forum.
   This commission attends to the complaints asking for compensation
   (i) Which is more than ₹ 5 lakhs
   (ii) Less than ₹ 20 lakhs.
   If the complainant is not satisfied with the judgment, the appeal can be made to the National Commission within 30 days.
3. **National Commission: Consists of 5 persons.**
   a. Sitting or past judge of Supreme Court.
   b. Four persons as described in the previous two committees.
   This commission handles complaints demanding more than ₹ 20 lakhs as compensation.

Consumer Protection Act also provides for:

a. State level consumer protection council.

b. Central consumer protection council for the purpose of
   (i) Protecting rights of the consumers,
   (ii) Promoting rights of the consumer's,
   (iii) Educating consumers

15.5 ADVANTAGES OF CONSUMER PROTECTION ACT

1. Doctors are accountable for their actions of:
   a. Omission
   b. Commission
2. Speedy justice to consumers.
3. Decisions are made on the basis of law, faith and fairness.
4. It encourages:
   a. Proper communication with patient's
   b. Proper documentation
   c. Better performance
   d. Reasonable charges.

15.6 DISADVANTAGES OF CONSUMER PROTECTION ACT

1. Medical services are personalized and cannot be standardized. Hence, there may be unnecessary complaints.
2. Doctors tend to practice defensive medicine by ordering more tests, ordering opinions, from other specialists and treating doubtful conditions vigorously.
3. Black mailing by patients, colleagues, lawyers and so called social workers.
4. Likely damage to the reputation.
5. Doctors may refuse to take up complicated cases.

15.7 INDENTITY INSURANCE FOR MALPRACTICE SUITS

In the event of dissatisfied consumer, i.e. patient claiming damages either through district forum, state commission, and national commission or through court of law alleging medical negligence or malpractice by the doctor, it becomes time consuming and expensive issue for the doctor to prove that there had been no negligence. If the judgment goes against the doctor, than payment of a very large sum becomes necessary. As the number of such litigations against doctors and hospitals is steadily increasing. It has become necessary for the doctor to have medical indemnity insurance.

At present there are some nationalized insurance companies having scheme for professional indemnity insurance for:

a. Doctor as an individual
b. Shared practice, i.e. partners
c. Diagnostic centers
d. Nursing homes
e. Laboratories
f. Hospitals
g. Blood banks etc.

In individual doctor's policy the policy holder can include the names of qualified assistants or qualifies employees mentioning their status. Hospitals can have comprehensive group policy which will cover all the staff employed by the hospital. If there are claims for compensation against an individual person or more persons of the hospital, the insurance company takes up the issue and if the act committed requires compensation, it is settled by the insurance company.

15.8 NURSING ASPECTS OF CONSUMER PROTECTION ACT

Safe nursing practice includes an understanding of the legal boundaries in which nurses must function. An understanding of the implication of the law supports critical thinking on the Nursing part. Laws are changing constantly to reflect changes in society, changes in the delivery of health-care and advancement in medical technology. The Supreme Court in November 1995 gave a judgment that patients who receive deficient services by medical profession and hospital are entitle to claim damages under Consumers Protection Act 1986. The concept of the Act is that if a wrong has been committed while giving service, the caregiver must pay for it. If it is a case of error in judgment then it has to be proved. According to the Act the consumer need not pay for appealing to consumer court. The act also prescribes penalties for negligence. However, the Act is not applicable to Government hospitals, clinics or health centers and to those who practice there. This is because services rendered in Government institutions are not charged.

CONCLUSION

The Consumer Protection Act of India is also quite specific about what a complaint is, under the law's definitions. First and foremost, the complaint must be made in writing and should concern an unfair action by a business or individual acting in a commercial setting. Defects in goods or unsatisfactory service can be the subject of written complaints, as can excessively high charges for goods or services. The Consumer Protection Act defines the obligation of traders and manufacturers as well as of service providers, and if the consumer feels that the goods provided or the services given are not to his satisfaction, are defective, and below the standards prescribed normally, he is entitled for what he has paid.

Section-5

Professional Adjustment

16 Autonomy in Nursing

16.1 INTRODUTION

Autonomy comes from the Latin auto meaning "self" and nomy which means "control". Individuals must be given the rights to assist in their own decision making. The central idea autonomy is self-rule. Autonomy that individuals are able to act for themselves to the level of their capacity. It is the right of individual to govern their actions according to their own purposes and reason. Respect for autonomy requires that persons honor another's right to govern him or her. The legal doctrine of informed consent is the direct reflection of autonomy. This ethical concept has led to the need for informed consent. Sometimes patients' religious or cultural beliefs lead them to make decisions regarding their own care that may seem controversial or even dangerous. However, the concept of autonomy gives them the right to make those decisions unless they are mentally impaired.

16.2 MEANING OF AUTONOMY

1. Autonomy referred to ethics means the autonomic choices and autonomous actions of an individual. Autonomy equate with power.
2. An autonomous decision is one that is based on the decision maker, values, utilizes adequate information and understanding and is free from coercion or restraint and is based on reason and deliberation.
3. Autonomous actions are those that stem from autonomous decision rather from the person being forced to act or restrained from acting in a certain way.
4. The broad principle of autonomy yields to many specific rules for healthcare providers. The best known of this is the rule of informed consent which specifies that we must obtain permission from the patient before doing any procedure on him/her.
5. Autonomy can also serve as the basis for duties of truth telling one way in which we can interfere with the person's right to make free choices is by deceiving the person in some way.
6. Autonomy incuse a specialized knowledge, authority, accountability and the independence. The autonomy real control of a profession over the structure and the condition of its work.

16.3 DEFINITION

1. Autonomy involves the right of self-determination, independence and freedom.
2. Autonomy is defined as accountability for patient care unit operations, and referred to the right to make decisions and the responsibility for outcomes.
3. Autonomous practice is the right to deliver or render professional duties in a self-determined manner while adhering to the legal ethical and practice standard of the profession.

16.4 PRINCIPLES OF AUTONOMY

The principle of autonomy is crucial to the study of ethics for three reasons:

1. Without some sense of person's as autonomous or free, rational decision makers, we have to basis for assigning responsibility for actions.
2. Impose some important duties on us, e.g. people have a right to make autonomous choices, we have a duty not to interfere with our choices. We can interfere with free choice by simply not permitting some one to make a choice, interference in our choices violate the principle of autonomy.
3. The third learn autonomy is a significant concept is ethics in that it provides a law of classifying actions that has important implications for other duties.

16.5 CHARACTERISTICS OF AUTONOMY

Autonomous describes an essential quality of person as well as a type of behavior. The autonomous person can be described as being rational unrestrained. This indicates that the person is self-governing and independent regarding his or her decisions and activity. Persons who are unaware or irrational may be unable to demonstrate autonomous behavior. However, autonomous remains an essential quality of their person, that is, a part of human character, integrity and holism. Preserving that autonomy becomes a concern for nurses as professional caregivers of such persons. When clients are not independent regarding either decisions or activity, nurses intervene. Nurses help persons do those things that they would do unaided if they had the necessary strength, will or knowledge. Nurses do this manner that enables the client to be as independent or autonomous as possible.

Self-awareness also helps to guard against exercising any personal need to control or have inordinate authority over others. Whenever students or graduate nurses find themselves labeling clients-calling them stubborn, uncooperative or noncompliant—it is instructive for them to take stock of their own expectations and behaviors. These situations are common warning signals that a power struggle may be developing; they are particularly inappropriate and suggest that nursing is not being practiced from a perspective that values client's abilities for self-care and autonomy.

16.6 AUTONOMY AS ATTITUDE AND STRUCTURE

Autonomy has both a personal or attitudinal dimension as well as a structural dimension. Autonomy is part of a nurse's attitude and is reflected in statements like these, "This nurse has a high personal sense of autonomy", and "This nurse is committed to an autonomy of practice," and "This nurse values autonomy of practice". Each of these statements reflects nurses who value, want, or embody an attitude of autonomy. If a nurse is to practice with autonomy, he or she must perceive and value the freedom to do so and be willing to exercise autonomy. If a nurse does not value autonomy or does not perceive the freedom to carry out autonomous acts, then the nurse will not be autonomous. Autonomy involves structure. Structure includes the structure of a health care agency, the scope of practice that is described in nurses' practice literature, nurses' license laws, nurse organization's professional practice standards, advanced practice certifications, and knowledge development within nursing science. Each will be briefly considered.

The structure of a healthcare agency reflects the degree of autonomy of nurses. Agencies vary enormously on the extent to which a nurse is encouraged, hired to do, and positively rewarded for carrying out discretionary and binding decisions and actions. If a nurse must seek permission for practice acts that are within his or her educational training before she or he carries them out, there is essentially no autonomy allowed by the agency. If, however, a nurse is promoted, given merit pay increases, and valued when she or he carries out discretionary and binding decisions for patient care, then the agency's structure supports and encourages autonomy.

Autonomy is affected by the scope of practice that is described in nurses' practice literature, license laws, and practice standards. These documents are essential for advancing and supporting autonomy in nursing. If the practice literature emphasizes nondiscretionary and nonbinding decisions, they are not supporting autonomy. One could even argue that they are holding back autonomy. Nurses' license laws should clarify the domains of knowledge and skills over which the nurse can make discretionary and binding decisions. Clear laws should reflect clarity on the nurse's assessment responsibilities, on binding decision-making responsibilities, and on delegated responsibilities. The literature should be examined and evaluated for text that discourages autonomy or encourages nurses' dependency on others for making most of the decisions for nurses. What do the license laws state about nursing actions? A review of these laws can be illuminating.

The text of these laws may include language that works against autonomy in nursing. For example, if the text of the practice law states that nurses must seek preapproval to initiate patient care plans, the law is working against autonomy. If the law states that nurses serve patients at the discretion of the physician, the law is working against autonomy. Functioning with autonomy as nurses is different than functioning collaboratively with physicians. Nurses do function collaboratively with physicians, but that does not preclude them from functioning autonomously within their scope of practice. These two issues should not be confused with each other.

16.7 AUTONOMY IN NURSING

Autonomy in nursing consists of making unconstrained decisions and being able to act on those decisions. Nursing has attempted to take back some control from the government in regulating its own practice through certification of the specialty practices. Many nurses feel that the bureaucracy of hospitals and healthcare organizations affects their autonomy. Most units do not give nurses freedom in scheduling and have numerous polices and procedures set by the hospital mandating nursing with the increased hiring of unlicensed personnel to take over nursing tasks. Professional autonomy includes controlling enter in to the profession establishing the standards for enter and training and influencing lawmakers through professional organizations.

16.8 THEMES OF AUTONOMY IN NURSING

The major three themes of autonomy in nursing are as:

1. Theme I: Ownership of practice.
2. Theme II: Emphasis of wellness and healing.
3. Theme III: Clients as partners.

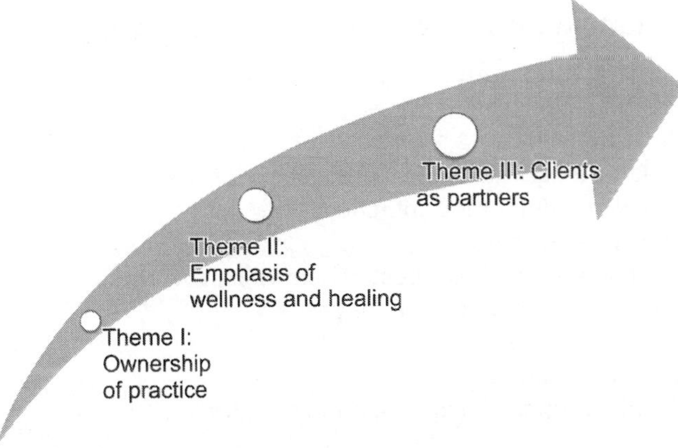

Fig. 16.1: Themes of Autonomy

Theme I: Ownership of practice: A sense of dignity about nurses as professionals, which we call ownership of practice. Ownership of practice includes many of the dimensions of autonomy. The dimensions of autonomy are: 1. Control over nursing practice, 2. The freedom to make decision, 3. The quality of professional exchange with colleagues that nurses always sought. Ability to use the nursing expertise to help others by becoming mentors and role models for less experienced and new nurse. The nurses recognize that autonomy is liked to power and that the many limits placed on our practice where simply a way to keep nurses in live.

Theme II: Emphasis of wellness and healing: The theme cooperates holistic theory and the concept of body mind connection in to the nursing practice. This concept helps the client to replace his fear and anxiety to the feeling of the safety and security. This enhances the client's cooperation for treatment and quick recovery from the diseases.

Theme III: Clients as partners: It means being to treat the clients as knowing subject rather than as an object of nursing care. The intervention becomes more and more caring when he see clients as partners.

16.9 SOURCES OF CONSTRAINS IN AUTONOMY

1. Nurses identified the following sources of constraints on their autonomy; they are society, the institutions where nurse work, members of other disciplines and nurse them.
2. The nurses must realize that the confidence with knowledge is held pride in that knowledge and correspondingly high valuation of self-related to possession of knowledge and skills in an important precursor to both autonomy and empowerment.
3. Nurses should resist establishment beliefs that limited their role and diminished our authority.

16.10 FACTORS ENHANCE AUTONOMY IN NURSING

While a nurse's scope of practice is legally defined based on educational qualifications and specific experiences, professional and organizational expectations determine the degree to which autonomous practice occurs. As described in the following section, strategies for enhancing autonomy are based on setting clear expectations for autonomous decision-making and providing support for increasing the knowledge and expertise of nurses.

1. Social or public contact.
2. Quality assurance.
3. Nursing audit.
4. Evaluation of nursing.
5. Evolvement in standard setting policy making.

Strategies for Enhancing Autonomy and Control Over Nursing Practice

I. Strategies for Enhancing Autonomy

a. Clarify expectations about clinical autonomy:
    1. Describe expected behaviors.
    2. Embed nursing knowledge into clinical practice processes.
    3. Recognize and reward autonomous practice.
    4. Role model expected behaviors.
    5. Coach Nurses not demonstrating expected behaviors.
    6. Provide manager support for autonomous practice.

b. Enhance competence in practice:
    1. Create a learning environment.
    2. Enable formal and informal educational opportunities.

II. Strategies for Enhancing Control over Nursing Practice

a. Establish participative decision-making:

1. Use an organized structure for nurse participation in decision-making.
2. Ensure authority for clinical decision making resides with direct care nurses.
3. Include nurses on organizational committees.
4. Minimize bureaucracy.
5. Support involvement by nurses on committees and workgroups.

b. Enhance competence in decision-making:

1. Teach nurses about the decision-making process.
2. Coach and support nurses through early decisions.
3. Teach facilitation skills to leaders.

III. Strategies for both Autonomy and Control over Nursing Practice

a. Ensure strong nurse leaders:

1. Create strong, visible, nurse leaders.
2. Ensure that nurses in supervisory positions are encouraging autonomy and CONP.
3. Have executives advocate for influential nursing practice.
4. Encourage new and innovative ideas.

b. Work upstream:

1. Influence social, political, and economic factors.
2. Publicly describe nursing's unique expertise and contribution.
3. Acknowledge nurses' contributions in all roles and practice settings.
4. Use political clout of professional organizations and nurses in leadership roles.

16.11 RESPECT FOR AUTONOMY

This principle states that an ethical theory should allow people to reign over themselves and to be able to make decisions that apply to their lives. This means that people should have control over their lives as much as possible because they are the only people who completely understand their chosen type of lifestyle. Each man deserves respect because only he has had those exact life experiences and understands his emotions, motivations and body in such an intimate manner. In essence, this ethical principle is an extension of the ethical principle of beneficence because a person who is independent usually prefers to have control over his life experiences in order to obtain the lifestyle that he enjoys.

There are, however, two ways of looking at the respect for autonomy. In the paternalistic viewpoint, an authority prioritizes a dependent person's best interests over the dependent person's wishes. For example, a patient with terminal cancer may prefer to live the rest of her life without the medication that makes her constantly ill. The physician, on the other hand, may convince the patient and her family members to make the patient continue taking her medication because the medication will prolong her life. In this situation, the physician uses his or her authority to manipulate the patient to choose the treatment that will benefit him or her best medically. As noted in this example, one drawback of this principle is that the paternalistic figure may not have the same ideals as the dependent person and will deny the patient's autonomy and ability to choose her treatment. This, in turn, leads to a decreased amount of beneficence.

A second way in which to view the respect for autonomy is the libertarian view. This standpoint prioritizes the patient's wishes over their best interests. This means that the patient has control over her life and should be content with her quality of life because she has chosen the path of life with the greatest amount of personal beneficence. Although, this viewpoint is more mindful of the patient's desires, it does not prevent the patient from making decisions that may be more harmful than beneficial.

16.12 AUTONOMY FOR NURSE PRACTITIONER

1. Nursing profession enjoy substantial freedom to practice their skills based on complete knowledge, with their guidelines established by their profession and without interference by the general public. They accept responsibility for standards of professional performance throughout their career.
2. An essential attribute of professional role is autonomy and staff control regarding the development and application of the body of generalized knowledge in which the professionals alone are experts.
3. The professional must have autonomy from administrative controlling determination occupation tasks and functions and do what ever will best serve the clients interest and welfare using standards of practice that are based on the application of specialized knowledge to the unique circumstances of the clients nurses can administer their functions and take decisions for the nurse care.

CONCLUSION

Ethics is a discipline involved with good and bad, moral duty, obligation, and values. Ethics also concerned with social and political philosophy and the philosophy of law. The professional use of the term ethics implies a high standard of moral quality of professional practice. The concept of client autonomy is recurring them in ethical issues. Autonomous means independent and self-governing. Many persons who seek the services of health professionals may believe that their dependency on other for care services. Two particular constrains that may be concerned are lack of ability and coercion. The current economics of healthcare, including constrains imposed on accessing some services and providers, may contribute to this belief.

17 Accountability in Nursing

17.1 INTRODUCTION

Accountability is the process that mandates that individuals are answerable for their actions and have an obligation to act. The concept of accountability has two major attributes: answerable and responsibility. A nurse is accountable to self, the client, the profession, the employer and society. To be accountable, the nurse practice with in the codes of profession. Accountability requires on evaluation of the nurses performance in providing quality care. Accountability can be better ensured and measured when quality care has been defined.

17.2 DEFINITION

1. American Nurses Association Code of Nurse defines, "accountability being answerable to someone for something one has done. It means providing an explanation to self, to the client, to the employing agency and to the nursing profession".
2. Accountability can be defined in terms of either of these attributes but answerability for how one has promoted, protected and net the health needs of the client.
3. A condition in which individuals who exercise power are constrained by external means and internal norms. Doctors and health professionals are accountable before the law, the Hippocratic Oath, peers, patients, and grant-giving agencies (if they do research), to the public, insurance carriers, and government agencies.
4. Taking responsibility for one's own actions and defending them to anyone who asks (e.g. to stakeholders, the general public, colleagues, partner agencies and policy makers). Organizational accountability includes the statutory responsibility of the NHS and Social Services Department in the UK.

17.3 MEANING OF ACCOUNTABILITY

1. Accountability involves assuring only the responsibility that are within one's scope of practice and not assuming responsibility for activities in which competencies has not been achieved.
2. Accountability involves admitting mistakes rather than blaming others and evaluating the outcomes of one's own actions.
3. Accountability includes a responsibility to the client to competent to render nursing services in accordance with standards of nursing practice and to adhere to the professional ethics code.

17.4 CHARACTERISTICS OF ACCOUNTABILITY

1. Accountability is the obligation to report back the results of responsibilities undertaken.
2. It is the liability for proper discharge of duties.

3. It is the personal answerability for results.
4. Accountability grows out of responsibility and goes hand in hand with it.

17.5 DOMAINS OF ACCOUNTABILITY

A profession undertakes, they require exercises of judgment in applying knowledge to the solution of problems and accept responsibility for the results. Accountability has always been acknowledged as one of the hallmarks of a professional nurse.

Table 17.1: Dimensions of accountability

S.N	Dimensions	Description
1	To the clients	The client is no longer blindly submissive, he is more aware of his rights, therefore he should be a full partner in decisions and actions regarding his health. The client has a right to receive the best possible quality in an equally knowledgeable manner through the application of sound judgment and appropriate values system. Nurse must know the importance of documenting their work and the progresses used in accomplishing goals.
2	To the society	Nursing is also accountable to society because profession has received society's authorization to practice by virtue a degree/diploma. Nursing is also accountable to the society in guarding against ill-prepared worker being certified to give nursing care.
3	To the profession	The profession of nursing has accountability towards itself in the performance of its duty to formulate its own policy and control its activities. Its standard for licensure and certification.
4	To self	Nurses must be responsible for their own mental and physical health for assuming that she keeps all aspects for her life in balance. Accountability to self also involves acknowledging her limitations and knowing when she is in need of further education in order to perform her role more fully and safely.
5	To employing agency	It is the last domain of nurses accountability. The agency is accountable to the public for the care provided, therefore in turn, it has the right to expect the nurses to be accountable to agency. The quality of nurses' work is one aspect in which she is accountable to agency.

17.6 ACCOUNTABILITY OF NURSING PERSONNEL

Nursing personnel are accountable for:

1. Proving safe and therapeutic environment for patients.
2. Delivering component and personalized care.
3. Maintaining adequate supplies of material and equipment for smooth functioning of the ward/unit.
4. Maintain accurate and up-to-date records and reports.
5. Maintaining good interpersonal relationship.
6. Protecting clients legal rights and privacy.
7. Working within legal and ethical boundaries.
8. Keeping pace with changing health needs and developing technology.
9. Developing care as per standards lay down by profession, statutory body and institution.
10. Delegating responsibility appropriately.
11. Contributing to development of the profession.

17.7 ACCOUNTABILITY IN NURSING

The concept of accountability is a concept closely aligned with public trust and confidence with a healthcare discipline. It is of vital importance to the discipline of nursing to define and examine the obligations and duties of professional nurse. The term is referred to and often defined through international and national professional codes of nursing and in standards of nursing practice documents. This column will begin exploration of the concept with offering a definition from a human becoming perspective.

Accountability is at the heart of nursing, weaving its way through nursing practice in all settings and at all levels. It is an energizing force throughout an organization, where a culture of accountability exists, people do what they say they'll do. Everyone builds credibility for themselves and for the organization by holding themselves and each other accountable.

17.8 WAYS TO MAINTAIN ACCOUNTABILITY

1. In order to maintain accountability, the nurse should know the code of ethics in nursing.
2. Providing quality nursing care, assures that the nurse maintains accountability.
3. To maintain accountability, the nurse should follow accurate technical skills and also should acquire knowledge through higher education.
4. The nursing profession itself regulates accountability through nursing audits and standards of practice.
5. Nurse should have sufficient knowledge about legal aspects in nursing. This enables her to maintain accountability towards the profession, client, team members also.

CONCLUSION

The person or position accountable for a task is responsible for insuring that it is completed on-time and in a manner which meets all expectations for it. The Accountable (A) person or position does not have to physically do the task. Accountability should be focused on the "Responsible" person whenever possible. Accountability must be assigned to each task. Accountability must never be used as a device for placing blame or designating a scapegoat. Developing accountability does not mean relinquishing accountability on management's part. It must be perceived as a partnership. In the beginning of a group's development, management usually carries the lion's share of the accountability burden, absorbing the brunt of any disappointments. However, as the group matures, members expect to be held more accountable for their own results.

18 Assertiveness in Nursing

18.1 INTRODUCTION

Assertiveness is an important issue in nursing practice. Educational programme in assertiveness knowledge and skills have been in vogue for some time in nursing because nurses have recognized the need for assertiveness in quality nursing care. Assertiveness is a tool for expressing ourselves confidently and a way of saying yes or no in an appropriate way. It is considered as healthy behavior foe all people against personal powerlessness and results in personal empowerment. Nursing has determined that assertive behavior among its practitioners is an invaluable component for successful professional practice.

18.2 MEANING OF ASSERTIVE BEHAVIOR

Assertive behavior means that a person stands up for himself or herself in a way that does not violate the basic rights of another; expresses true feelings in an honest, direct manner; does not let others take advantage of him or her; shows respect for others rights, needs, and feelings; and takes responsibility for the consequences of those actions; is able to accept compliments and criticism; and acts in a way that enhances self-respect.

18.3 DEFINITION

Assertiveness is a style of behavior to interact with people while standing up for the rights. Assertive manner certainly means that we will feel more empowered and more in control of circumstances. However, it is definitely not a strategy to get our own way more frequently.

18.4 ASSERTIVENESS MODEL

Assertiveness model: A-S-E-R-T Model:

S.N	Model	Description
1	A	Ask for god's help-pray to god to guide you through scriptures and his spirit.
2	S	State the problem-think over state the facts of the problem.
3	E	Express your-self- state your feeling, do not judge.
4	R	Request change and feedback–specify one behavior change. Then listen to the other person's thoughts and opinions.
5	T	Talk it out—paraphrase their ideas. Discuss the consequences, considerations and opinions.

18.5 AIMS OF ASSERTIVENESS

1. The aim of assertiveness is to find the best possible solution for all people. It is about finding win-win solutions. Assertiveness sees every one as equal rights and responsibilities.
2. Assertiveness increases the chances of our needs being met.
3. Assertiveness allows us to remain in control.
4. Assertiveness brings greater self-confidence.
5. Assertiveness lets us have greater confidence in others.
6. Assertiveness people have more friends.
7. Reduced stress.

18.6 BENEFITS OF ASSERTIVENESS

1. It helps to create healthy and meaningful relationship.
2. It helps for lessen the friction and conflict.
3. There is increased self-respect as well as request from others.
4. Our self-esteem is enhanced and we always feel in control.
5. Our productivity at work and in the home increases.
6. It decreases the work stress and increases the overall well-being.
7. It helps to express our emotion appropriately and also improves the physical and emotional health.

18.7 GUIDELINES OF ASSERTIVENESS

I. Respect your feelings.
1. Understand the difference among thinking, feeling and communicating your feelings.
2. Learn to listen to your feelings.
3. Have the courage to act on your feelings.
4. Learn to express your feelings.
5. Learn to listen to others and their feelings.

II. Know your rights as a human being.
1. To judge your own behavior, thoughts and emotions.
2. To offer no excuses for justifying your behavior.
3. To judge if you are responsible for finding solutions to other people's problems.
4. To change your mind.
5. To make mistakes -- and be responsible for them.
6. To say "I don't know".
7. To be independent of the goodwill of others before coping with them.
8. To say "I don't understand".
9. To say "I don't care".
10. To attempt to achieve objectives and feel good about doing so, so long as you don't hurt others in the process.

III. Know your responsibilities to yourself.
1. Your actions.
2. Self-improvement.
3. Your state of mind.

IV. Look change in the eye.

18.8 ADVANTAGES

1. Lets other people know what you feel, what you need and what you are thinking.
2. Helps you feel good about yourself.
3. Allows you to treat others with respect.
4. Reflects confidence.
5. Indicates decisiveness.
6. Leads to a more satisfying life.

18.9 DISADVANTAGES

1. At times if not properly conveyed, then one considers it to be rudeness.
2. It can also reflect over-confidence.
3. Can prove to be counter-productive.
4. One may appear to be arrogant.

18.10 ASSERTIVENESS IN NURSING

Assertiveness is considered healthy behavior. When present fights against personal powerlessness and results in personal empowerment. Assertive behavior among nurses is an important component for successful professional practice. Self assertion will eventually lead to further personal and professional empowerment. It is all about valuing yourself and your profession. Becoming more assertive can lead to increased respect and recognition as a person and as a nurse. It can get you more of what you want. Becoming more assertive is a process. It's not something that happens overnight. As nurses work in different situations they have to be assertive in order to meet the challenges and to win the cooperation from others.

Assertiveness is an important behavior for today's professional nurse. As nurses move away from traditional subservient roles and perceived stereotypes it is increasingly being recognized that a nurse needs to behave in an assertive manner. Assertiveness is necessary for effective nurse/patient communication, and it is suggested that its development may also aid the confidence of the profession as it develops. Assertive behavior may be encouraged through educational methods. It is preferable that nurses receive this educational preparation during undergraduate programes. Nurse educators have an important role in the development and implementation of assertiveness training/education programmes for undergraduate nursing students.

CONCLUSION

Assertiveness is an important behavior for today's professional nurse. As nurses move away from traditional subservient roles and perceived stereotypes it is increasingly being recognized that a nurse needs to behave in an assertive manner. Assertiveness is necessary for effective nurse/patient communication, and it is suggested that its development may also aid the confidence of the profession as it develops. Assertive behavior may be encouraged through educational methods. It is preferable that nurses receive this educational preparation during undergraduate programes.

19 Discipline in Nursing

19.1 INTRODUCTION

The word 'discipline' comes from the Latin term 'disciplina' which means teaching, learning and growing. When employees are unsuccessful in meeting organizational goals, managers must attempt to identify reasons for their failure and counsel employees accordingly. If employees fail because they are unwilling to follow rules or established policies and procedures, or they are unable to perform their duties adequately despite assistance and encouragement, the manager/administrator has an obligation to discipline the employee.

19.2 MEANING OF DISCIPLINE

Discipline can be defined as a training or molding of the mind and character to bring about desired behaviors. Thus, discipline allows one individual to have some control over another. It is a necessary and positive tool in promoting subordinate growth. Constructive discipline uses discipline as a means of helping the employees to grow, not as a punitive measure. Punishment is frequently included when defining discipline but it also can be defined as training, educating and/or molding. The primary emphasis in constructive discipline is assisting employees to behave in a manner that allows them to be self-directive in meeting organizational goals. Discipline refers to working in accordance with certain recognized rules, regulations and customs, whether they are written or implicit in character. Human performance is greatly influenced by the state of discipline in any organization.

19.3 ADVANTAGES OF DISCIPLINE

The discipline has following advantages for employees as well as an organization.

1. Discipline creates a climate under which individual excellence is encouraged, group I performance improved and harmonious working is developed.
2. Discipline sets a pattern to acceptable behavior and performance on the part of human beings, i.e. it provides a code of conduct for the guidance of the group.
3. Good discipline promotes individual growth, develops human capacity and stimulates will to perform effectively, i.e. it helps in morale building.

19.4 CAUSES OF INDISCIPLINE IN STAFFING

1. Discipline is imposed when indiscipline steps in the organization. The causes of indiscipline and suggestion are given below. Faulty disciplinary actions taken by the authorities may lead to indiscipline. It has been suggested that disciplinary actions must be consistent enough to provide equal justice to all concerned, for which managerial actions in regard to discipline must be free from any bias, privilege or favoritism.

2. Neglect of employee's grievances: Neglecting or deferring the settlement of employees grievances cause indiscipline such as strikes, agitation and others. It has been suggested that the grievances of the employees should be settled by enquiring as early as possible. Otherwise it leads to poor performance, poor morale and serious indiscipline.
3. Wrong placement and promotions or remunerations also leads to indiscipline.
   Taking prompt decision for right placement, timely promotion and proper remuneration helps to reduce such indiscipline.
4. Deficiency of well-defined code of discipline also leads to indiscipline. The code of discipline should encompass sufficient rules, regulations, customary practices for the guidance and information to employees.
   Hence, proper code of discipline should be formulated and circulated and communicated in clear and simple language to all employees.
5. Divide and rule policy in the organization also leads to indiscipline. This type of behavior on the part of the administration or management should not be practiced at any cost in the interest of the organization.
6. Improper attitude towards employee's problem leads to indiscipline. Basically attitudes influence human beings and their activities; moreover discipline itself is a byproduct of attitude. Understanding of the employees' personal problems and individual difficulties helps to maintain discipline.
7. Ill-equipped supervisor may cause indiscipline. As the maintenance of discipline is the case of supervisory responsibilities, indiscipline may spring from the want of the right type of supervision.

19.5 DEALING WITH DISCIPLINARY PROBLEMS

When dealing with disciplinary problems. It is better to conduct disciplinary conference. While conducting disciplinary conference both directive and nondirective interview techniques can be used. To guide the discussion in the conference, the manager should begin with clear statement of the broken behavior rule, i.e. gives description of the specific rule broken by the employee.

1. Should describe corrective action expected by the employees, i.e. action that employee should take to correct the problem.
2. Should specify the time allowed to employee to remedy his shortcomings, i.e. amount of time allowed the employee to correct his or her behavior.
3. Further discipline to result if specified behavior change is not made.
4. See that disciplinary conference documented and included in employment record.

19.6 ERRORS IN DISCIPLINE

While administering discipline, there are some common management failures come across by the managers refer to errors in discipline as follows:

1. Delay in administering discipline.
2. Ignoring rule violation in hope that it is an isolated event.
3. Accumulation of rule violations causing irritated manager to 'blow up'.
4. Administering sweetened discipline.
5. Failure to document disciplinary actions accurately.
6. Failure to act within time limits set by grievance procedure.
7. Imposing discipline disproportionate to the seriousness of the offence.
8. Disciplining inconsistently.

As stated above, failure to follow due process in disciplinary procedures results in unfair, inappropriate or ineffectual disciplinary action.

19.7 MANAGEMENT IN DISCIPLINARY ACTION

To apply due process in disciplinary actions the manager must ensure that:

1. There is an agency rule or standard that governs the behavior under consideration.
2. The employee was aware of the rule or standard governing her or his problem behavior.
3. The employee did, in fact, violate the agency rule or standard.
4. The penalty imposed is appropriate to the rule or standard violated.

In recent days, some of the managers in industry and healthcare have stimulated employees to aim for the 'higher ideal' of organization by employing what is known as 'positive discipline' or discipline without punishment. The positive discipline is based on the assumption that an employee with self-respect, respect for authority and interest in the job will adhere to high quality work standards.

The positive discipline consists of the following steps:

1. Friendly oral reminder to employee of first violation.
2. For repeated violations, written statement of problem and work goals to employee.
3. Development by manager and employee of action plan to improve employees' behavior.
4. Repeat violation, one-day paid leave to reflect on commitment to agency goals.
5. Submission by employee of written statements of intent to stay and improve or leave agency.
6. Employee notified that failure to meet commitments with result in termination. For maintenance of effective discipline in the organization following four practices are essential.
   a. Condonation of past offences.
   b. Agreement as to disciplinary rules.
   c. The discipline committee.
   d. Investigation by the human resource management.

19.8 ROLE AND FUNCTIONS OF ADMINISTRATOR IN DISCIPLINE

The following are the roles and functions of administrator/manager in discipline.

1. He or she encourages employees to be self-disciplined in conforming to established rules and regulations.
2. Assists employees to identify themselves with organizational goals, their increasing the likelihood that the standards of conduct deemed to be accepted by the organization and will be accepted by its employees.
3. Humanistically uses discipline as a means of promoting employee growth.
4. Periodically assesses the need for existing rules and regulations and suggests modifications as necessary.
5. Is self aware regarding the power and responsibility inherent in having formal authority to set rules and discipline employees?
6. Demonstrates sensitivity to the environment in which discipline is given.
7. Serves in the role of coach in performance deficiency coaching.
8. Ensures that rules and regulations are clearly written and communicated to subordinates.
9. Discusses rules and policies with subordinates, explaining the rationale for their existence and encouraging questions.
10. Enforces established rules in a fair and consistent manner.
11. Judiciously uses formal authority to take progressively stronger forms of discipline when employees continue to fail to meet expected standards of achievement.
12. Carefully documents employees behavior(s) that prompts disciplinary action and any attempts to counsel the employee.
13. Uses developed communication skills to do the following, clearly explain the nature or seriousness of disciplinary problems.

a. Allow employees feedback in the disciplinary process.
   Explain disciplinary actions to be taken and why
b. Describe expected behavioral changes and what the consequences of failure to change, will be.
c. Reach agreement and acceptance of the disciplinary plan with the employee.

14. Disciplines union employees in accordance with the steps, penalties and time frames established in the union contact.
15. Advises employees in seeking disciplinary action redress through informal and formal grievance procedure.

CONCLUSION

Discipline may be the self-controlled discipline or enforced discipline. In the case of self- controlled discipline, the employee brings her or his behavior into agreement with the organizations' official behavior code, i.e. the employees regulate their own activities for the common good of the organization. As a result, human beings are induced to work for a peak performance under self-controlled discipline. In the case of enforced discipline, a managerial action enforces employee compliance with organization's rules and regulations, i.e. it is a common discipline imposed from the top here, and the manager exercises his authority to compel the employees to behave in a particular way.

20 Confidentiality

20.1 INTRODUCTION

The ethical codes of healthcare profession also embrace confidentiality of health information as a major principle. Confidentiality refers to the ethical, professional and legal obligation of a physician not to disclose what is communicated to him/her within physician-patient relationship. The basic elements of the confidentiality includes respect for patient privacy and autonomy, prevention of harm to patient fiduciary relationship between patient and physician, service to common goods etc.

Medical confidentiality is a concern as old as the practice of medicine itself. The Hippocratic Oath, which new medical school graduates around the world must swear to uphold, states "whatever in connection with my professional practice, or not in connection with it, I see or hear in the life of men, which ought not to be spoken of abroad, I will not divulge as reckoning that all such should be kept secret"(Thirumoorthy, T. 2001).

The essence of medical confidentiality is the nondisclosure of personal information gathered in the course of the practice of medicine. Since, medical practitioners deal with the most intimate physical and mental data concerning the people they treat, it is not hard to understand why patients would not want potentially embarrassing facts or conditions divulged to others without their consent. Furthermore, the information may also be used to persecute, discriminate against, or harm the individual involved—especially if they suffer from a hot button disease like Human immunodeficiency virus (HIV)/Acquired immunodeficiency syndrome (AIDS).

20.2 DEFINITIONS

1. "Confidentiality is something that is confidential and is meant to be kept secret."-Oxford dictionary.
2. Dimond (2002) defines confidentiality as one of the values of good care practice that is concerned with protecting private information about the patient and clients obtained during the period of professional practice.
3. The NMC code of conduct, performance and ethics for nurses and midwives' (NMC, 2008) states firstly one must respect people's right to confidentiality. Professionals must ensure people are informed about how and why information is shared by those who will be providing their care.
4. The ethical principle or legal right that a physician or other health professional will hold secret all information relating to a patient, unless the patient gives consent permitting disclosure.
5. Confidentiality has been defined by the International Standards Organization (ISO) as "ensuring that information is accessible only to those authorized to have access".

20.3 DEFINING KEY TERMS OF CONFIDENTIALITY

1. Confidentiality is a term that indicates preserving the privacy of the persons in which you care for. This will mean that all information related to them will be kept in strict confidence for use

only by the team of care providers. This includes information gained verbally or from resident or client records.

All information is considered confidential when it pertains to medical care and client records.

2. Breach of confidentiality is sharing information verbally or in written form regarding a resident or client with someone who is not on the care team of the resident or client, or who does not have a release of information form from the resident or client.
3. Indiscretion is an action in which you inadvertently share confidential information. There is no bad intent associated with an indiscretion.
4. Informed consent is when a resident or client acknowledges and allows the release of information to other parties. This permission is given by filling out a legal consent form, which becomes part of the resident or client's permanent record.
5. Private is defined as not available for public viewing or knowledge.
6. Privileged information is a term that refers to all information shared between an attorney and his client. This information is considered confidential and is not admissible in court.

20.4 MEANING OF CONFIDENTIALITY

1. Confidentiality is the duty to respect privileged information. The principle of confidentiality provides that caregivers should respect a patient need for privacy and use personal information about him or her only to improve care.
2. Nurses should practice confidentiality to decrease patient vulnerability and share from widespread knowledge of personal information divulged during care.
3. Confidentiality is both a legal and an ethical concept. It is legal in the sense that several sections of state law now address the subject. It is an ethical concept in that the codes of ethics for all professional associations address the subject.
4. Confidentiality is a part of the information security triad of "Confidentiality, Integrity and Availability." Information possesses confidentiality when it is accessible only to those who are authorized to access it. Conversely, information lacks confidentiality to the extent that it is available or disclosed to unauthorized persons or processes.
5. Confidentiality (in the context of personal information for example) is vital to protect vulnerable people and information from general viewing by people to whom the information has no bearing. An example would be a person's bank account.
6. Confidentiality covers all medical records (including x-rays, lab-reports, etc.) as well as communications between patient and nurse, and it generally includes communications between the patient and other professional staff working with the doctor.
7. The duty of confidentiality continues even after patients stop seeing or being treated by their nurse. Once the nurse is under a duty of confidentiality, they cannot divulge any medical information about their patients to third persons without patient consent. There are, however, exceptions to this rule.

20.5 HISTORICAL PERSPECTIVES OF CONFIDENTIALITY

1. "I win respect the secret which are confined in me even after the patient has died"

   - Geneva Declaration
2. Except when obligated by the law of the country concerned, a doctor shall not disclose, without the consent of the patient information which he has obtained in the course of his professional relationship with the family".

   - International Code of Medical Ethics
3. Hippocratic Oath states, "Whatever in connection with my professional practice or not in connection with it, I see or hear in the life of men, which ought not to be spoken of abroad, I will not divulge as reckoning that all such should be kept confidential".

4. Thomas Percival, a physician and philosopher in England during the early 1800's, wrote and published his Code of Medical Ethics. The concept of confidentiality, or secrecy, was covered in that early code, which supposedly formed the basis for the American Medical Association's first formal Code of Ethics in 1847. From the beginning, it should be noted, the ethical principle of confidentiality was not absolute.

20.6 CONCEPTS CONCERING CONFIDENTIALITY

1. **Do no harm:** In regard to gathering, recording and sharing verbal or written information, "do no harm" means that the resident and healthcare provider will have an honest relationship in which sensitive data should be and shall be disclosed at no risk to the resident or client that there will not be a breach in confidential issues. In regard to privacy, "do no harm" means that the resident/client will not be unnecessarily exposed or intentionally embarrassed while physically examined or treated.
2. **Be honest:** Deal honestly with residents and families, and also your peers. Don't be afraid to admit a mistake.
3. **Use information proactively:** Information shared will be used for the sole purpose of being accurate in diagnosis, prescribing the best recommended treatment, and providing the best care.
4. **Irreversible:** Information once shared cannot be unshared, erased, or deleted. Think about what you are saying before words fall out of your mouth.

Threat of self destruction: A claim of confidential or private matters cannot be honored if concealment poses a threat to the resident or client. For example, most everything is shared in confidence, but lets say for example a person threatens suicide. You would not be able to honor privacy as you would have to share this information to prevent a possible threat to harm oneself.

Table 20.1: Concept of confidentiality

S.N	Concept	Description
1	C	Creating trust with patient relationship.
2	O	Opening the details of patient to other after proper judgment.
3	N	Not revealing the documents of the patient to others.
4	F	Following the ethics of trust, faith in maintaing the patients records.
5	I	Integrating sincerity, honesty, towards patient care.
6	D	Decision-making with nurse leaders before revealing the confidential details of patient's families.
7	E	Engaging the patient in all confidential matters of patient care.
8	N	Not openly taking to other coworkers about patient information.
9	T	Trustworthiness should create confidentiality; help to gain cooperation to do quality patient care.
10	I	Intelligent way of handling the ethical issues will safeguard not only the nurse but also the patient.
11	A	Alertness among the nurses are the expected quality during recording the patients document.
12	L	Leading the entire nursing team abide the rules of confidentiality.
13	I	Interacting the patient's details in the court is allowed for the nurse to reveal the confidentiality report of patient with the permission of medical officer.
14	T	Thorough knowledge about ethics and importance of confidentiality is needed for the nurse to give high quality care.
15	Y	Yelling and gossiping about patient's problems inform of patients and others should be avoided.

20.7 TYPES OF CONFIDENTIALITY

Confidentiality concerns a host of different businesses, organizations and laws. The actual meaning of confidentiality covers the secrets that you tell to a service that must remain between you and the person being told. Different types of confidentiality are recognized by the legal system.

1. **Doctor-Patient confidentiality:** Doctor-patient confidentiality goes as far back as the Hippocratic Oath taken by doctors. The oath states that a doctor will not disclose anything pertaining to a patient to any unauthorized person. The Hippocratic Oath also states that those things that are sacred shall not be imparted on anyone other than persons that are sacred. In simpler terms, a doctor will not discuss a patient's condition or any medical background to anyone other than a person that the patient has formally released information by signing an authorization form.
2. **Attorney-Client confidentiality:** Attorney-client privilege is covered by the American Bar Association, which outlines the ethical duty of attorneys to their clients. Basically, an attorney may not discuss anything with other individuals. An attorney who represents a client must withhold any information disclosed to him by a client or prospective client. Any information garnered from the client during interviews or during representation must not be released to any other person without the written consent of the client.
3. **Confidentiality agreements:** Businesses require that most employees working in confidential areas of the company sign confidentiality agreements. These type of confidentiality agreements are primarily used when a company has a secret ingredient, product in development or new research on existing products in development. The protection of sensitive technical information or other vital information that if disclosed will harm the company, concerns this type of confidentiality agreement.
4. **Pastoral confidentiality:** One of the most unrecognized types of confidentiality is the pastoral confidentiality that exists between a clergy and congregation or person disclosing information to a clergy member in private. A lot of states do not recognize this type of confidentiality, but most religious organizations do permit clergy members to withhold any information told to them by individuals. In recent years, people have sued clergy members for disclosing information given to them in private. Most of these lawsuits have been won by the individual and not the church. Private conversations between individuals and their pastor, minister, priest or clergyman must be kept confidential.

20.8 CONFINDENTIALITY IN NURSING

1. The code of conduct will define confidentialities importance to nursing profession and professional code of conduct. It will further look at the possible dilemmas that could arise in interaction between the nurse colleagues and their relatives and how to ensure confidentiality and legislation governing access to confidential information.
2. The term "confidential patient information" as used in this statement refers to individually identifiable health and personal information, and recognizes a patient's expectation of and right to privacy in the maintenance of this information. Such information would include, but is not limited to: information related to the past, present or future physical or mental health of an individual and treatment; and any information that identifies the individual or in which there is a reasonable basis to believe that the information can be used to identify the individual.
3. Patient privacy is important in the field of medicine, and nurses are frequently the ones to maintain it. Maintenance of confidentiality affects most aspects of nursing, including record-keeping, discussing the medical issues of patients with others, and the manner in which nurses interact with the patients themselves. The nurse should inform patients of the limits of confidentiality protections and allow the patients to decide whether treatment outweighs

the risk of the disclosure of sensitive information. A patient expects to have his or her privacy respected by the physician and should not be disappointed. If a record must be released, the patient should sign an appropriate release authorizing the disclosure of information in the medical record. General releases will not suffice for records containing HIV or other sensitive material.

The nurse should become familiar with laws involving the duty to maintain confidentiality. Any breach in confidentiality—even one that seems minor—can result in mistrust and, possibly, a lawsuit and/or disciplinary action.

20.9 IMPORTANCE OF CONFIDENTIALITY

The major importance of confidentiality is to protect you and the patient. It protects the patient in the sense that their personal information is not getting out to random people and they won't have to be embarrassed about what ever they have (e.g. STDs. Would you want random people knowing about it?). It also protects you from possible lawsuits from sharing the information.

The ethical and legal principle of confidentiality is anchored in a set of values and assumption about the treatment relationship and the consequences of disclosing private information. It is central to trust between the doctor and patient, 'under which the patient puts trust and confidence in doctor to act in faith for his/hers best interest. Without assurance about the confidentiality, the patient may be reluctant to give doctor the information they need in order to provide best care.

The healthcare team involved in patient care is ethically bound to respect the confidentiality of health information of each patient because it is the natural desire of human being to be protected from social embarrassment, disapproval, discrimination and stigmatization. It encourages the free exchange of information which is essential for effective medical intervention, public health and preventing harm to others.

20.10 QUALITIES OF A NURSE IN CONFIDENTIALITY

Developing an environment of trust is another key factor. Trust develops when patients see a facility's commitment to protecting privacy and confidentiality. Staff should handle medical records carefully. Be sure to never leave them open or unattended in public areas where others can have access to them. Seek informed consent whenever health information needs to be released. This included Medication Administration Records (MARs) and Treatment Administration Records (TARs), which need to be closed when not in use, and removed from the tops of medication carts and treatment carts when not in use as well.

1. Understand your facility's "need to know policy". Healthcare staff should only have access to information needed for their job. It is important to keep evaluating what information really needs to be known.
2. Ask yourself, "Do I want to know this information or do I NEED to know it?" "Do I have a right to know this information?"
3. Use Good Sense.... Along with following your facility's policies and procedures, using common sense is one of the most important ways to help protect patient privacy and confidentiality.
4. For example: Think before you speak, Be aware of whether others can over hear your conversation, If you think that certain information might be confidential, treat it as such.
5. Show courtesy and respect.

This is a key part of protecting patient privacy and confidentiality. It is important to treat all patients with respect, Handle patients' medical records with the same care that you would want your own medical records handled.

Respect every patient's right to privacy.

20.11 PRINCIPLES OF CONFIDENTIALITY

1. Confidentiality is central to trust between nurse and patients. Without assurances about confidentiality, patients may be reluctant to seek medical attention or to give nurse the information they need in order to provide good care. But appropriate information sharing is essential to the efficient provision of safe, effective care, both for the individual patient and for the wider community of patients.
2. The nurse should make sure that information is readily available to patients explaining that, unless they object, their personal information may be disclosed for the sake of their own care and for local clinical audit. Patients usually understand that information about them has to be shared within the healthcare team to provide their care. But it is not always clear to patients that others who support the provision of care might also need to have access to their personal information. And patients may not be aware of disclosures to others for purposes other than their care, such as service planning or medical research.

20.12 THE CONFIDENTIALITY MODEL

The model outlines the requirements that must be met in order to provide patients with a confidential service. Record holders must inform patients of the intended use of their information, give them the choice to give or withhold their consent as well as protecting their identifiable information from unwarranted disclosures. These processes are inter-linked and should be ongoing to aid the improvement of a confidential service. The four main requirements are:

a. Protect—look after the patient's information.
b. Inform—ensure that patients are aware of how their information is used.
c. Provide choice—allow patients to decide whether their information can be disclosed or used in particular ways.
   To support these three requirements, there is a fourth:
d. Improve—always look for better ways to protect, inform, and provide choice.

Protect patient information: Patients' health information and their interests must be protected through a number of measures:

a. Procedures to ensure that all staff, contractors and volunteers are at all times fully aware of their responsibilities regarding confidentiality.
b. Recording patient information accurately and consistently.
c. Keeping patient information private.
d. Keeping patient information physically secure.
e. Disclosing and using information with appropriate care.

Inform patients effectively—no surprises: Patients must be made aware that the information they give may be recorded, may be shared in order to provide them with care, and may be used to support clinical audit and other work to monitor the quality of care provided. Consider whether patients would be surprised to learn that their information was being used in a particular way—if so, and then they are not being effectively informed.

In order to inform patients properly, staff must:

a. Check where practicable that information leaflets on patient confidentiality and information disclosure have been read and understood. These should be available within each National health service (NHS) organization.
b. Make clear to patients when information is recorded or health records are accessed.
c. Make clear to patients when they are or will be disclosing information with others.
d. Check that patients are aware of the choices available to them in respect of how their information may be disclosed and used.

e. check that patients have no concerns or queries about how their information is disclosed and used.
f. answer any queries personally or direct the patient to others who can answer their questions or other sources of information.
g. respect the rights of patients and facilitate them in exercising their right to have access to their health records.

Provide choice to patients: Patients have different needs and values—this must be reflected in the way they are treated, both in terms of their medical condition and the handling of their personal information. What is very sensitive to one person may be casually discussed in public by another—just because something does not appear to be sensitive does not mean that it is not important to an individual patient in his or her particular circumstances.

Staff must:

a. Ask patients before using their personal information in ways that do not directly contribute to, or support the delivery of, their care.
b. Respect patients' decisions to restrict the disclosure or use of information, except where exceptional circumstances apply.
c. Communicate effectively with patients to ensure they understand what the implications may be if they choose to agree to or restrict the disclosure of information.

Improve wherever possible: It is not be possible to achieve best practice overnight. Staff must:

a. Be aware of the issues surrounding confidentiality, and seek training or support where uncertain in order to deal with them appropriately.
b. Report possible breaches or risk of breaches.

20.13 DISCLOSURE OF HEALTH INFORMATION

Confidentiality is a time-honored principle of medical ethics and it is extended after death and is fundamental to the doctor-patient relationship, the doctor must not disclose the information from the medical records to any person without the consent of the patient. The principle of disclosure states that the patient information can be disclosed to the spouse/family, third party payers and others after getting the written consent from the patient. The consent should be written, original and addressed to the concerned doctor.

The medical information can be disclosed when the question of benefit of the patient arises, i.e. during the time of emergency, patient incompetency, when the care is shared among the professional and to prevent harm to the patient.

When the patient is suffering from infectious disease and there is risk of infection to others and if there is a question of public safety, e.g. person having infectious disease handling food, or bus driver with color blindness.

The information contained in the health records is a matter of confidentiality but in case of malpractice or negligence and when the court of law asks for the information from the health records of the patient, the hospital should provide the complete and original records without any delay.

Need to Safeguard from Unauthorized Disclosure

All medical records in whatever format and wherever kept, must be safeguarded and protected from unauthorized disclosure. All the personnel involve in patient care should follow the principle of disclosure; because unauthorized disclosure of health information to the third party may lead to the breach of confidentiality, defamation and invasion of privacy. Before disclosing the medical records information, the healthcare providers as well as health records personnel should analyze the type of requisition and the extent of information to be released. All patient-identifiable health data, whether written, computerized, visually or audio recorded or simply held in the memory of health professionals, is subject to the rules of confidentiality.

When the confidentiality is critical?

Professional ethics will sometime require confidentiality to be breached, for ethically and legally justifiable reason, e.g. cases in which the healthcare professional knows or suspect that an individual is acting illegally harming others, might harm to others in future, harming themselves, or being exploited or abused by others.

20.14 BREACH OF CONFIDENTIALITY

There are two types of outcomes related to breach of confidentiality.

Outcome can be positive or negative.

Positive Outcomes

1. Suspected abuse or neglect can be investigated.
2. Possible future abuse and neglect may be avoided or prevented.
3. A suicide or attempted suicide may be prevented.
4. Appropriate interventions may be initiated for a resident or client to get help in appropriate related areas.

Do not ever assume that someone else will take care of getting the information to the proper person. Take the initiative to make sure the bases are covered and the resident or client receives appropriate interventions as needed. Remember to always respect information given to you with high regard to confidential matters unless it is in the best interest of the resident or client for this information to be shared with appropriate resource personnel.

Negative Outcomes

1. The facility or agency may reprimand a healthcare worker, such as disciplinary action against the employee for breaching confidentiality related to patient care issues.
2. The resident or client may suffer embarrassment and emotional distress.
3. Irreversible damage may be done to the caregiver/care receiver relationship.
4. The resident or client may file charges against the healthcare worker, staff, and facility. They may be able to sue and win compensation for breach of confidential matters.

Remember, often times it is not WHAT we say, But rather HOW we say it, and more importantly. WHO we say it to. Never forget that lives are affected by breaching confidentiality.

20.15 RESPONSIBILITIES OF A NURSE WITH PRIVATE AND CONFIDENTIAL INFORMATION

Guidelines for protecting private and confidential information include the following:

1. Discuss resident and client information ONLY in a place that is away from other residents, families and visitors.
2. Report should not be given at the nurse's station, as this is not a private area, with much opportunity for information to be overheard.
3. Never discuss patients in an elevator, in a hallway, cafeteria, or any other public place within or outside of the facility.
4. Discuss resident information only with appropriate staff. Do not ever release information to media or newspapers.
5. Don't release information to the police without first alerting a supervisor. Instead refer them to an appropriate manager.
6. Do not keep a copy or make copies of resident information.
7. Destroy all ends of shift report sheets after use.

8. Any item with a residents name or identifying medical information should NEVER be placed in general trash receptacles. They should be shredded for appropriate disposal of confidential information.

Responsibilities Regarding Private and Confidential Information Include:

1. Know your expected limits: Check your job description. Ask your supervisor to clarify anything you do not understand. Never discuss information that you are unsure of, and be sure of who you are sharing this information with. Not all friends and family are authorized to know information regarding your resident or client's condition.
2. Be on the alert for "breaks" or "leaks". Be particularly mindful of when private information becomes casual chatting.
3. Practice care that is private and behavior that guards confidence.
4. Report to your supervisor. The best working relationships are those in which you keep your supervisor well-informed and on top of things that are going on. Keep open lines of communication between your superior and yourself.

Patient Privacy and Confidentiality Generally Refers to a Patient's Right to:

1. Decide what personal health information can be shared with others.
2. Decide how that information can be shared, and with whom it may be shared.
3. Not have information about resident or client discussed in areas where others could overhear.
4. Privacy also refers to the right to have physical privacy (curtains pulled).
5. Patient confidentiality generally refers to a patient's trust that health information will only be shared with those who need to know, and in order to provide appropriate care.
6. Protecting patient privacy and confidentiality is vital to your organizations mission. It helps increase patient's satisfaction and sense of dignity. It helps ensure that patients get the most effective care.

20.16 CONFIDENTIALITY IS A CHALLENGE

Protecting Patient Privacy and Confidentiality can be a Challenge

New technology and the growing use of computers help improve healthcare. These also make it easier than ever for patient data to be wrongfully shared.

For example, staff must take care to protect patient privacy and confidentiality when using modern technology such as:

1. Fax machines.
2. E-mail and other computer networks.
3. Electronic records.
4. Telephones and voice mail systems.

Ethics and Standards

Ethics and Standards for professional behavior are very important in healthcare. For example, security measures can protect patient data only if staff use them correctly and consistently.

Breach of confidentiality and patient privacy can result in costly lawsuits for healthcare providers and facilities. By understanding and following your facility's policies and guidelines, you can help prevent legal action.

20.17 AGENCIES THAT MONITOR PATIENT PRIVACY

1. **Joint Commission on Accreditation of Healthcare Organizations (JCAHO):** This national organization accredits healthcare facilities that meet JCAHO standards. Patient confidentiality and privacy is an important part of these standards. If JCAHO surveyors evaluate your

organization, they will expect you to know your organizations mission, your organizations policies for protecting confidentiality, what efforts your department is making to improve patient privacy and confidentiality, and how your job relates to all of these.

2. **National Committee for Quality Assurance (NCQA):** This National organization evaluates managed care plans. It also accredits managed care organizations. NCQA teamed up with JCAHO to develop special recommendations to help managed care organizations protect patient privacy and confidentiality. Areas that these recommendations address include: staff education, patient consent, and systems to ensure confidentiality.
3. **Health Care Financing Administration (HCFA):** HCFA is a part of the US Department of Health and Human Services. It administers Medicare, Medicaid and Child Health Insurance Programs. HCFA's responsibilities include: ensuring that Medicare, Medicaid and the Child Health Insurance Programs are properly run by state agencies. HCFA also plays a part in evaluating healthcare facilities and services.

Healthcare facilities and providers must meet strict guidelines to be certified by HCFA. These include guidelines related to patient privacy and confidentiality.

20.18 CONFIDENTIALITY AND HIV/AIDS

Every state requires reporting of HIV positive status and AIDS cases. While the data is used for infection control purposes, the requirement is controversial. That is because in some states, facilities must report a patient's name, address or other identifying information.

It's very important to protect HIV/AIDS information. Anyone who improperly releases a patients HIV/AIDS status can face serious legal action, as well as severe reprimand by the Board of Nursing.

Other Related Rules Regarding Confidentiality

In many states, minors can give consent for certain medical care. This includes care for pregnancy, sexually transmitted diseases, and drug dependency. Some minors, such as those who are married or in the armed forces, can make all their own decisions about medical care.

Mental health or substance abuse treatment, in general, for these types of treatment, special laws and policies apply to the release of patient information. Staff needs to be aware of how any laws and policies affect release of information to the patient and others.

CONCLUSION

Patient confidentiality and privacy are a very important aspect within our jobs in the healthcare industry. Each and every day we place our trust into the hands of our patients. Maintaining confidentiality will ensure quality care by showing that your patients can count on you for maintaining privacy and respect for their care and their medical records. With legality issues so much on the rise today, we should always be ever so mindful to the problems at hand when confidentiality issues are violated. Smart charting and adherence to company policy and procedures will go along way in protecting you legally as you do your best to give high quality care to your patients. Confidentiality issues are also a standard of practice related to ethical and professional healthcare.

21 Morale

21.1 INTRODUCTION

Morale is concept that describes the attitude of the employees collectively towards all aspects of their work, their job, the institution, working conditions, fellow worker, and supervisors and so on. It is the attitude of the collective body. Attitude is a predescription to respond positively or negatively to different aspects of a job. A greater presence of positive attitudes indicates high morale. While a greater presence of negative attitude indicates low morale. Morale is a mental condition or attitude of individuals and groups which determine their willingness to cooperate. Good morale as defined by management is evidenced by employee enthusiasm, voluntary conformance with regulations and orders and a willingness to cooperate with others in the accomplishment of an organizational objectives. Poor morale is evidenced by surliness, cases of insubordination, discouragement and dislike for the job, company and associates.

21.2 MEANING OF MORALE

1. Morale is a feeling of enthusiasm, zeal, confidence in an individual or group which will motivate employees to cope with the task assigned to them
2. It is feeling, emotions, sentiments, attitudes and motives combine together and lead to a particular type of behavior which is called morale.
3. It is a sum of affects production of satisfaction expressed by an employee on account of his job and as member of work team.
4. Morale also affects production, quality of product costs, cooperation, enthusiasm, discipline, initiative and other ingredients of success.
5. Morale is an attitude of mind, an esprist de corps a state of well-being and an emotional force which affects the employee and executives in their interventions.
6. Morale is a group attitude towards persistence, determination etc., and it reflects the acceptance of group goals by group members and their interest for achieving the goals.
7. Morale is social or group oriented and it emphasized the feeling of a team as a whole.
8. In the industrial situation, morale is concerned with an employee's attitude towards the kind of work he does, to his fellow worker to maintain his prestige and status and his employer's status.

21.3 DEFINITION

1. Morale is the sum of total of several psychic qualities which include courage, fortitude, resolution and above all confidence. Mooney
2. Morale is the capacity of group of people to pull together persistently and consistently in purpose. AA Leighton

3. Morale may be described as a readiness to cooperate warmly in the task and purpose of a given organization. EFL Brech
4. Morale may be defined as an attitude of satisfaction with the desire to continue in and willingness to strive for the goals of a particular group organization. MS Viteless
5. Programs that aim at keeping the general run those employees happy, have gone about as far as they can go-but there is still plenty of mileage to be got out of a clearer recognition that morale, in the final analysis is an individual affair. Carl E Gregory

21.4 MORALE COMPOSED OF 5 W'S

1. What is morale? It is an attitude of mind, spirit of cooperation, state of well-being and an emotion force.
2. What does it do? It affects output, quality, cost, cooperation, discipline, enthusiasm, initiative etc.
3. Where does it reside? It resides in minds, attitudes and emotions of a worker and the group also.
4. Whom does it affect? It affects immediate employees, executives, supervisors in their interactions and ultimately consumers, business units and the community.
5. What does it affect? It affects the will to work and team spirit in the best interests of the enterprise and in turn individuals themselves.

21.5 PRINCIPLES OF MORALITY

Immanuel Kant's work on morality and ethics primarily comes from his "Grounding for the Metaphysics of Morals," which describes the history of the way in which people have traditionally thought about morality and Kant's amendments to the prevailing theories of his time. In "Grounding for the Metaphysics of Morals," Kant argues against empirical reasoning for morality and approaches moral questions a priori, or dealing with concepts instead of observing human beings and behavior. In the course of his work, he sets up three basic principles that define morality.

Defense of a Priori approach: Although, Kant's defense of using an a priori approach is not explicitly one of his moral principles, it underlies all of his analyses and conclusions. He approaches ethics and morality without using empirical data but instead dealing with concepts, because all concepts of morality deal with certain values, such as "duty," "justice," "good will," and "obligation". Serious consideration of moral issues, for Kant, must first deal with the ways in which these concepts are understood. Thus, he approaches moral questions a priori, from the perspective of the concepts.

Universal Law: The first of Kant's principles of morality may be called the universal law or maxim. Kant claims that the basic principle of morality should be that individuals should act in such a way that they could want their maxim (motivation for acting) to be universal. This led Kant to describe such a universal maxim as a "categorical imperative". This simply means that all individuals should act in such a way that they would wish all others to follow the same guiding principle.

Treat humans as ends: The second of Kant's principles claims that a person should never treat another person as a means to an end. He separates individuals and objects into two categories: means and ends. Humans, he claims, should always be thought of as ends, or autonomous individuals with their own goals and desires. Treating others as ends promotes equality, because each person recognizes the other as an individual.

Everyone is a rational agent: Because all of Kant's moral conclusions came from reasoning and a priori conclusions, he felt that all rational beings ought to be able to come to the same moral conclusions that he did. Therefore, his third moral principle is that his moral conclusions are universally available to all rational agents, who can use mental faculties to come to the same principles. Kant argued that all humans should be thought of in this way, as capable of arriving at moral conclusions through the process of reasoning.

21.6 FACTORS INFLUENCING MORALE

Morale, being complex phenomenon, is influenced by the factors like job, supervision, objectives of the company, working conditions, compensation to worker' family, likes of employees and so many other factors.

Table 21.1: Factors influencing morale

S.N	Factors	Description
1	The organization	The organizational objectives, goals and structure influence morale. If they are acceptable to employee, high morale prevails in him and it results in improved productivity and development of good image for the organization.
2	Nature of work	The attitude of the employees is influenced by the nature of work of an employee. forced dress code, repeating the task in the short cycles, large interpersonal organizational restructure, unachievable organizational goals etc.
3	Job satisfaction	Employees working condition have impact on job satisfaction, job related value system such as opportunity to learn a job, steadiness of employment, supervision, pay, cooperativeness, or otherwise of coworker, working conditions, working hours, cleanliness, communication, recognition, group relationship outside the job etc., have relevance to job satisfaction.
4	Perceptions of employee	The perceptions of employees of themselves like lack of self-confidence, attitude towards organizational environment, perception of past rewards and future opportunities and such other perceptions influence the morale.
5	Age of employee	Age also influences employee morale. they are have direct relationship. As age passes they perceive the qualities like stability, serious attitude towards jobs more reliability, less absenteeism, proved steady work habits and a sense of responsibility and loyalty.
6	Educational level	The higher educational level of an employee, lower the satisfaction. Because hr compares his attainments with those of others.
7	Others	Occupational level, employee's activities also influence morale of the employee. The confidence level of individuals each member's confidence in a group, group confidence, organizational efficiency etc., cause disturbances in the individual thinking and will have its impact on the morale.

21.7 TYPES OF MORALE

There are two types of morale: high morale and low morale. High morale in an organization prevails when employee attitudes are favorable to the total situation of the organization. If one can observe, zeal, enthusiasm, team spirit, persistence to frustration etc., in a work place, the morale of the organization is said to be high.

High employee morale is important because:

1. It governs plant productivity and efficiency of operations.
2. It governs harmonious industrial relations, i.e. absence of labor unrest and conflicts.

21.8 EFFECTS OF HIGH MORALE

1. Willing cooperation from employees.
2. Loyalty to the organization and leadership.
3. Good voluntary obedience, disciple and conformity to rules, regulations and orders.
4. Strong organizational health and stamina in crisis.
5. High degree of employee interest in the job and the organization.

6. Display of initiative.
7. Pride in the organization.

Dimensions of morale: There are four dimensions of morale:

1. Job satisfaction.
2. Satisfaction with wages and promotional opportunities.
3. Identification with the company, i.e. a feeling of belonging to the company.
4. Pride in the work.

Morale and productivity: The relationship between morale and productivity is not absolute. An increase in morale may cause increase or decrease in morale. A research finding states the following combination of morale and productivity.

1. High morale-high productivity.
2. High productivity-low morale.
3. Low morale-low productivity.
4. Low morale-high productivity.

Symptoms of low morale:

1. Poor attendance and absence from work.
2. Nature and frequency of accident.
3. High labor turnover.
4. Internal mobility as shown by transfer and promotion.
5. The prevalence of employee complaints and grievances.

21.9 MORALE BUILDING MEASURES

Table 21.2: Morale building measures

S.N	Measures	Description
1	Unity of interest	Integration of worker goals with company objectives will create workers confidence in the purpose and objectives for which they are called upon to work.
2	Leadership confidence	Manager must adopt appropriate managerial style. Manager who are firm but fair and impartial in their dealings with employees and who are sincere, sympathetic and democratic in attitudes towards worker can easily establish confidence in their leadership.
3	Managerial set-up	Sound organization and efficient managerial set-up constitute the best foundation for peaceful work environment and rising of morale.
4	Sound wage structure	Complete wage plan incorporates guaranteed wage base, incentive for productivity, merit rating, profit sharing, cost of living adjustment and other fringe benefits together with social security and labor welfare.
5	Favorable work environment, working conditions etc.	These will create ease of work, both mental and physical, job satisfaction as well as security and we shall have minimum labor turnover and labor absenteeism.
6	High-order need satisfaction	Worker should be motivated by giving ample opportunities to satisfy their social and egoistic wants at the plant levels as well as other management levels.
7	Lower participation	When educated, trained labor is offered opportunity to take intelligent interest in the affairs of the business through different forms of participation. It can develop sense of belonging, team spirit in the job enterprise.
8	Other measures	Employee counseling, sound promotion policy, grievance procedure, proper selection techniques, induction training, collective bargaining are some of the other measures to enhance employee morale.

21.10 ADVANTAGES OF GOOD MORALE

1. Job satisfaction.
2. High productivity.
3. Employee stability.
4. Employee identification with the institution.
5. The employee initiative and involvement.
6. The employee's willingness to accept responsibility.

21.11 IMPACT OF POOR MORALE

1. Fatigue and monotony.
2. High labor turnover.
3. Work stoppages.
4. High absenteeism.
5. Disciplinary problems.
6. Restrictions of output.
7. Increase in grievances.
8. Apathy and noninvolvement.

21.12 METHODS OF MEASURING MORALE

There are various methods of appraising morale:

1. Supervisors and executives impression.
2. An analysis of production and other records.
3. Guided interviews.
4. Unguided interviews.
5. The listening in process.
6. The questionnaire.
7. By combining any two of the above methods.

The most common practice of personnel administration to determine the current employee's morale is to conduct morale or aptitude survey among the employees. Generally, morale is indicated by various attitudes and behaviors of the employees such as action, expression, oral comments, criticism, suggestion and answers to questions.

The management should measure employee attitude and morale pertaining to factors about which they can take remedial actions. Hence, they must be interested in the direction of intensity, inter relations and attitudes. Interestingly managers are resorting to the attitudes of morale survey using various techniques in gathering data on employee morale or as referred to above.

I. The group approach:

1. Settlements (both long-term and short-term with union).
2. Proper wage salary administration.
3. Unbiased and merit based promotion polices.
4. Retirement plans.
5. Cultural and recreational programmes.
6. Employee's service like canteen, shelter, rest-room etc.
7. Group insurance and social security etc.

II. Individual approach:

1. Job placement.
2. Job training.
3. Job rotation.

4. Job enlargement.
5. Job description.
6. Job evaluation.
7. Job analysis.
8. Performance self-appraisal.
9. Counseling.
10. Profit sharing and incentives.
11. Rewards for individual suggestions.
12. Psychological services etc.

CONCLUSION

Morale is a concept, which is essentially a group concept that describes the attitudes of employees collectively towards all aspects of their work, their job, the company, working conditions, fellow-workers, supervisor and other psychological issues. It is a feeling of enthusiasm, zeal and confidence in an individual or group. Group morale exhibits spirit de corps. It is a reflection of collective group of personalities. High morale improves productivity and low morale disturbs organizational activities. Morale is a sentiment activity and motivation is an energy mobilization activity and both are to be complimentary to each other.

Section-6

Trends in Nursing

22 Trends in Nursing

22.1 INTRODUCTION

Trends denote general directions and tendencies especially of events, of opinion. Nursing trends refer to direction towards which the different nursing events have moved or are moving, as well as the opinions in and around nursing and tendencies that are found in and about nursing profession. Trends in nursing mean changes currently taking place in any area of nursing which influence the profession as a whole. These do not occur independently but each one has a basis of related changes in other fields. These are: If we are aware of current trends it will help us plan for developments in nursing education and nursing services as well as controlling the direction in which the profession moves. A global perception will enable nurses to rise to higher levels in their knowledge, skills and improved performance both in India and around the globe.

22.2 FACTORS INFLUENCING TRENDS

The factors influencing the trends in nursing:

1. **Changes in society:** For the past five decades, five social factors have greatly influenced present trends in nursing. These are:
   a. Intensive efforts of government to meet the health needs of people.
   b. Gradual improved literacy level of the people with the growing awareness of health needs.
   c. Advanced scientific technology.
   d. The changing role of women.
   e. The continuing growth of population.
2. **Changes in other professions:** Trends in the nursing profession have always been closely related to those in the medical profession. Growing specialization in medical field is resulting in a trend towards increased specialization in nursing. The development of new diagnostic procedure and equipments make specialization even more necessary.
3. **Patients' Bill of Rights** After the development of the "Patients' Bill of Rights", the nurses is also accountable for patients care and have legal responsibilities for the patient.
4. **Developments in other discipline:** Developments in other discipline other than medicine also influence trends in nursing profession. Nursing is moving towards more specific nursing functions as other members of health team like dieticians, social workers and physiotherapists are more available and more highly specialized.
5. **Leadership within the profession:** Leadership within the profession also influences the trends in nursing. Nursing is moving towards professionalism due to the untiring efforts of nurses who have been dedicated to achieve the aim.
6. **Working and studying in abroad:** Working and studying in abroad is influenced by many factors within India and in other countries. Shortage of nurses in other countries, higher salary paid in abroad is the main causes for the working of Indian nurses in abroad.

7. **Greater specialization in nursing education and practice:** Greater specialization in nursing education and practice is a trend related to that in the medical profession and the growing amount of scientific knowledge available.
8. **Working conditions:** Working conditions for nurses are also changing. There is a gradual change towards shorter and more convenient hours of duty, better accommodations and higher salaries.
9. **Trends in other countries:** Trends in other country also influence the trends in the nursing profession in India. The rapid development of the degree programme has promoted the same emphasis and development here for professional nursing.

22.3 ISSUES RELATED TO NURSING PROFESSION

Issues refer to the items for consideration or questions for discussion. Various issues in nursing profession maybe related to profession, education, practice and nurses themselves.

Various issues related to nursing profession are:

1. Status of nursing in society in healthcare delivery system.
2. Values reflected in our nursing performances.
3. Attitudes, humane approach and concern shown in the behavior patterns of nurses.
4. Quality in nursing hand in hand between education and practice.
5. Unique functions of nursing.
6. Different levels of nurses required in the country.
7. Emphasis from traditional to primary healthcare approach.
8. Evidence based nursing research and nurses in administration.
9. Expanded and extended roles of nurses.
10. Globalization in the profession.
11. Nursing leadership in bringing changes in health scenario according o community demands.

22.4 FUTURE CONCERN FOR NURSES

In the near future, the issues of concern for the nursing practice involve autonomy and independent practice among nurses, quality of care in community setting and homes, and development of nurse as leaders in the health care field. Various challenging health care issues are patients refusal towards healthcare, euthanasia, patient advocacy by nurses, cost effective quality nursing care, competency in nursing practice Nurses need to look at these issues, professional values and expectations they face and decide. Once these issues are identified, strategies for promoting the quality care nursing can be delineated.

22.5 EXTENDED ROLE OF NURSE

The nurses in India are also prepared and more privileged to face the changes and ready to accept the challenging roles and functions of the nurse as perceived in the globe because of the development in the education and training system. The following roles and positions perceived as in the globe are given below.

1. **Nurse educator** works in schools of nursing, staff development departments. They provide the educational programme for student's nurses and nurses, teach clients about the self-care and home care.
2. **Clinical nurse specialist** specializes in managing specific diseases and they function as clinicians, educators, managers, consultants and researchers.
3. **Nurse practitioners** are certified to provide healthcare to clients in out-patient or community settings.

4. **Certified nurse-midwife** is certified by the American College of Nurse-Midwives to provide independent care for women during normal pregnancy, labour and delivery.
5. **Nurse anesthetist** having advance training in anesthesiology, provides surgical anesthesia to the client under the supervision of an anesthesiologist during minor surgery with baccalaureate degrees or master's degree.
6. **Nurse administrators** manage client care within the healthcare agencies in a middle level or upper level management position.
7. **Nurse researcher** with Doctoral degree investigate nursing problem to improve care and to define and expand the scope of nursing practice.

Advancements in science increase health needs of the society and thereby expect changes in the role of nurses and thus increases the scope for nurses.

22.6 TRENDS IN NURSING EDUCATION

The form of teaching has remained unchanged for centuries. The needs of society. The practical side of the matter has been left to chance, whereas specific features of the situation of each country are changing more rapidly. Unfortunately, little or no account has been taken in to consideration for the training of health personnel, but following traditional systems in teaching. What is required now is to make sure that the educational program is relevant?

No educational system can be effective unless its purposes are clearly defined.

The members of health team must be trained specially for the task they will have to perform taking into account the circumstances under which they will work, so defining the professional task of health personnel to be trained is the very basis of the educational objectives of training centers/institutions and must be shaped selectively in terms of the goal to be achieved. If the goal is modified in the course of time the program also to be modified accordingly.

Definition of professional task must proceed from a study of needs, availability of resources, various category of personnel be called upon to do their professional career in a given type of health services. In nursing education, depending upon the needs of the country we need to deicide whom we would like to prepare, the type of health services to be provided and to achieve the institutional goal and educational objectives.

For example, generalist or specialist such as graduate midwives, lactation consultants, birth spacing consultants, etc. Depending on this professional task to be identified and prepare the suitable educational objectives and educational programmers as pre-registration nursing courses for diploma level and post-registration courses for the higher education framework with the pathways leading towards an honors degree or masters and doctoral degree.

22.7 TRENDS IN NURSING PRACTICE

Definition of professional task becomes precondition for ensuring that the training program is really designed to meet the population health needs. The training programs, professional profile and educational program objectives should provide basis for nursing practice in all three levels of healthcare, such as primary, secondary and tertiary healthcare. The advancement to adopted and develop professional skill as specialist is essential. So, that the nurses can be prepared as clinical consultants, administrators and as researches in the various fields of nursing practice in order to make both nursing education and practice identical three principles are fundamental importance. It must be oriented towards the community as well as the individuals taking account of the needs of each particular activity, i.e. education must be community oriented. The education must be learner centered. If educational objectives are based on faulty principles, then the "best system" of training may give "bad results".

The support system which should support health systems are:

1. The political system.
2. The structure and authorities of the administrative system.
3. The general system/general infrastructure.
4. The education system. Unfortunately, most of the time these systems act as obstacles rather than support. Based upon these trends the following issues need to be looked into before developing curriculum.

CONCLUSION

Trends denote general directions and tendencies especially of events, of opinion. Nursing trends refer to direction towards which the different nursing events have moved or are moving, as well as the opinions in and around nursing and tendencies that are found in and about nursing profession. Trends in nursing mean changes currently taking place in any area of nursing which influence the profession as a whole. These do not occur independently but each one has a basis of related changes in other fields. These are: If we are aware of current trends it will help us plan for developments in nursing education and nursing services as well as controlling the direction in which the profession moves. A global perception will enable nurses to rise to higher levels in their knowledge, skills and improved performance both in India and around the globe.

23 Development and Trends in Nursing Education

23.1 INTRODUCTION

The Nursing Council Act came into existence in 1948 to constitute a council of nurses who would safeguard the quality of nursing education in the country. The mandate was to establish and maintain uniform standards of nursing education. Today, the Indian Nursing Council is a statutory body that regulates nursing education in the country through prescription, inspection, examination, certification and maintaining its stand for a uniform syllabus at each level of nursing education. They have also ensured easier measures for equivalence, exchange and practice for nurses in any part of the country. On the other hand, the strive for maintenance of a uniform standard and pattern of nursing education has curbed creative development and experiments for expansion of nursing into newer horizons of caring and function.

23.2 LEVELS OF NURSING EDUCATION

There are six levels of nursing education in India today. They are:

1. Multipurpose health worker female training (ANM or MPHW-F).
2. Female health supervisor training (HV or M PHS-F).
3. General nursing and midwifery (GNM).
4. BSc (N).
5. MSc (N).
6. M Phil and PhD.

The first 3 MPHW (f) training, female health supervisor training and general nursing are conducted in schools of nursing. The last 3 are university level courses and examinations are conducted by the respective universities. Besides, there are several certificate and diploma courses in specialties.

23.3 TRAINING SCHOOL

The first Mid-wives School was started at the government hospital in 1871.

The formal schools of nursing was started for conducting diploma in general nursing and midwifery programmes for a duration of 3 ½ years in Madras and in other parts of Tamilnadu. Schools of nursing offering diploma program increased slowly (there were 9 schools of nursing and 4 midwifery schools till 2001) conducted by government of Tamilnadu. The number of schools conducted by government of Tamilnadu is now increased to 17 in 2003 and now the government executed to start one school of nursing in every district hospitals. The numbers of private schools have also increased. Multipurpose health worker schools are also functioning in many places in Tamilnadu conducted by government and private bodies.

23.4 COLLEGE OF NURSING

A teachers training program running for duration of one year was functioning in government hospital. In 1967 an integrated 2½ years Bachelor Science degree nursing program attached to Madras Medical College (for trained nurses) commenced replacing the then existing diploma program. In 1980, diploma in community nursing program was started.

In 1983, Bachelor of Science Nursing, 4-year program was started in College of Nursing, attached to Madras Medical College.

In 1995, Master of Science (Nursing) program was started in the College of Nursing, attached to Madras Medical College.

In 2001, a post of Principal for the College of Nursing was sanctioned and started functioning. Dr. Sumathi Kumarswamy was appointed as the first Principal.

Many candidates have completed Doctoral degree in nursing.

In 2003, a College of Nursing at Madurai started functioning by the government Services the cadre strength of nursing increased slowly and many categories in nursing services prompted up.

In 1962, a post of Assistant to Director of Medical Services was created and filled at the state level. A post of Deputy Director of Nursing at the state level was created in 1986, and Dr Sumathi Kumaraswamy was appointed as the first Deputy Director of Medical Education in Nursing in 1992.

23.5 AUXILIARY NURSE MIDWIFE

The Development of Auxiliary Nurse Midwife Training (Rural Health Services)

During the Second World War, there was a great demand for nursing personnel in the military hospitals as well as in the civil hospitals. So, auxiliary nurses midwife services was founded in 1942.

This course was simple and the duration of training period was shorter than the nursing course. The nurses under this course were posted to do useful work under supervision in the hospital, or in the health center and to give domiciliary care. Auxiliary nurse midwives were prepared to meet the demands of the health personnel in the community development programmes. After the independence and in the Second Five Year Plan, it was decided to prepare 6000 auxiliary nurses and midwives. The private hospitals also were requested to cooperate with the Government to start such training institution. The government hospitals were given facilities to train the auxiliary nurse midwife since 1955.

Today the auxiliary nurse midwife has a vital role in the health services of the rural health centers such as primary health center, family welfare center, and Maternity and Child Health centers. They can work as a midwife and a health worker in the community. They are also given opportunity to be trained as health visitors or as nurses if they have the basic educational requirements.

The practice of the auxiliary nurse midwife in the rural center had helped to improve the health status of the people, by health teaching, domiciliary care, and regular follow-up of patients and families. Auxiliary nurse midwife in the present health care delivery system functions as a Multipurpose Female Health Worker. With the present introduction of vocational courses such as nursing in the academic stream as one of the options, it is believed that it will contribute towards the basic nursing care of individuals, families and community for health and happiness. It will also be a foundation course for future diploma and degree programs in nursing.

23.6 MULTIPURPOSE HEALTH WORKER (F) TRAINING

The training grew out of the earlier auxiliary nursing and midwifery (ANM) course. The ANM training was for 2 years and mainly covered maternal and childcare and family welfare. In keeping with the policies of the Government of India to have multipurpose health workers, the Indian

Nursing Council revised the ANMs syllabus in 1977 and reduced the duration to 18 months. The focus of training is on community health nursing. At the end of the course candidates are eligible for working in health subcentres. There are nearly 500 schools offering this course in India at present. The MPHA (M) training course is also conducted in some states with duration of 18 months to render healthcare services at community.

23.7 FEMALE HEALTH SUPERVISOR TRAINING

This course was initially meant as a health visitor training course. It went through several modifications and finally became metamorphosed into the current six months promotional training. The female health supervisor or MPHA (f) course is being conducted in 21 centers in the country. Besides this basics course, several states have their own promotional training courses as requirement for ANMs to be qualified for promotion to supervisors.

23.8 GENERAL NURSING AND MIDWIFERY

The general nursing and midwifery (GNM) course is conducted in 477 centers in the country. The syllabus has undergone many revisions according to the changes in health plans and policies of the Government and changing trends and advancements in education, nursing, health sciences and medical technology. The latest revision of the general nursing syllabus by the INC in 1988 has reduced the duration of the course from three and half years to three years. The basic entrance qualification has become intermediate or class XII instead of the earlier 10th class. Both science and arts students are eligible. The focus of general nursing education is care of the sick in the hospital. Schools of nursing are therefore usually attached to teaching hospital. Three Board examinations are conducted, one at the end of each year. On passing, the candidates are registered as nurses (RM) and as Midwives (RM) by the respective state nursing councils.

23.9 GRADUATE NURSING EDUCATION

There are two types of graduate nursing education in India-one is of 4-year basic course for fresh entrants and the second is a condensed post basic course for those who have undergone the GNM course.

1. **Four-year BSc (N):** Graduate nursing education started in India in the year 1946 in CMC, Vellore and in the RAK College of Nursing at Delhi University. At present several universities in India offer the course. The entry qualification is intermediate with biological sciences, physics, and chemistry. Some universities also give admission to those who have arts background.

   The course focuses on preparation of professional nurses for working at the bedside and for taking up leadership roles in public health nursing. Besides nursing and medical subjects the syllabus includes humanities, arts and allied sciences. The course also includes managerial and teaching subjects to prepare graduates to take up first level teaching and administrative jobs in the hospital. An introductory course in research is also given. Overall, the graduate nursing course in the country offers a broad base in both arts and sciences and lays the foundation for a holistic perspective to health and caring.
2. **Two-year Post-basic BSc (N):** A 2-year degree course in nursing is offered in several universities in India. This course was specially designed to provide higher educational opportunities for practicing nurses. The entry requirement is that they should have completed the general nursing course and class XII (usually with science). Most places also ask for at least 2 years experience after completing the diploma (GNM) course. Two exams are conducted by the university—one at the end of the year, and the other at the end of the 2nd year.

3. **Degree in Nursing through Distance Education:** Distance education in post-basic nursing has also been started by Indira Gandhi National Open University (IGNOU) in 1994. This has provided an opening for diploma nurses all over the country to undertake higher education. The IGNOU offers courses through its study centers throughout the country.

23.10 POSTGRADUATE NURSING EDUCATION

MSc (N) course is presently being offered in about ten universities in the country. The 2-year course is designed to prepare clinical and community health nursing specialists. Besides clinical specialization the students are also taught to conduct research in nursing. A thesis is submitted by each student in partial fulfillment of the requirements for the degree. Courses in education and administration are given to prepare the students to take up responsible administrative and teaching jobs in nursing and allied health areas. The entrance requirement is BSc (N) and 2 years experience as nurses. The candidates also have to pass an entrance test. University exams are conducted at the -end of the first and second years or at the end of each semester.

23.11 MPHIL AND PhD IN NURSING

Till a few years ago nurses had to travel abroad to study PhD course or seek admission in allied disciplines. In the 80s RAK College of Nursing started an M Phil program as a regular and part-time course. Since, then several universities started registering candidates for PhD in nursing. Prominent among these are: MGR Medical University, Rajiv Gandhi University of Health Sciences, SNDT University and Delhi University. The Manipal Academy of Higher Education (MAHE) has started both MPhil and PhD programmes in nursing. The INC has recently initiated a project on starting a PhD program in nursing through support from the WHO.

However, nurses keen to obtain doctorate degrees continue to seek admission into universities and departments with related disciplines such as community health, nutrition, social sciences. The Jawaharlal Nehru University at New Delhi, the Padmavathi Mahila University, Tirupathi, and the Centre for Development Studies, Trivandrum and the Centre for Economic and Social Sciences, Hyderabad are some of the universities and institutes where nurses seek to obtain higher degrees.

23.12 VOCATIONAL NURSING (AT 10+2 LEVEL)

Since, independence India has assumed wide economic and social responsibilities in attempting to provide the security of an adequate standard of living for its people. Investment in education is necessarily a long-term on begins to yield results after a generation and in some cases even after a long period. In developing countries like India, due to financial constraints and low gross national product levels, it is difficult to finance universal university education.

Gandhiji had rightly visualized the magnitude of the problem and recommended village upliftment through basic education and development of basic craft in consonance with national growth, most of the youth out of school are workers. The base through which they can earn their livelihood and extend support to their families at grass root level. JP Naik in his paper on new policies, priorities and programmes stated that in addition to the existing full time courses of vocational education, it should be possible for a person to transfer himself from general vocational courses and vice versa and carry on credits with him. To meet the health needs of the population especially at grass root level, multipurpose health worker programme was introduced in 1978, to carry on various tasks relevant to promotion of health and prevention of disorders with special emphasis on maternal and child health services. This course of 2 years duration is designed for the candidate with 10th class certificate Staff selection commission (SSC).

CONCLUSION

The form of teaching has remained unchanged for centuries. The needs of society. The practical side of the matter has been left to chance, whereas specific features of the situation of each country are changing more rapidly. Unfortunately, little or no account has been taken in to consideration for the training of health personnel, but following traditional systems in teaching. What is required now is to make sure that the educational program is relevant? No educational system can be effective unless its purposes are clearly defined. The members of health team must be trained specially for the task they will have to perform taking into account the circumstances under which they will work, so defining the professional task of health personnel to be trained is the very basis of the educational objectives of training centers/institutions and must be shaped selectively in terms of the goal to be achieved. If the goal is modified in the course of time the program also to be modified accordingly.

24 Leadership in Nursing

24.1 INTRODUCTION

Leadership represents an abstract quality in a man. It is a psychological process of influencing followers or subordinates and providing guidance to them. Thus, the essence of leadership is follower ship. It is the followers who make a person as leader. An executive has to earn followers. He may get subordinates because he is in authority but he may not get a follower unless he makes the people to follow him only willing followers can and will make him a leader.

24.2 DEFINITION

1. Leadership is the ability to influence other people. *–Lansdale*
2. Leadership is the ability of a manager to induce subordinate to work with zeal confidence. *–Koontz and O' Donnell*
3. Leadership as the ability to secure desirable actions from a group of followers voluntaril, without the use of coercion. *–Afford and Beaty*
4. Leadership is the process of influencing the behavior and work of others in group effort towards the realization of special goal in a given situation.
5. Leadership is the activity to persuade others to seek defined objectives enthusiastically. It is the human factor which binds a group together and motivates it towards goals. *–Keith Davis*
6. Leadership is interpersonal influence exercise in a situation and directed through communication process, towards the attainment of a special goal or goals.

24.3 CHARACTERISTICS OF LEADERSHIP

1. **Leadership implies the existence of followers:** We appraise the quality of a person's leadership in practice by studying his followers. We ask: How many and what kind of followers does he have? How strong is their commitment as a result of his leadership? How long will their commitment last? By answering questions of this nature we get to know the quality of leadership. We must not, however, forget that leaders within organizations are also followers. The supervisor works for a branch head, who works for a division manager, who works for the vice-president of a department and so on. Thus, in formal organizations of several levels, a leader has to be able to wear both hats gracefully, to be able to 1relate himself both upward and downward.
2. **Leadership involves a community of interest between the leader** and his followers. In other words, the objectives of both the leader and his men are one and the same. If the leader strives for one purpose and his team of workers for some other purpose, it is no leadership. In the words of G.R. Terry, "Leadership is the activity of influencing people to strive willingly for mutual objectives".

3. **Leadership involves an unequal distribution of authority among leaders** and group members. Leaders can direct some of the activities of group members; that is the group members are compelled or are willing to obey most of the leader's directions. The group members cannot similarly direct the leader's activities, though they will obviously affect those activities in a number of ways.
4. **Leadership implies that leaders can influence their followers or subordinates** in addition to being able to give their followers or subordinates legitimate directions. In other words, leaders not only tell their subordinates what to do by way of command but also influence by their behavior and conduct. The use of command by leaders succeeds only in bringing about a temporary behavioral change in the followers. Permanent attitudinal change in followers comes through the use of influence only. According to Hersey and Blanchard leadership of the first type though successful is not effective. The second type of leadership is both successful and effective.

24.4 CHARACTERISTICS OF LEADER

1. It is a personal quality of character and behavior in man which enables him to exert internal personal influence.
2. It is concerned with the lying down group objectives and polices for the followers, motivating them coordinating their efforts to accomplish the objectives.
3. It pre-supposes the existence of a group followers.
4. Its style may differ from situation to situation.
5. It is the ability to perused others and motivate them to work for accomplishing certain objectives.
6. It is process of influencing exercised by leader on members of a group.
7. It involves an unequal distribution of authority among leaders and groups.

24.5 QUALITIES OF GOOD LEADER

1. **Integrity:** Integrity is expected of health care professional. Patients, colleagues, and employers all expect nurses to be honest, law —abiding and trust worthy.
2. **Courage:** Sometimes, being a leader means taking some risks.
3. **Initiative:** Good ideas are not enough. To be leader, you must act on those good ideas. This requires initiative on your part.
4. **Energy:** Leadership also requires energy. Both leadership and management are hard satisfying endeavors that require effort on your part.
5. **Optimism:** When the work is difficult and one crisis seems to follow another in rapid succession, it is easy to become discouraged. However, it is important not to let discouragement keep you and your coworkers from seeking ways resolve your difficulties.
6. **Perseverance:** Effective leaders to not give up easily. In seated, they persist, continuing their efforts when others tempted to give up the struggle.
7. **Balance:** In our effort to become the best nurses we be, we may forget that other aspects of life are equally important.
8. **Ability to handle stress:** There is some stress in almost every job. Coping with stress in as positive and healthy a manner as possible helps you conserve your energy model for others.
9. **Self awareness:** People who do not understand themselves are limited in their ability to understand the motivations of other people.

24.6 DIFFERENCE BETWEEN LEADERSHIP AND MANAGEMENT

From the above definitions and characteristics of leadership, it can be observed that leadership and management are related but they are not same. A person can be an effective manager, a leader, both or neither.

1. **Leadership deals with vision:** Keeping the mission in sight and with effectiveness and results. Management deals with establish structure and system to get those results. It focuses on efficiency, cost benefit analysis, logistics, methods procedures and politics.
2. **Leadership focuses on the top line:** Management focuses on the bottom line leadership derives its power from values and correct principles. Management organizes resources to serve selected objectives to produce the bottom line.
3. **Leadership inspires and motivates people** to work together with a common vision and purpose. Management involves controlling and monitoring results against plans, identify deviations and then planning and organization to solve the problems.
4. **Leadership emphasis transformational aspect** and, therefore transformational leadership emerges.

24.7 IMPORTANCE OF LEADERSHIP

Leadership is an important factor for making any type of organization successful. Through the history, it has been recognized that the difference success and failure, whether in a war, a political movement, business or a team game, can be attributed largely to leadership.

1. **Motivation employee:** Motivation is necessary for work performance. Higher the motivation, better would be the performance.
2. **Creating confidence:** A good leader macerate confidence in his followed by directing them advice, and getting through the good results in the organization.
3. **Building morale:** Morale is expressed as attitude of employee towards organization, management, and voluntary cooperation offers their ability to organization follows.

24.8 LEADERSHIP TECHNIQUES

Leadership is to be effective in nursing. The nurse has to poses certain qualities of leader and has to apply certain techniques as:

1. Planning and organizing the work schedule according to availability of personal and materials.
2. Assigning work to subordinates should be defined and recorded with clear-cut directions.
3. Proper teaching and guidance to subordinates.
4. Good communication is needed for proper understanding, cooperation and unified action.
5. Cooperations and coordination between superior and subordinates.
6. Identifying talented subordinates and involving them in planning.
7. Democratic supervision.
8. Evaluation of performance of subordinates and self.
9. Awareness of responsibilities and account.

CONCLUSION

The heart of management is dealing with people in order to achieve the organizational goals. Therefore, the success of every organization depends upon the leadership qualities of its managers. Good leadership is to win the support of the people. It is to direct and co-ordinate the personnel in an organization. Every leader may not be a good manager, but every manager must be a good leader. The leadership process comprises of various factors such as personality of the leader, attitudes and needs of the followers, the structure and maturity of the group and the situational or task factors.

25 Nursing Research

25.1 INTRODUCTION

Nursing research is a detailed systematic study of a problem in the field of nursing. Nursing research is practice or discipline-oriented and is essential for the continued development of the scientific base of professional nursing practice. Nursing research is research that provides evidence used to support nursing practices. Nursing, as an evidence-based area of practice, has been developing since the time of Florence Nightingale to the present day, where many nurses now work as researchers based in universities as well as in the health care setting.

25.2 DEFINITION

1. **American Nurses Association:** Nursing research develops knowledge about health and promotion of health over the full life span, care of persons with health problems and disabilities and nursing actions to enhance the ability of individuals to respond effectively to actual or potential health problems.
2. **International Nurses (Benolie) 1984:** Nursing research supports the need for nursing research as a means of improving health and welfare of the people. Nursing research is a way to identify new knowledge, improve professional educational practice and use of resources effectively.
3. **JW Best:** Research may be defined as the systematic and objective analysis and recording of controlled observations that may lead to the development of generations, principles, theories, resulting in predictions and possible ultimate control of events.
4. **Polit and Hungler:** Research is a process in which the researcher scientifically collects data to be used in the clinical administrative or instructional area in order to find solutions to nursing problems, evaluating nursing practices, procedures, policies or curriculum, assess the needs of the patients, staffs or students and or make decisions to change or continuous various nursing process which in turn advances the scientifically knowledge in Nursing field.
5. **French-Ruth M (1968):** Research essentially in a problem solving process, a systematic, intensive study directed towards full, scientific knowledge of the subject studied.

25.3 GOALS OF RESEARCH IN NURSING

The importance of nursing research cannot be stressed enough. Some of the goals for conducting research are to (a) promote evidence-based nursing practice, (b) ensure credibility of the nursing profession, (c) provide accountability for nursing practice, and (d) document the cost effectiveness of nursing care. One goal of research in nursing is to provide a basis for decision-making at all levels of the profession.

1. Schlotfeldt adds another dimension. "The primary task of nursing research is the development and refinement of nursing theories which can be organized into a body of scientific nursing knowledge".

2. The major reasons for doing research in nursing are providing the profession with a body of scientific knowledge and identifying and developing nursing theories. Even though much of nursing research can be carried out in manner similar to educational and social science research, new techniques will be needed as nursing and general knowledge grow, as findings are analyzed, as insight is gained into these findings and as evaluation is carried out. It may be necessary to develop new methods and techniques in patient care as nursing responsibilities change and expand.
3. Nursing research should provide the foundation for the changes in nursing.
4. Nursing research is needed because there are so many questions of vital importance to nursing that require a trained investigator. Nursing decision can then be based on facts rather than on surmise.
5. There is a need for nursing research because nursing has moved into an era of substantial independence. Nurses have begun to question, to creative, to think analytically and to systematically solve some of the problems facing them. The National Commission or study has stated it is regrettable that so little research has been conducted to determine the relative effectiveness of various nursing inventions.
6. Only through research we can begin to determine and fully exploit the capabilities of nurses to contribute to the health system. The National Commission cites research among the basic problems in nursing.
   a. Increased research into both the practice of nursing and the education of nurses.
   b. Enhanced educational system and curricula based on the results of that research.
7. The Pan-American Regional group, which held its first meeting in Caracas, Venezuela in November 1970, included the need for research as one of its recommendations. "There is a need to carry out research in every country to identify the needs of nursing and available resources in order to increase the number of schools at basic and university level".

25.4 CHARACTERISTICS OF NURSING RESEARCH

1. Research discrete towards the solution of a problem.
2. Research emphasizing the development of generalizations of principles or theories. Research is more than information retrieval, i.e. the simple gathering of information's.
3. Research based upon observable experience or empirical evidence. Research rejects revelation methods of establishing knowledge and accepts only what can be verified by observation.
4. Research demands accurate observation and description.
5. Research gathering new data from primary or first hand source or existing data for a new purpose.
6. Research carefully designed.
7. Research requiring expertise.
8. Research striving to be objective and logical.
9. Research monitoring the quest for answer to solve the problems.
10. Research characterized by patience and unhurried activity.
11. Research carefully recorded and reported.
12. Research some time requires courage.

25.5 SCOPE OF NURSING RESEARCH

1. To improve the standard of nursing care.
2. To redefine the existing theories and discovering new theories.
3. To discover new measures for nursing practice.
4. To foster a commitment to client.

5. To provide basis for professional accountability.
6. To impart professionalism in nursing.
7. To help in decision-making.
8. To improve standards in nursing education.
9. To help in documentation.
10. To bridge the gap between knowledge and practice.
11. To build the body of knowledge in nursing profession.
12. To validate improvement in nursing profession.
13. To make healthcare efficient and cost effective.
14. To act as a basis for standard setting and quality assurance.
15. To find solution on immediate practical problems of nursing.
16. To discover new facts about a known phenomenon.
17. To discover new message for nursing practice.
18. To identify the role of the nurse in changing society.

25.6 IMPORTANCE OF NURSING RESEARCH

Nursing profession is accountable to society for providing high-quality care patients and families. The healthcare provided by nurses must be constantly evaluated and improved based on new information. Nursing scientific knowledge base is expanding rapidly with the generation of new findings by nurses and other health professional using a variety of research methods. The knowledge generated through research is essential to provide a scientific basis for description, explanation prediction and control of nursing practice.

1. **Descriptive:** It involves identifying the nature and attributes of nursing phenomena and sometimes the relationship among these phenomena (Chinn and Kramer 1995). These studies are often called descriptive or explanatory. This descriptive research is essential ground work for studies that will focus on explanation, prediction and control of nursing phenomena.
2. **Explanation:** Relationship among variables is clarified and the reasons why certain events occur are identified. Explanation determining relationships among variables provides a basis for conducting studies for the purpose of predicting and controlling patient outcomes.

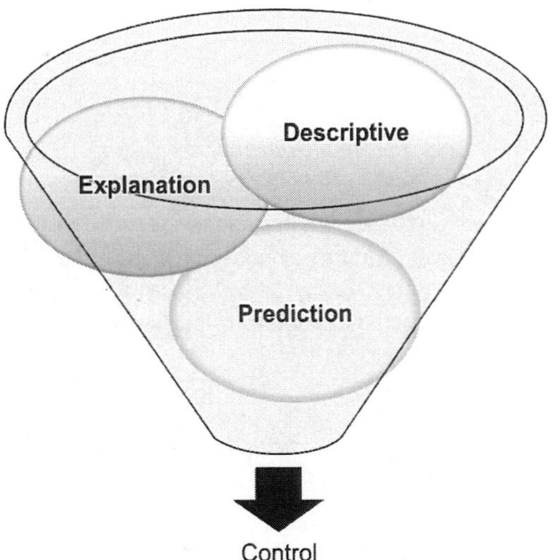

Fig. 25.1: Importance of research

3. **Prediction:** Through prediction, one can estimate the probability of a specific outcome in a given situation (Chinn and Kramer 1995). Health promotion research is being conducted to predict the effects of healthy behaviors such as exercising regularly, eating a balanced diet and not smoking on health status and longevity.
4. **Control:** It can be described as the ability to write a prescription to produce the desired results. Control involves imposing condition on the research situation so that biases and confounding factors are minimized. Based on the research of Meek (1993), nurses could prescribe slow stroke back massage to promote comfort and relaxation in hospice patients.

25.7 OBJECTIVES OF CONDUCTING RESEARCH IN NURSING

1. **Improvements in nursing care:** The nursing profession exists to provide a service to society, and this service should be based on accurate knowledge. Scientific research has been determined to be the most reliable means of obtaining knowledge. Clinical nursing research parallels the nursing process. Research finding enable the nurse to describe, explain, predict and control phenomena related to the health of clients.
2. **Credibility of the nursing profession:** Nursing has traditionally borrowed knowledge that is distinct from the natural and social sciences, and only in recent years have nurses concentrated on establishing a unique body of knowledge that would allow nursing to be clearly identified as a distinct a unique body of knowledge that would allow nursing to be clearly identified as a distinct profession. The most valid means of developing this knowledge base is scientific research.
3. **Accountability for nursing practice:** As nurses have become more independent in making decisions about the care of clients, their independence has brought about a greater need for accountability. Nurses must have sound rationales for their actions, based on knowledge that is gained through scientific research. Nurses have the responsibility of keeping their knowledge base current and one of the best sources of current knowledge is the scientific literature.
4. **Documentation of the cost:** Nursing services can consume a large percentage of a hospital's budget. With prospective payment systems determining the amount of reimbursements that hospitals receive, nursing care services are being closely examined. There are many studied in the literature that demonstrates the cost—effectiveness of nursing care. Ventura et al. (1985) conducted a study to examine the cost saving of nursing interventions with patients with peripheral vascular disease.

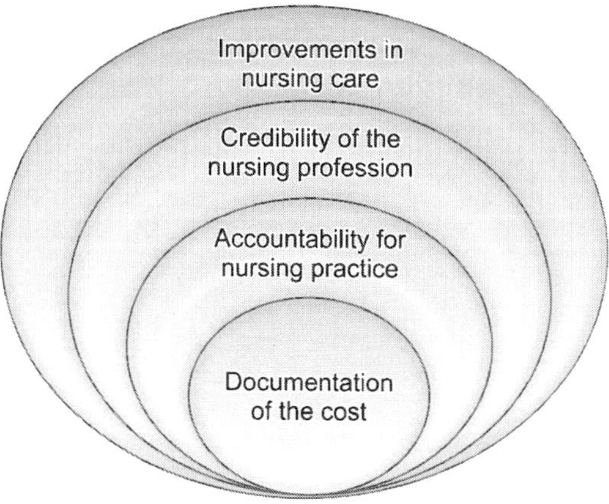

Fig. 25.2: Objective of conducting nursing research

25.8 AREAS OF NURSING RESEARCH

1. **Nursing education:** Research in nursing education may include study of effectiveness of educational programs, strength and weakness of teaching learning process.
2. **Nursing Administration:** The study includes effectiveness and efficiency of nurse's roles and functions, development of nursing standards, study of planning for nursing manpower, strategies to strengthen nurse's knowledge and performance.

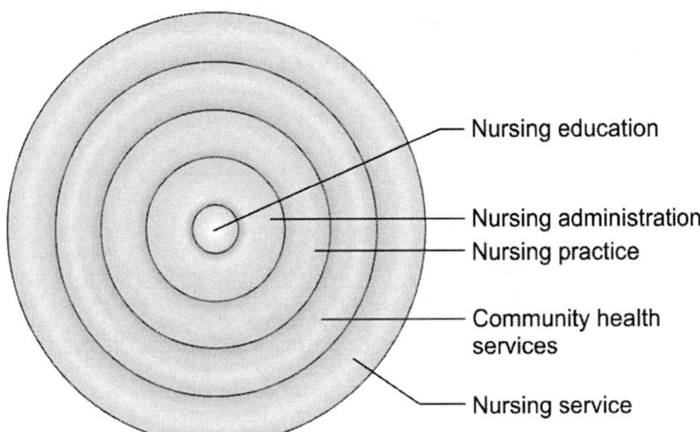

Fig. 25.3: Areas of nursing research

3. **Nursing practice:** Research enables nurses to describe the characteristics of a particular nursing situation. It explains the phenomena that must be considered in planning nursing care or to predict the probable outcomes of certain nursing decisions made in relation to client care.
4. **Community Health Services:** Several studies are conducted especially relevant to primary healthcare concepts. The spiraling cost of healthcare and the cost containment practices being instituted in healthcare facilities. Nurses are being asked more than ever to document the relevancy and the efficiency of their nursing practice to other, such as consumers of nursing care, administrators of healthcare facilities and government agencies.
5. **Nursing service:** Research has important in nursing service, where the nurses are able to answer the professional questions by which the profession is affected. Nursing research uplift the areas of administration and nursing care. Nursing research seeks to understand the nature of human behavior in health and illness and it identify interventions that nurse can use to enhance response.

25.9 RESEARCH RELATED ACTIVITIES IN NURSING

1. Organizing Journal club in a practice setting, which involves regular meeting among nurses to discuss and critique research articles.
2. Attending research presentations at professional conferences.
3. Formal evaluation of completed research, for its possible utilization in the practice setting.
4. Discussion with clients about the implications and relevance of research findings.
5. Providing assistance in collection of research information.
6. Review of proposed methods for gathering research information with respect to their feasibility in a clinical setting.

7. Contribution in the development of an idea for a research project.
8. Participation on an institutional committee whose mission is to review the ethical aspects of proposed research before it is undertaken.
9. Incorporation of research findings in to nursing practice or nursing education.

25.10 NEED OF RESEARCH IN NURSING

The ultimate goal of any profession is to provide its clients with maximum effective and efficient services. A profession seeks to improve the practice of its members and to enhance its professional stature for the continual development of a relevant body of knowledge. Nursing research represents a critically important 'tool' for the nursing Profession to acquire such knowledge.

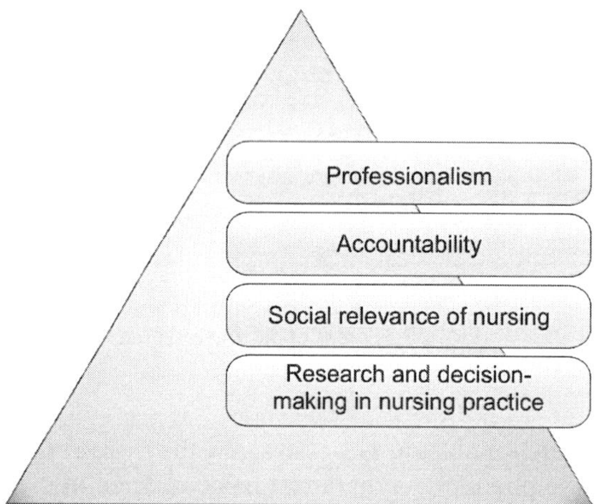

Fig. 25.4: Need of nursing research

1. **Professionalism:** Nurses increasingly recognize the need to extend the base of nursing knowledge as part of professional responsibility and endorse research investigations as a way to achieve this objective. Moreover nurses are committed to the evolution of a fairly distinct body of knowledge that separates nursing from other profession. Nursing is only one of the several professions involved in the delivery of healthcare. Information from nursing investigation helps to define better the unique role that nursing plays.
2. **Accountability:** During the 1970's nursing, leaders pointed out that the quality of nursing care cannot be improved until information based accountability becomes as much part of nursing tradition as humanitarianism. Nurses who corporate research evidence into their clinical decisions are being professionally accountable to their clients and are also helping nursing to achieve its own professional identity.
3. **Social relevance of nursing:** Nurses today are being asked more than ever before to document their role in the delivery of health services. People are recognizing healthcare as a right rather than a privilege and with spiraling costs, are asking various groups of health professionals how their service contribute to the total delivery of healthcare. This increased interest in examining healthcare practices makes it essential for nurses to evaluate the efficacy of their practices and to modify or abandon those practices shown to have no effect on client health.

4. **Research and decision-making in nursing practice:** Many nurses use the standards of clinical nursing practice published by the American Nurses Association (1991) both as theirs of clinical practice and to evaluate the quality of their nursing process requires nurses to engage in many decision-making
   What will be assessed?
   What nursing diagnoses result from the assessment?
   What plan of care is most likely to produce the desired outcomes?
   What nursing interventions are necessary?
   How will the result be evaluated in terms of their effectiveness?

Research conducted by nurses can potentially play a pivotal role at raise of the nursing process by helping nurses to make more informed decisions.

25.11 ROLE OF NURSE IN RESEARCH

Nurses act as principal investigators, members of research teams, identifiers of researchable problems, evaluators of research findings, users of research findings, client advocates during studies, and subjects/participants in research. Research utilization focuses on the implementation of findings from specific research studies.

1. **Principal investigator:** Nurses can and should serve as principal investigators in scientific investigations. To be a principal investigator, special research preparation is necessary.
2. **Members of a research team:** Nurses may act as data collectors or administer the experimental intervention of the study. As nurses increasingly participate in research, it is possible that interest and enthusiasm to conduct their own investigations may grow.
3. **Evaluator of research findings:** All nurses should be involved in the evaluation of research findings. As research consumers, nurses have the obligation to become familiar with research findings and determine the usefulness of these findings in the practice area. The evaluation of research is not an easy task.
4. **User of research findings:** After evaluating research findings, nurses should use relevant finding in their practice. The primary goal of nursing research, as has been mentioned, is the improved care of clients. However, nurses must be judicious in their use of research findings.
5. **Client advocate during studies:** Nurses have the responsibility to act as client advocates when clients are involved in research. Nurses can help answer questions and explain a study to potential participants before the study begins. They also can be available during the study to answer questions or provide support to study participants.
6. **Subject in studies:** Nurses also can act as subjects in research. Many nurses are involved in a long-term survey study that is being conducted by researcher at Harvard Medical School, with funds provided by the National Institute of Health.

CONCLUSION

Research has importance in nursing service also where the nurses are able to answer the professional questions by which the profession is affected. Nursing research uplift the areas of administration and nursing care. Nursing research seeks to understand the nature of human behavior in health and illness and it identify interventions that nurse can use to enhance responses. The nurse researcher investigates problems to improve nursing care and to further define and expand the scope of nursing practice. The nurse researcher may be employed in an academic setting, hospital, or independent professional or community-service agency. The minimum educational requirement is now a doctoral degree, with at least a master's degree in nursing.

26 Evidenced-Based Nursing Practice

26.1 INTRODUCTION

Evidence-based practice (EBP) is a problem-solving approach to the delivery of health care that integrates the best evidence from studies and patient care data with clinician expertise and patient preferences and values. Healthcare that is evidence-based and conducted in a caring context leads to better clinical decisions and patient outcomes. Gaining knowledge and skills in the EBP process provides nurses and other clinicians the tools needed to take ownership of their practices and transform healthcare. Key elements of a best practice culture are EBP mentors, partnerships between academic and clinical settings, EBP champions, clearly written research, time and resources, and administrative support.

26.2 DEFINITION

1. Evidence-based practice is an integration of the best evidence available, nursing expertise and the values and preferences of the individuals, families and communities are served.

   –Chris Jordan
2. Evidence-based practice is a continuous interactive process involving the explicit, conscientious and judicious consideration of the best available evidence to provide care.

   –Canadian Nurses Association
3. Evidence-based practice is a problem solving approach to the delivery of healthcare that integrates the best evidence from studies and patient care data with clinician expertise and patient preferences and values. *–Fineout Overholt*
4. Evidence-based practice nursing is the practice of health care in which the practitioner systematically finds, appraises and uses the most current and valid research findings as the basis for clinical decisions. *–Mosby*
5. Evidence-based practice is the conscientious use of current best evidence in making clinical decisions about patient care.

26.3 PURPOSES OF EBP

1. To provide the highest quality and most cost-efficient nursing care possible.
2. To advance quality of care provided by the nurses.
3. To increase satisfaction of patients.
4. To focus on nursing practice away from habits and tradition to evidence and research.

26.4 STEPS INVOLVED IN EBP

1. Select a topic and correct appropriate reviews.
2. Analyze data for clinical practice and design interventions based on evidence.

3. Predict and analyze outcomes and examine the pattern of behavior and outcomes.
4. Identify gaps in EBP and evaluate projects to determine and implement best practices.

26.5 LIMITATIONS OF EBP

1. Resistant to change in nursing practice.
2. Ability to critically appraise research findings in nursing.
3. Poor administrative support in nursing.
4. Fear of stepping on one's toes in nursing.
5. Lack of continuing educational programmes in nursing.

26.6 EVIDENCE-BASED NURSING

Evidence-based nursing or EBN is an approach to making quality decisions and providing nursing care based upon personal clinical expertise in combination with the most current, relevant research available on the topic. EBN implements the most up to date methods of providing care, which have been proven through appraisal of high quality studies and statistically significant research findings. The goal of EBN is to improve the health and safety of patients while also providing care in a cost-effective manner to improve the outcomes for both the patient and the healthcare system. EBN is a process founded on the collection, interpretation, appraisal, and integration of valid, clinically significant, and applicable research. The evidence used to change practice or make a clinical decision can be separated into seven levels of evidence that differ in type of study and level of quality. To properly implement EBN, the knowledge of the nurse, the patient's preferences, and multiple studies of evidence must all be collaborated and utilized in order to produce an appropriate solution to the task at hand. These skills are taught in modern nursing education and also as a part of professional training.

26.7 STEPS OF EVIDENCED-BASED NURSING

Cultivate spirit of inquiry: A spirit of inquiry refers to an attitude in which questions are encouraged to be asked about existing practices. Cultivating a spirit of inquiry allows healthcare providers to feel comfortable with questioning current methods of practice and challenging these practices to create improvements and change. A culture that fosters this should have a philosophy that incorporates EBP, access to tools that can enhance EBP, and administrative support and leadership that values EBP.

Ask Clinical Question (PICOT): PICOT formatted questions address the Patient population, Issue or intervention, Comparison group, Outcome, and Time frame. Asking questions in this format assists in generating a search that produces the most relevant, quality information related to a topic, while also decreasing the amount of time needed to produce these search results. An example of a quality PICOT question would be: In total knee arthroplasty patients (Population), what is the effect of nerve blocks (Intervention) compared to opioid pain medication (Comparison) in controlling postoperative pain (Outcome) within the first 24 hours after surgery (Time)?

Search for and collect relevant evidence: To begin the search for evidence, use each keyword from the PICOT question that was formed. Once results have been found on the intervention or treatment, the research can be rated to determine which provides the strongest level of evidence. There are seven levels of evidence, with a level I being of the strongest quality and a level VII being of the weakest quality:

1. **Level I:** Evidence from systematic reviews or meta-analysis of randomized control trials.
2. **Level II:** Evidence from well-designed randomized control trials.
3. **Level III:** Evidence from well-designed control trials that are not randomized.

4. **Level IV:** Evidence from case-control or cohort studies.
5. **Level V:** Evidence from systematic reviews of descriptive or qualitative studies.
6. **Level VI:** Evidence from a single descriptive or qualitative study.
7. **Level VII:** Evidence from expert opinions the strongest levels of evidence, systematic reviews and meta-analyses; summarize evidence related to a specific topic by finding and assessing studies that specifically relate to the question being asked. Meta-analyses are systematic reviews that also use quantitative measures such as statistics to summarize the results of the studies analyzed.

Critically appraise the evidence: To begin the critical appraisal process, three questions may be asked to determine the validity, reliability, and applicability of the evidence found. The three questions are:

1. Are the results of the study valid? In order to be valid, the results of the study must be as close to the truth as possible. Also, the study must be conducted using best available research methods.
2. What are the results? This question measures the reliability of the study. In an intervention study, reliability consists of: whether the intervention worked, how large the effect was, and whether a clinician could repeat the study with similar results. For a qualitative study, reliability would be measured by determining if the research accomplished the purpose of the study.
3. Will the results be applicable in caring for patients? The study may be used in practice when caring for patients if the subjects are similar to the patients being cared for, the benefit outweighs the harm, the study is feasible, and the patient desires the treatment. After asking these three questions, evidence appraisal continues by creating an evidence synthesis. This synthesis compares multiple studies to see if they are in agreement with each other.

Integrate the evidence: After appraising the evidence, it is necessary to integrate it with the provider's expertise and patient's preferences. The patient is encouraged to practice autonomy and participate in the decision-making process. Therefore, even if the study had successful outcomes, the patient may refuse to receive a treatment. Assessment findings and patient history may reveal further contraindications to a certain evidence-based treatment. Lastly, availability of healthcare resources may limit the implementation of a treatment even if it is found to be effective in a study.

Evaluate outcomes: The next step in the evidence-based practice process is to evaluate whether the treatment was effective in terms of patient outcomes. It is important to evaluate the outcomes in a real-world clinical setting to determine the impact of the evidence-based change on healthcare quality.

Disseminate outcomes: The last step is to share the information especially if positive outcomes are achieved. By sharing the results of evidence-based practice process, others may benefit. Some methods to disseminate the information include presentations at conferences, rounds within one's own institution, and journal publications.

26.8 BARRIERS TO PROMOTE EVIDENCE-BASED PRACTICE

The use of evidence-based practice depends a great deal on the nursing student's proficiency at understanding and critiquing the research articles and the associated literature that will be presented to them in the clinical setting. According to, Blythe Royal, author of Promoting Research Utilization in nursing: The Role of the Individual, Organization, and Environment, a large amount of the preparation requirements of nursing students consists of creating care plans for patients, covering in depth processes of pathophysiology, and retaining the complex information of pharmacology. These are indeed very important for the future of patient care, but their knowledge must consist of more when they begin to practice. Evidence based nursing in an attempt to facilitate the management of the growing literature and technology accessible to healthcare providers that can potentially improve patient care and their outcomes. Nancy Dickenson-Hazard states, "Nurses have the capacity to serve as caregivers and change agents in creating and implementing community and population-focused health systems". There is also a need to overcome the barriers to encourage the use of research by new graduates in an attempt to ensure familiarity with the process. This will help nurses to feel more confident and be more willing to engage in evidence based nursing. A survey that was established by the Honor Society of Nursing and completed by registered nurses proved that 69% have only a low to moderate knowledge of EBP and half of those that responded did not feel sure of the steps in the process. Many responded, "lack of time during their shift is the primary challenge to researching and applying EBP". There is always and will always be a desire to improve the care of our patients. The ever increasing cost of healthcare and the need for more accuracy in the field proves a cycle in need of evidence-based healthcare. The necessity to overcome the current issues is to gain knowledge from a variety of literature not just the basics. There is a definite need for nurses, and all practitioners, to have an open mind when dealing with the modern inventions of the future because these could potentially improve the health of patients.

There are many barriers to promoting evidence based practice. The first of which would be the practitioner's ability to critically appraise research. This includes having a considerable amount of research evaluation skills, access to journals, and clinic/hospital support to spend time on EBN. Time, workload pressures, and competing priorities can impede research and development. The causes of these barriers include nurse's and other professional practitioners lack of knowledge of research methods, lack of support from professional colleagues and organizations, and lack of confidence and authority in the research arena. Another barrier is that the practice environment can be resistant to changing tried and true conventional methods of practice. This can be caused because of reluctance to believe results of research study over safe, traditional practices, cost of adopting new practices, or gaining momentum to rewrite existing protocols. It is important to show nurses who may be resistant to changes in nursing practice the benefits that nurses, their patients, and their institutions can reap from the implementation of evidence-based nursing practice, which is to provide better nursing care. Values, resources and evidence are the three factors that influence decision-making with regard to healthcare. All registered nurses and healthcare professionals should be taught to read and critically interpret research and know where to find articles which relate to their field of care. In addition, nurses need to be more aware of how to assess the information and determine its applicability to their practice.

Another barrier to implementing EBN into practice is lack of continuing education programs. Practices do not have the means to provide workshops to teach new skills due to lack of funding, staff, and time; therefore, the research may be tossed dismissed. If this occurs, valuable treatments may never be utilized in patient care. Not only will the patients suffer but the staff will not have the opportunity to learn a new skill. Also, the practitioners may not be willing to implement change regardless of the benefits to patient care. Another barrier to introducing newly learned methods for improving treatments or patients' health is the fear of "stepping on one's toes". New nurses might feel it is not their place to suggest or even tell a superior nurse that newer, more efficient methods and/or practices are available.

26.9 IMPACT OF EVIDENCED-BASED NURSING PRACTICE

The impact of evidence-based practice (EBP) has echoed across nursing practice, education, and science. The call for evidence-based quality improvement and healthcare transformation underscores the need for redesigning care that is effective, safe, and efficient. In line with multiple direction-setting recommendations from national experts, nurses have responded to launch initiatives that maximize the valuable contributions that nurses have made, can make, and will make, to fully deliver on the promise of EBP. Such initiatives include practice adoption; education and curricular realignment; model and theory development; scientific engagement in the new fields of research; and development of a national research network to study improvement. This article briefly describes the EBP movement and considers some of the impact of EBP on nursing practice, models and frameworks, education and research. The article concludes with discussion of the next big ideas in EBP, based on two federal initiatives, and considers opportunities and challenges as EBP continues to support other exciting new thinking in healthcare.

In spite of many significant advances, nurses still have more to do to achieve EBP across the board. A recent survey of the state of EBP in nurses indicated that, while nurses had positive attitudes toward EBP and wished to gain more knowledge and skills, they still faced significant barriers in employing it in practice. One example of implementation of EBP points to the challenges of change. The evidence-based program, Team Strategies and Tools to Enhance Performance and Patient Safety carries with it proven effectiveness of reducing patient safety issues and the program is available with highly-developed training and learning materials. Yet, because of the change necessary to fully implement and sustain the program across the system supported by organizational culture, a sophisticated implementation plan is required before the evidence-based intervention is adopted across an institution.

26.10 IMPACT ON NURSING MODELS AND FRAMEWORKS

Early in the EBP movement, nurse scientists developed models to organize our thinking about EBP. A number of EBP models were developed by nurses to understand various aspects of EBP. These frameworks guide the design and implementation of approaches intended to strengthen evidence-based decision-making. Forty-seven prominent EBP models can be identified in the literature. Once analyzed, these models can be grouped into four thematic areas: (1) EBP, research utilization, and knowledge transformation processes; (2) Strategic/Organizational change theory to promote uptake and adoption of new knowledge; and (3) Knowledge exchange and synthesis for application and inquiry. Listed among models in Category 1 is the ACE Star Model of Knowledge Transformation; this model is the exemplar for the present discussion of the impact of EBP on nursing models and frameworks (Fig. 26.1).

The ACE Star Model of Knowledge Transformation was developed to offer a simple yet comprehensive approach to translate evidence into practice. As explained in the ACE Star Model, one approach to understanding the use of EBP in nursing is to consider the nature of knowledge and knowledge transformation necessary for utility and relevance in clinical decision-making. Rather than having clinicians submersed in the volume of research reports, a more efficient approach is for

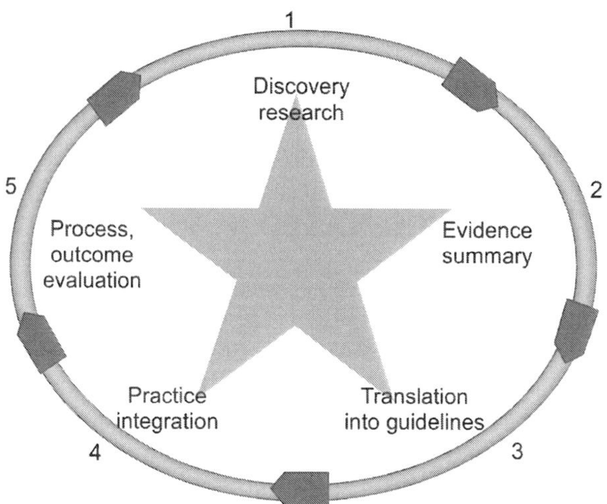

Fig. 26.1: ACE star model of knowledge transformation

the clinician to access a summary of all that is known on the topic. Likewise, rather than requiring frontline providers to master the technical expertise needed in scientific critique, their point-of-care decisions would be better supported by evidence-based recommendations in the form of clinical practice guidelines.

The ACE Star Model of Knowledge Transformation highlights barriers encountered when moving evidence into practice and designate solutions grounded in EBP. The model explains how various stages of knowledge transformation reduce the volume of scientific literature and provide forms of knowledge that can be directly incorporated in care and decision-making. The ACE Star Model emphasizes crucial steps to convert one form of knowledge to the next and incorporate best research evidence with clinical expertise and patient preferences thereby achieving EBP. Depicted in figure, the model is a five-point star, defining the following forms of knowledge:

Point 1—discovery, representing primary research studies;

Point 2—evidence summary, which is the synthesis of all available knowledge compiled into a single harmonious statement, such as a systematic review;

Point 3—translation into action, often referred to as evidence-based clinical practice guidelines, combining the evidential base and expertise to extend recommendations;

Point 4—integration into practice is evidence-in-action, in which practice is aligned to reflect best evidence; and

Point 5—evaluation, which is an inclusive view of the impact that the evidence-based practice has on patient health outcomes; satisfaction; efficacy and efficiency of care; and health policy.

26.11 IMPACT ON NURSING EDUCATION

Following the influential *Crossing the Quality Chasm* report, experts emphasized that the preparation of health professionals was crucial to bridging the chasm. The *Health Professions Education* report declared that current educational programs do not adequately prepare nurses, physicians, pharmacists or other health professionals to provide the highest quality and safest healthcare possible. The conclusion was that education for all health professions were in need of "a major overhaul" to prepare health professions with new skills to assume new roles. This overhaul would require changing way that health professionals are educated, in both academic and practice settings. Programs for basic preparation of health professionals were to undergo curriculum revision in order to focus on evidence-based quality improvement processes. Also, professional development programs would need to become widely available to update skills of those professionals who were already in practice. Leaders in all health disciplines were urged to come together in an effort for clinical education reform that addresses five core competencies essential in bridging the quality chasm: All health professionals should be educated to deliver patient-centered care as members of an interdisciplinary team emphasizing evidence-based practice, quality improvement approaches, and informatics.

26.12 IMPACT ON NURSING RESEARCH

Nursing research has been impacted by recent far-reaching changes in the healthcare research enterprise. Never before in healthcare history has the focus and formalization of moving evidence-into-practice been as sharp as is seen in today's research on healthcare transformation efforts. Nascent fields are emerging to understand how to increase effectiveness, efficiency, safety, and timeliness of healthcare; how to improve health service delivery systems; and how to spur performance improvement. These emerging fields include translational and improvement science, implementation research, and health delivery systems science.

Investigation into uptake of evidence-based practice is one of the fields that has deeply affected the paradigm shift and is woven into each of the other fields. Investigation into EBP uptake is equivalent to investigating Star Point 4 (integration of EBP into practice). Several notable federal grant programs have evolved to foster research that produces the evidential foundation for effective strategies in employing EBP. Among the new research initiatives are the Clinical Translational Science Awards and the Patient-Centered Outcomes grants.

26.13 PATIENT-CENTERED OUTCOME RESEARCH

Another recent and swooping change in healthcare research emerged with a focus on patient-centered outcomes research (PCOR). As evidence mounted on standard medical metrics (mortality and morbidity), it was noted that metrics and outcomes of particular interest to patients and families (such as quality of life) were understudied. In 2010, attention was drawn to the need to produce evidence on patient-centered outcomes from the perspective of the patient. Congress founded and heavily funded the newly-formed Patient-Centered Outcomes Research Institute (PCORI) with the following mission: "The Patient-Centered Outcomes Research Institute (PCORI) helps people make informed healthcare decisions, and improves healthcare delivery and outcomes, by producing and promoting high integrity, evidence-based information that comes from research guided by patients, caregivers and the broader healthcare community".

Likewise, some of the most recent calls for research from the Agency for Healthcare Research and Quality (AHRQ) are also focusing on PCOR. These calls encourage early and meaningful engagement of patients and other stakeholders in stating the research question, conducting the study, and interpreting results. This new direction in healthcare research will produce evidence that is coinvestigated by patients and families in partnership with health scientists, increasing relevance so that EBP reflects the patient's viewpoint.

26.14 OPPORTUNITIES AND CHALLENGES

Those leading clinical practice have willing partners from the academy for discovering what works to improve healthcare. Such evidence to guide clinical management decisions is long overdue. While there are benefits to both as the evidence is gathered and applied, the true benefit goes to the patient. Clinical leaders have unprecedented opportunity to step forward to transform healthcare from a systems perspective, focusing on EBP for clinical effectiveness, patient engagement, and patient safety.

Those leading education have great advantages offered from a wide variety of educational resources for EBP. The rich resources offer students a chance to meaningfully connect their emerging competencies with clinical needs for best practices in clinical and micro system changes. As they emerge from formal education, students will see great enthusiasm for employing EBP in today's clinical environments.

Those leading nursing science have access to new funding opportunities to develop innovative programs of research in evidence-based quality improvement, implementation of EBP, and the science of improvement. Readiness of the clinical setting for academic-practice research partnerships brings with it advantageous access to clinical populations and settings and an eagerness for utilization of the research results. The challenges for moving EBP forward spring from two sources: nurses becoming powerful leaders in interprofessional groups and nurses becoming powerful influencers of change. Therefore, adopting the following habits hold promise for moving us ahead:

1. Redesigning and/or investigating the redesign of healthcare systems through creativity and mastery of teamwork.
2. Persistence in educating the future workforce, and retooling the current workforce, with awareness, skills, and power to improve the systems of care.

3. Laying aside comfortable programs of research and picking up programs of systems research.
4. Insistence on multiple perspectives and sound evidence for transforming healthcare.

The nursing profession remains central to the interdisciplinary and discipline-specific changes necessary to achieve care that is effective, safe, and efficient. New in our vernacular and skill set are systems thinking, microsystems change, high reliability organizations, team-based care, transparency, innovation, translational and implementation science, and, yes, still evidence-based practice. Let us move swiftly to make these new ideas and skills common place.

CONCLUSION

Evidence-based nursing practice was started in 1800s with Florence Nightingale. It is a problem-solving approach to clinical decision making. It is the process of integrating clinical knowledge, judgment, proficiency skills with the best available clinical evidence, such as nursing practice into patient care. Gaining knowledge and skills in evidence-based practice provides nurses and other clinicians the tools needed to take ownership of their practice and transform healthcare in a comprehensive manner.

27 Futuristic Nursing

27.1 INTRODUCTION

Nursing continue to be challenged and rewarded by both new and changing opportunities and constraints. Professional image continues to be major challenge for all nurses individually and collectively. A number of forces that have affected the development of professional nursing still continue to affect significant issues which includes:

1. Societal images and expectation of nurses.
2. Degree of the nursing professions control over the quantity and quality of practitioners.
3. Impact of technology and theory on nursing practices roles and setting.
4. Professional self image of nurses.
5. Sources of financing for healthcare services.

Predicting the future is an occupation fraught with peril in a society and world that are changing rapidly. The changes that seem likely to occur in due course will be changes in the demographics, the deteriorating environment, risky life styles, and economics of healthcare and governmental regulation of healthcare. The changes will be accomplished by changes in both nursing practice and nursing education.

27.2 NURSING PRACTICE

I. **Demographical changes:** The trends important to future of nursing includes rising number of elderly people, continuing increase in poverty an increasing in cultural diversity in the population and a continued trend urbanization. Each has implication or nursing.
   1. Many older persons are healthy, but the likelihood of illness becomes greater as people age. It indicates clearly nurse of the future must be prepared to work affectively with rising number of elderly persons.
   2. The number of people living below the poverty lines increasing, particularly among children and elderly. When basic needs for food, clothing and shelter are unmet or uncertain, health care becomes a luxury.
   3. Immunizations, for children's parental care for pregnant woman, nutritious meals and other health maintaining factors are neglected even though some care has been taken on these issues.
   4. Poor people tend to put off seeking care until illness advanced and thus harder to treat.
   5. Preventable conditions are often not prevented due to lack of education lack of sanitation, crowded living conditions. Improper shelter, homelessness, and host of other poverty related factors.
   6. Nursing as a profession, is committed to provide care to all peoples, regardless of social and economic factors to take challenges to meet these issues.
      a. Cultural diversity refers to the array of people from different racial, religious, social and geographic backgrounds who make up a particular entity, cultural beliefs and practices of

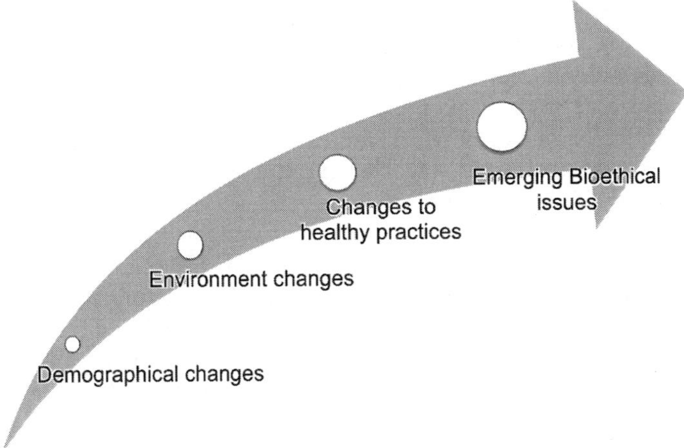

Fig. 27.1: Nursing practice

the citizens are quite different. Each groups has its own health beliefs, folk remedies and conventional wisdom about health and sickness.

b. Nurses increasingly need to take these beliefs into considerations when planning and implementing nursing care for individuals of diverse cultural backgrounds.

7. Urbanization, that is, people moving from rural farming areas to cities has increased since the time of industrial revolution. The trend continues today and is expected to continue in the future. This will create more social problems (homelessness, drugs, gangs, mental illness, violence, crime). These spread over into suburbs and rural areas, creating further social change. Nurses of the future will be increasingly confronted with health problems created by these social phenomena.

II. **Environment changes:** Major environmental tragedies such as nuclear power plant accident, burning oil wells, Tsunami, gradual decline in the qualities of the air, water, plant and animal life of the universe leads to many social and health problems. Depletion of the ozone layer, accidental lead and mercury poisonings, pesticides spilling into streams and rivers and accidental releases of radioactive steam from nuclear power plants, are all leads to health problems. The related problems of environmental deterioration and over population are health care issues that future nurses will undoubtedly have to face.

III. **Changes to healthy practices:** Obesity is predisposing cause of number of illnesses is due to unhealthy dietary habits, lack of exercise, stress, having contact with Multipartner for sex, AIDS. Substance abuse which in another unhealthy habit leads to many problems. Given the predominance of these unhealthy lifestyle factors, it is clear that nurses will play an increasingly important role in educating people about wellness and self-care. Nurses will also play an instrumental in educating the public about how to be involved in the development of sound public policies concerning these issues. Nursing, through its professional association, will become powerful player in the National Health Care politics. Nurses will form coalition with customer groups. Individual nurse become politically active as voters, campaign workers, community health activities, and political candidate. As nursing's public profits profile becomes higher, public scrutiny of the profession will increase. Consumers of nursing services will exercise their political power to pressurize nursing to provide quality health care.

IV. **Emerging bioethical issues:** Bioethics related to those ethical issues that are raised because of new technologies advancement in medicine and biological sciences.

1. Issues related to birth involve processes that prevent conception or terminate pregnancy prematurely as well as processes that enable conception and pregnancy to occur through technological intervention the fetal. Development sterilization, contraception and abortion on the one hand, and "test tube" conception, and artificial inseminations on the other, evoke strong feelings from various groups and individuals.
2. Each of these issues had its own ethical ramification, risks and consequences which must be weighed against the desired outcomes
3. Issues related to life or death, which includes that with the invention of life saving apparatus such as the kidney dialysis unit, artificial respirator, heart and lung machine, and fetal monitor and with the development of new surgical procedures (ex. Fetal surgery, organ transplantation, etc.) and new technology (ex. Genetic research, fetal research), it has become necessary to redefine the terms of life and death as new technology emerges, new issues will arise, and nurses must be prepared to confront them with Doth changing technical skills and value system that adapts to the demands of society.

27.3 NURSING EDUCATION

In the future, the nurses will need broad based education, assessment skills, technical competence, and the ability to deal with rapid change. The knowledge base and technology used in providing nursing care will continue to increases as well as nurses need for skill and ability in:

1. Intensely acute aspects of care.
2. Diagnostics and decision-making.
3. Client teaching.
4. Coordination of less-skilled workers.
5. Collaboration with client and healthcare professionals to improve the quality of health.

In earlier days, entry level for profession was certificate level and diploma level. Now changing circumstances people are thinking that undergraduate (BSc Nursing degree) as entry level of professional nursing. Entry to nursing could conceivably occur at one of four level Diploma, (DGNM), Bachelors Degree level (UG-BSc Nursing), Masters Level (PG-MSc Nursing) or the doctoral degree (PhD Nursing).

The current pattern, entry at diploma level, with professional education at the UG Level (Bachelors degree) might be perpetuated. There are some who propose that education for entry to professional nursing be moved to the master's level rather than basic degree level. This level of education would prepare the student for combination of specialized and generalized practice appropriate for developing healthcare delivery system. All students would need prior general education and possible a bachelor's degrees for entry into nursing, which would strengthen the liberal arts and science base for practice. Since, in India predegree course (PUC) included liberal arts and science concepts, human education PUC is made as entry into nursing both diploma and degree courses in nursing. So, it is better that after PUC-science, students can join BSc nursing degree courses. After few years of experience in bedside nursing or community health nursing, they can join the Master degree courses in nursing. After they can think of doing doctoral degree courses in nursing in their respective interest in the field of nursing.

As the coming decades sees nursing practice become more exciting and autonomous than ever, the need for strong, differentiated educational preparation for nurses at all levels will be crucial. More nurses will recognize the value of bachelor's degrees for beginning professional practice and masters degrees for specialty practices. More will pursue doctoral degrees to prepare for research and theory development. In response, colleges of nursing will expand flexible educational programmes to improve access. They will also develop differentiated levels of nursing education that correspond to differentiated levels of practice.

The major challenge for nursing education in the future will be to produce a steady supply of well-prepared nurse's graduates in the face of an aging faculty, rapidly changing technology, increasing cultural diversity of students and patients and budgetary constraints in higher education. So, meeting continuing or advanced education needs is an individual responsibility of every nurses. It is the obligation of nurses who are responsible for their patients care, to maintain current and relevant knowledge and skills in their field. It is important for each nurse to realize that the attainment of a certificate or a degree is not an end itself. Rather, it is to be viewed as a beginning foundation upon which to build their nursing knowledge.

27.4 NURSING RESEARCH

Today almost all nursing leaders and nursing organization offer professional nurse perhaps both the greatest demands and greatest rewards for nursing research. Research opportunities and needs await interested professionals in nursing. Professionals nurses are obligated both to ask the significant questions that need to be answered and to use research findings on the basis of nursing practice. Research in nursing generates the knowledge that is used in practice, while practice generates ideas of research. Nurses need to understand research as legitimate scientific enquiry. To fulfill the professional obligations in healthcare delivery system, the nurses have to keep following objectives. Nursing education will develop programs to educate practitioners skilled in scientific inquiry at all levels of practice:

1. Nursing research will be an integral part of nursing education and nursing practice.
2. Nursing practice will establish an environment receptive to inquiry and professional practice.

Most nurses' today would probably agree that a practice based on research is desirable. Capitalizing on that agreement, the profession could begin to present different images to the public. To help actualize the motivation to base nursing practice on research, education programs need to prepare students in scientific inquiry whole also preparing them to apply theory in the conduct of professional roles.

CONCLUSION

In the near future, the issues of concern for the nursing practice involve autonomy and independent practice among nurses, quality of care in community setting and homes, and development of nurse as leaders in the healthcare field. Various challenging healthcare issues are patient's refusal towards healthcare, euthanasia, patient advocacy by nurses, cost effective quality nursing care, competency in nursing practice Nurses need to look at these issues, professional values and expectations they face and decide. Once these issues are identified, strategies for promoting the quality care nursing can be delineated.

Section-7

Issues in Nursing

28 Independent Nurse Practitioner

28.1 INTRODUCTION

The nurse practitioner (NP) role, which originated in the United States (US), is now recognized as an enhanced nursing role working in partnership with clients, rather than just an extended nursing role with delegated medical tasks.

Ageing populations, rising expectations of patients, and reforms that shift care from hospitals to the community has led to the increased demand for general practitioners' services in many Western countries. Many countries have sought to shift care from general practitioners to other health professionals, notably nurses, to accommodate this expansion in workload. The presumption is that aspects of care provided by general practitioners could be provided by nurses instead.

28.2 DEFINITION OF NURSE PRACTITIONER

A nurse practitioner (NP) is a registered nurse (RN) who has completed advanced education (a minimum of a Bachelor degree) and training in accessories and management of common including care of chronic illnesses. Nurse practitioners provide a broad range of healthcare services. They provide some of the same care provided by physicians and maintain close working relationships with physicians. An NP can serve as a patient's regular health care provider. Nurse practitioners see patients of all ages. The core philosophy of the field is individualized care. Nurse practitioners focus on patients' conditions as well as the effects of illness on the lives of the patients and their families. In addition to healthcare services, NPs conduct research and are often active in patient advocacy activities.

28.3 SCOPE OF NURSE PRACTITIONER

Because the profession is regulated by each country and states within, care provided by NPs shall vary. A nurse practitioner's duties may include the following:

1. Collaborating with physicians and other health professionals as needed, including providing referrals.
2. Counseling and educating patients on health behaviors, self-care skills, and treatment options.
3. Diagnosing and treating acute illnesses, infections, and injuries.
4. Diagnosing, treating, and monitoring chronic diseases (e.g. diabetes, high blood pressure).
5. Obtaining medical histories and conducting physical examinations.
6. Ordering, performing, and interpreting diagnostic studies [e.g. lab tests, X-rays, electrocardiogram (EKGs)].
7. Prescribing medications.
8. Prescribing physical therapy and other rehabilitation treatments.
9. Providing prenatal care and family planning services.

10. Providing well-child care, including screening and immunizations.
11. Providing health maintenance care for adults, including annual physical assessment.
12. Nurse practitioners provide high-quality, cost-effective individualized care that is comparable to the healthcare provided by physicians, and usually the NP services are covered by insurance providers.

28.4 ROLE OF NURSE PRACTITIONER

Nurses can undertake much of the health promotion work of general practice and have a leading role in the routine management of chronic diseases such as asthma, diabetes, and coronary heart disease. Depending on the complexity of tasks, degree of autonomy, and level of training, care may be provided by nurse practitioners, practice nurses, or care assistants. A review of available research has shown that nurses can achieve health outcomes that are as good as those of general practitioners and that they may have superior interpersonal skills. Advanced practice roles for nurses in tomorrow's healthcare systems emerge as an outcome of the felt need for care shift.

This recent emergence of new healthcare providers such as nurse practitioners and physician assistants has initiated a re-examination of the healthcare division of labor. Professional organizations, legislatures, and hundreds of practices where new healthcare providers are employed are into the discussions and negotiations over these new roles. Emergence of NP has become a subject of much debate. This debate is a complex one and involves competing images of healthcare as well as issues of professional and economic self- interest, but two fundamental issues which can be identified are: (1) the specific tasks which should constitute the NP's role, and the (2) questions of professional autonomy. The former issue revolves around the question of which specific healthcare delivery tasks ought to be performed by NPs, and the latter issue is primarily concerned with the relationship of NP to physicians.

The issue of appropriate tasks for NPs is influenced by the intra-as well as interprofessional disagreement, much of which focuses on aspects of the NP's role overlapping with functions traditionally reserved for physicians. A recent report of a survey of nurse practitioner preparatory programs which describes them as reflecting "the broadest possible range" with respect to program content reflects the lack of standardized definitions of NP functions. There is still a good deal of flux and ambiguity in the field in general even though some types of NPs, such as nurse-midwives and pediatric nurse practitioners have enjoyed a relatively long tradition.

28.5 AREAS OF NURSE PRACTITIONER

Several attempts to gain legislative sanction for increased independence for these new healthcare providers, specific to the proper relationship of NPs to physicians-reflecting the issue of professional autonomy have been made. Virtually all still perpetuate "the traditional view that in the overlap between medicine and nursing the nurse acts in a dependent capacity," but this issue is far from settled, and questions about the proper measure of autonomy for NPs continue to be raised. Now, the question arises" Who should be called as Nurse Practitioner? What is the roles/function? And, what should be the licensure and certification criteria for a Nurse Practitioner?

Various setting of clinical nurse practionner: The institutions in which NP's may work include the following:

1. Community clinics and health centers.
2. Health departments.
3. Health maintenance organizations (HMOs).
4. Home.
5. Healthcare agencies.
6. Hospitals and hospital clinics.

7. Hospice centers.
8. Nurse practitioner offices.
9. Nursing homes and nursing schools.
10. Physician offices.
11. Private offices.
12. Public health departments School/college clinics.
13. Veterans Administration facilities.
14. Walk-in clinics.

Most NPs specialize in a particular field of medical care, and there are as many types of NPs as there are medical specialties.

NPs and women's health: Women with serious conditions, especially those that require surgery, need the services of a physician. But when women have typical healthcare needs, an NP can serve as the healthcare provider.

CONCLUSION

The nurse practitioner provides healthcare to clients, usually in an outpatient, ambulatory care, or community-based setting and comprehensiveness of care. A significant percentage of primary care encounters extend beyond the boundaries of medicine and demand the expertise of the nurse. The nurse practitioner is able to establish a collaborative provider-client relationship. The major nurse practitioner categories are adult, family, pediatric, obstetrics-gynecology, and geriatric nurse practitioner. A nurse practitioner has the knowledge and skills necessary to detect and manage limited acute and chronic stable conditions. The nurse practitioner's educational preparation includes a practitioner program or a master's degree in nursing.

29 Holistic Nursing

29.1 INTRODUCTION

The holistic nurse is an instrument of healing and a facilitator in the healing process. Holistic nurses honor each individual's subjective experience about health, health beliefs, and values. Holistic nurses may integrate complementary/alternative modalities (CAM) into clinical practice to treat people's physiological, psychological, and spiritual needs. Doing so does not negate the validity of conventional medical therapies, but serves to complement, broaden, and enrich the scope of nursing practice and to help individuals access their greatest healing potential. Florence Nightingale, who believed in care that focused on unity, wellness, and the inter relationship of human beings and their environment, is considered to be one of the first holistic nurses.

29.2 DEFINITION

Holistic nursing is defined as "all nursing practice that has healing the whole person as its goal" (American Holistic Nurses' Association, 1998, Description of Holistic Nursing). Holistic nursing is a specialty practice that draws on nursing knowledge, theories, expertise and intuition to guide nurses in becoming therapeutic partners with people in their care. This practice recognizes the totality of the human being—the interconnectedness of body, mind, emotion, spirit, social/cultural, relationship, context, and environment.

29.3 HOLISTIC TREATMENT MODALITIES

I. Whole Medical Systems

1. **Homeopathy:** A system of medicine which stimulates healing through the administration of substances prescribed according to three basic principles: (1) like cures like, (2) the more a remedy is diluted, the greater the potency; and (3) illness is specific to the individual. Homeopathy is based on the belief that symptoms are signs of the body's effort to get rid of disease; treatment is based on the whole person, rather than on the symptoms.
2. **Osteopathic medicine:** A form of medicine that focuses on the relationship between the structure of the body and its function, and recognizes that both structure and function are subject to a range of disorders. In treatment of the individual, osteopaths use various forms of physical manipulation, to facilitate the body's self-healing mechanism, as well as more conventional medical therapies. Osteopaths are fully licensed to diagnose, treat, and prescribe.

II. Manipulative and Body-based Practices

1. **Acupressure:** Use of finger and hand pressure over specific points on the body to relieve pain and discomfort and to influence the function of internal organs and body systems. Various approaches are used to release tension and restore the natural flow of energy in the body.

2. **Acupuncture:** Use of fine-gauged needles inserted into specific points on the body to stimulate or disperse the flow of energy. This ancient Oriental technique is used to alleviate pain or increase immunity by balancing energy flow. Massage, herbal medicine, and nutritional counseling are often used in conjunction with acupuncture.
3. **Alexander technique:** A series of lessons in rebalancing the body through awareness, movement and touch. As the student explores new ways of reorganizing neuromuscular function, the body is reacquainted with relaxed, healthy posture and direct, efficient movement.
4. **AMMA therapy:** Amma is a form of oriental massage that focuses on the balance and movement of energy within the body.
5. **Aromatherapy:** Use of essential oils extracted from plants and herbs to treat physical imbalances, as well as to achieve psychological and spiritual well-being. The oils are inhaled, applied externally, or ingested.
6. **Body work:** Any therapy that involves touch and/or pressure on the body. Often the term is used as an umbrella to describe the use of two or more therapies by a single practitioner, either in separate sessions or during a single session, according to the needs of the client.
7. **Breema bodywork:** Breema incorporates simple, playful bodywork sequences along with stretch and movement exercises that help create greater flexibility, relaxed body, clear mind, and calm, supportive feelings.
8. **Chiropractic medicine:** A healthcare system emphasizing structural alignment of the spine. Adjustments involve the manipulation of the spine and joints to re-establish and maintain normal nervous system functioning. Some chiropractors employ additional therapies, such as massage, nutrition, and specialized kinesiology.
9. **Cranial osteopathy:** Gentle and almost imperceptible manipulation of the skull to re-establish its natural configuration and movement. Such correction can have a positive influence on disorders manifested throughout the body.
10. **Cranio-sacral therapy:** Diagnosis and treatment of imbalances in the cranio-sacral system. Subtle adjustments are made to the system through light touch and gentle manipulations.
11. **Dance therapy:** Therapy in which dance and music combine to allow the body, mind, soul, and spirit to be refreshed, uplifted, and experience the freedom that natural bodily movement allows.
12. **Feldenkrais method:** A method of instruction, through movement and gentle manipulation, to enhance self-image and restore mobility. Students are taught to notice how they are using their bodies, and how to improve their posture and move more freely.
13. **Jin Shin jyutsu:** A bodywork technique which balances body energy as it travels along specific pathways. Specific combinations of healing points are held with the fingertips to restore balance and harmony.
14. **Lymphatic therapy:** A vigorous form of massage that helps the body release toxins stored in the lymphatic system-excellent for the immune system and rebuilding the body.
15. **Massage:** The use of strokes and pressure on the body to dispel tension, increase circulation and relieve muscular pain. Massage can provide comfort and increased body awareness, and can be an excellent method of releasing emotional as well as bodily tension.
16. **Movement therapy:** A guided series of movements and body work to open energy pathways and facilitate healing.
17. **M technique:** A registered method of gentle, structured touch suitable for the very fragile or actively dying or when the giver is not trained in massage. It was created by a nurse for nurses.
18. **Neuromuscular therapy:** A massage therapy in which moderate pressure over muscles and nerves, as well as on trigger points, is used to decrease pain and tension.
19. **Physical therapy:** The treatment of physical conditions of body malfunction, damage or injury, using procedures designed to reduce swelling, relieve pain, strengthen muscles, restore range of motion and return functioning to the patient.

20. **Qi Gong:** An internal Chinese meditative practice that uses breathing techniques, gentle movement, and meditation to cleanse, strengthen, and circulate the life energy.
21. **Shiatsu:** An energy-based system of bodywork using a firm sequence of rhythmic pressure held on specific points, designed to awaken acupressure meridians.
22. **Trigger Point therapy:** A method of compression of sensitive points in the muscle tissue, along with massage and passive stretches, for the relief of pain and tension. Treatment decreases swelling and stiffness and increases range of motion. Exercises may be assigned.

III. Body Mind Medicine

1. **Art therapy:** Use of basic art materials to discover how to restore, maintain or improve physical and mental health. Through observation and analysis, the art therapist is able to formulate treatment plans specific to the individual.
2. **Color therapy:** The use of electronic instrumentation and color receptivity, according to the work of Jacob Lieberman, to integrate the nervous system and body-mind. It increases well-being, and can be helpful for many acute and chronic ailments.

IV. Counseling/Psychotherapy

A broad category of therapies which treat individuals as a whole. Treatments and sessions are focused on integrated care on all levels, for individuals, families or groups.

1. **Eye Movement desensitization and reprocessing (EMDR):** An accelerated information processing method using alternating stimuli—either eye movements or sounds--to desensitize and reprocess emotional wounds or install a healthier belief system. EMDR is effective with post traumatic stress syndrome, childhood trauma, depression, addictions, compulsions, unhealthy patterns and future-oriented solutions.
2. **Guided imagery:** This holistic modality assists clients in connecting with their inner knowledge at the thinking, feeling, and sensing levels, promoting their innate healing abilities. Together, guide and client cocreate an effective way to work with: pain, symptom, grief, and stress management; conflict resolution; self-empowerment issues; and/or preparing for medical-surgical interventions.
3. **Hypnotherapy:** The use of a state of focused attention, achieved through guided relaxation, to access the unconscious mind. Hypnosis is used for memory recall, medical treatment, and skill enhancement or personal growth.
4. **Interactive imagery:** Fosters active participation, disease prevention and health promotion, returning the focus of wellness to the individual. See also Guided imagery.
5. **Meditation:** A method of relaxing and quieting the mind to relieve muscle tension and acilitate inner peace. There are numerous forms of meditation, taught individually or in group settings, and it is thought that prayer for the self might have an effect similar to meditation. The nonsectarian form of prayer, which is akin to meditation and used for stress reduction, has long been recognized by clinicians to improve one's sense of well-being. Studies by Dr. Herbert Benson of Harvard University have shown that inducing a relaxed state of mind is good both for the health and immune-system response. Prayer may work partly in this way.
6. **Music therapy:** An expressive art form designed to help the individual move into harmony and balance. Through the use of music, individuals explore emotional, spiritual and behavioral issues. Musical skill is not necessary, as the process, rather than technique, is emphasized.
7. **Neuro-linguistic programming (NLP):** A systematic approach to changing behavior through changing patterns of thinking.

IV. Psychotherapy

1. **Stress management:** Any therapy or educational practice with the objective of decreasing stress and enhancing one's response to the elements of life that cannot be changed. This broad category may include bodywork, energy work, visualization and counseling.

2. **Tai Chi (Chuan):** A movement practice, and Chinese martial art, which enhances coordination, balance and breathing, and promotes physical, emotional, and spiritual well-being. Tai Chi is taught in classes or as private lessons, and requires home practice to be effective.
3. **Yoga therapy:** The use of yoga postures, controlled breathing, relaxation, meditation, and nutrition to release muscular and emotional tension, improve concentration, increase oxygen levels in the blood, and assist the body in healing itself.

V. Biologically Based Therapies

1. **Biofeedback:** A relaxation technique involving careful monitoring of vital functions (such as breathing, heart rate and blood pressure) in order to improve health. By conscious thought, visualization, movement or relaxation, one can learn which actions result in desirable changes in these vital functions. Biofeedback is used for medical problems related to stress and for conditions such as incontinence, irregular heartbeat and epilepsy.
2. **Herbal therapy:** The use of herbs and their chemical properties to alleviate specific conditions or to support the function of various body systems. Herbal formulas have three basic functions: elimination and detoxification, health management and maintenance, and health building.
3. **Hydrotherapy:** The use of water, ice, steam, and hot and cold temperatures to maintain and restore health. Treatments include full body immersion, steam baths, saunas, and the application of hot and/or cold compresses.
4. **Nutritional counseling:** A practitioner who uses diet and supplementation therapeutically as the primary or adjunctive treatment for illness, as well as for maintaining good health. Nutritionists employ a variety of approaches, including food combining, macrobiotics, and orthomolecular theory.

VI. Energy Medicine

1. **Chi Kung healing touch:** A method of healthcare involving breath and gentle movements which follows the Chinese five-element theory and works with the meridian system.
2. **Energy work:** A broad category of body work influencing the seven major energy centers (chakras) and the flow of energy around and through this field. As the body's energy field is balanced and strengthened, healing occurs simultaneously on the physical and nonphysical levels.
3. **Healing touch:** An energy-based therapeutic approach to healing. Touch is used to influence the energy system, affecting physical, emotional, mental and spiritual health and healing. The goal of treatment is to restore harmony and balance, promoting self-healing.
4. **Magnetic therapy:** The use of magnets to generate controlled magnetic fields which can benefit the functioning of the nervous system, organs and tissues, and stimulates healing.
5. **Prayer:** Prayer is considered by National Center for Complementary and Alternative Medicine (NCCAM) to belong in the category of putative energy fields (also called biofields). Therapies involving putative energy fields are based on the concept that human beings are infused with a subtle form of energy. This vital energy or life force is known under different names in different cultures, such as qui in traditional Chinese medicine, the vital energy or life force proposed to regulate a person's spiritual, emotional, mental, and physical health and to be influenced by the opposing forces of yin and yang.
6. **Reiki:** The use of hands and visualization to direct energy to various parts of the body to facilitate healing and relaxation. Reiki can promote mental, emotional, physical, and spiritual balance.
7. **Therapeutic touch:** A technique for balancing energy flow in the body through human energy transfer. Therapeutic touch is based on the principle that in balance there is health and in health there is growth, order and wholeness.
8. **Touch for health:** A science of energy-balancing encompassing aspects of applied kinesiology, acupressure, massage and nutrition to maximize physical and emotional health. Touch for

Health emphasizes the uniqueness of the individual, and uses measurement of muscle strength as a biofeedback mechanism to determine the unique needs of the individual.

29.4 HOLISTIC NURSING PRACTICE

Holistic nursing embraces all nursing practice that has enhancement of healing the whole person from birth to death as its goal. Holistic nursing recognizes that there are two views regarding holism: that holism involves identifying the interr elationships of the bio-psycho-social-spiritual dimensions of the person, recognizing that the whole is greater than the sum of the parts; and that holism involves understanding the individual as a unitary whole in mutual process with the environment. Holistic nursing responds to both views, believing that the goals of nursing can be achieved within either framework.

1. The holistic nurse is an instrument of healing and a facilitator in the healing process. Holistic nurses honor the individual's subjective experience about health, health beliefs, and values. To become therapeutic partners with individuals, families, and communities, holistic nurses draw on nursing knowledge, theories, research, expertise, intuition, and creativity. Holistic nursing practice encourages peer review of professional practice in various clinical settings and integrates knowledge of current professional standards, law, and regulations governing nursing practice.

Practicing holistic nursing requires nurses to integrate self-care, self-responsibility, spirituality, and reflection in their lives. This may lead the nurse to greater awareness of the interconnectedness with self, others, nature, and God/LifeForce/Absolute/Transcendent. This awareness may further enhance the nurse's understanding of all individuals and their relationships to the human and global community, and permits nurses to use this awareness to facilitate the healing process.

29.5 ROLE OF NURSE IN HOLISTIC NURSING

The goal of holistic nursing is to treat and heal the whole person—by recognizing the interconnectedness of body, mind, spirit, and environment. Use Holistic Nursing as a place to discuss ways to incorporate nursing knowledge, theories, complementary/alternative modalities, expertise, and intuition to guide nurses in becoming therapeutic partners with people in their care, treating their physiological, psychological, and spiritual needs.

The practice of holistic nursing requires nurses to integrate self-care, self-responsibility, spirituality, and reflection in their lives. This may lead the nurse to greater awareness of the interconnectedness with self, others, nature, and spirit. This awareness may further enhance the nurses understanding of all individuals and their relationships to the human and global community, and permits nurses to use this awareness to facilitate the healing process.

Also called Complementary Health Nurses, Holistic Nurses use alternative medicine, sometimes combined with traditional Western medicine, to care for patients. This field of nursing is based on the premise that you cannot treat a patient's physical health without addressing the "whole" person—including their mental, spiritual and emotional wellbeing. This approach to nursing is much different than other, more traditional specialties, and an increasingly sought-after, niche field.

CONCLUSION

Holistic nursing is a medical specialty that takes the entire being of the patient into consideration, rather than just diagnosing specific physical symptoms. Holistic nurses often recommend complementary medical treatments to assist patients in attaining better health. The nurse becomes a partner with patients by forging interpersonal and lasting relationships. Nurses who are trained in holistic healthcare practices often work in hospice settings and long-term care facilities. A philosophy of nursing practice that takes into account total patient care, considering the physical, emotional, social, economic and spiritual needs of patient's, their response to their illnesses, and the effect of illness on patient's abilities to meet self-care needs.

30 Nursing Standards

30.1 INTRODUCTION

Nurses have been leaders in the field of standards development. Since nursing is the largest health profession providing care to individuals, families, groups, communities and populations in a multiplicity of settings, standards have an important role in guiding nursing practice. One of the characteristics of a self-regulating profession is the development of standards of practice, based on the values of the profession nurses. Regulatory bodies for nursing have the legal requirement to set standards of practice for registered nurses to protect the public in their province or territory. Together, the code of ethics and standards provide the basis for nursing practice in Canada. Therefore, the provincial/territorial regulatory bodies establish, monitor and enforce standards of professional practice and conduct. Below are links to jurisdictional standards currently available.

30.2 DEFINITIONS

1. Standards are professionally developed expressions of the range of acceptable variations from a norm or criterion. *-Donabedian*
2. Standards may be defined as "Benchmark of achievement which is based on a desired level of excellence.
3. Standard setting includes establishing fundamental definition in using and determining qualifications for education and practice. Administration encompasses interpreting these standards, developing mechanisms and tools for their enforcement and conducting the actual processes for regulation. *-ICN-1986*
4. According to American Nurses Association, a standard is described as a criterion used by general agreements as acceptable level of practice or an established norm.
5. Nursing practice standards are descriptive statements that affect that nature of current nursing practice current knowledge and current quality of nursing care.

30.3 MEANING OF STANDARDS

Standards are as broad statement of quality. It is a definite level of excellence or adequately required, aimed at possible. It agreed upon achieved level of performance, considered proper and adequate for a specific purpose against which actual performance is compared. So, standard is an acknowledge measure of comparison for quantative or qualitative value, criterion, norm.

Standard are an established rules or basis of comparison in measuring or judging capacity, quality context and value of objects in the same category. The term norm is frequently used synonymously with standard in the literature. Selected standards are reliable and relevant for the category being compared.

30.4 IMPORTANCE OF STANDARDS

1. Standards give direction and provide guidelines for performance of nursing staff.
2. Standards provide a baseline for evaluating quality of nursing care, ranging from excellent care to unsafe care.
3. Standards help improve quality of nursing care, increases effectiveness of care and improve efficiency.
4. Standards may help to improve documentation of nursing care provided, i.e. maintaining record of care.
5. Standards may help to determine the degree to which standards of nursing care maintained and take necessary corrective action in time.
6. Standards help supervisors to guide nursing staff to improve performance.
7. Standards may help to improve basis for decision-making and devise alternative system for delivering nursing care.
8. Standards may help justify demands for resources association.
9. Standards may help clarify nurse's area of accountability.
10. Standards may help nursing to define clearly different levels of care.

30.5 CHARACTERISTICS OF STANDARDS

1. Standard statement must be broad enough to apply to a side variety of settings.
2. Must be realistic, acceptable and attainable.
3. Nursing care must be developed by members of nursing profession, preferable nurses practicing at the direct care level with consultation of experts in the domain.
4. Should be phrased in positive and indicate acceptable performance.
5. Nursing care must be express what desirable optional level is.
6. Must be based on current knowledge and scientific practice.
7. Must be reviewed and revised periodically.
8. May be directed towards an ideal, i.e., optional standards or may only specify the minimal care that must be attained, i.e. minimum standard.

30.6 SOURCES OF STANDARDS

The standards can be established developed, reviewed to enforce by variety of sources.

1. Professional organization, e.g. Associations TNAI, GNAK.
2. Licensing bodies, e.g., Statutory bodies INC, MCI, DCI etc.
3. Institutions/healthcare agencies, e.g. NIHFN, University hospitals, health centers.
4. Department of institutions, e.g. Department of Nursing.
5. Patient care units, e.g. Specific patient's units.
6. Government units at National, State and Individual, e.g. Personal standards.

30.7 CLASSIFICATIONS OF STANDARDS

Nursing care standards can be divided into ends and means standards. The ends standards are patient oriented, they describe the change as desired in a patient's physical status or behavior. The means standards are nursing oriented, they describe the activities and behavior designed to achieve the ends standards. Ends standards require information about the patients. A means standard calls for information about the nurse's performance. Standards are expected to understand achievable and measurable.

Standards can be classified and formulated according to frames of references relating to nursing structure, process and outcome, because standard is a descriptive statement of desired level of performance against which to evaluate the quality of service structure, process or outcomes.

1. **Structure standard:** The structure is related to the framework, that is care providing system and resources that support for actual provision of care. Evaluation of care concerns nursing staff, setting and the care environment. The use of standards based on structure implies that if the structure is adequate reliable, and desirable, standard will be met or quality care will be given.
2. **Process standards:** Process standards describe the behaviors of the nurse at the desired level of the performance. The criteria that specify desired method for specific nursing intervention are process standards. A process standard involves the activities concerned with delivering patient care. In process standard, there is an element of professional judgment, i.e. determining the quality of the degree of skill. It includes nursing care techniques, procedures, regimens, processes.
3. **Outcome standards:** Descriptive statements of desired patient care results are outcome standards, because patient's results are outcomes of nursing interventions. Here outcome as a frame of references for setting of standards refers to description of the results of nursing activity in terms of the change that occur in the patient. An outcome standard measures change in the patient health status. In quality assurance, outcomes are stated in positive terms as the nursing goal is to improve the health status of client.

30.8 GOOD NURSING STANDARDS

1. All standards of practice provide a guide to the knowledge, skills, judgment and attitudes that are needed to practice safely.
2. They reflect a desired achievable level of performance against which actual performance can be compared. Their main purpose is to promote, guide and direct professional nursing practice.
3. Standards are necessary to demonstrate to the public, government and other stakeholders that a profession is dedicated to maintaining public trust and upholding the criteria of its professional practice.
4. Standards is an established rule or basis of comparison or judging capacity, quantity contact and value of objects in the same category.
5. Standard is a broad statement of quality. It is a definite level of excellence or adequately required, aimed at or possible. It agreed upon achieved level of performance, considered proper and adequate for a specific purpose against which actual performance is compared.
6. Standards are a benchmark against which to plan, implement and assess quality of services and to show that nursing is accountable to society, to consumers of nursing service and to government, as well as to the profession of nursing itself and individual members.

30.9 IMPORTANCE OF STANDARDS

1. The standard is a practice that enjoys general recognition and conformity among professional or an authoritative statement by which the quality or practice, service or education can be judged.
2. The standards will be measured and have the primary responsibility for seeing that the standard are enforced.
3. It promotes guides and directs professional nursing practice—important for self-assessment and evaluation of practice by employers, clients and other stakeholders.
4. It provides nurses with a framework for developing competencies aids in developing a better understanding and respect for the various and complimentary roles that nurses have.
5. A standard is a means of determining what something should be in the case of nursing practice, standards are the established criteria for the practice of nursing.

6. Standards are statements that are widely recognized describing nursing practice and are seen as having permanent value. A nursing standard is a descriptive statement of described quality against which nursing care is evaluated in guidelines.

30.10 PURPOSES OF STANDARDS

Table 30.1: Purposes of standards

S.N	Purposes	Description
1	Communication	Communication provides for sharing of common language with nursing professional which can cross barriers between special.
2	Research	The standards provide a framework for further investigation, so that current practices are no longer based on intention or word of mouth but are derived from theory developed by authorities with the nursing profession.
3	Legal implication	The nursing profession must be self-regulating to maintain credibility as a profession. The court use the professional standards as a yard stick to determine whether hospitals and healthcare professionals have provided quality patient care according to rationally acceptable standards.
4	Quality assurance	Standards can be used as the criteria of quality assurance studies to assess the current levels of practice rendered by the healthcare services provided by the organization or both.
5	Professional accountability	Standards set guidelines for nursing practice, providing uniform basis for collecting a convention with an established assurance programme and performances appraisal system.
6	Decision-making	Standing also helps in decision-making and choosing alternatives for delivering of healthcare, help in supervision and improving performance.

30.11 PROFESSIONALIZATION OF NURSING

Professionalization is the process by which an occupation achieves professional status. The status of nursing as a profession is important because it reflects the value society places on the work of nurses and the centrality of this work to the good of society. A profession is characterized by prolonged education that takes place in a college or university. Values, beliefs, and ethics relating to the profession are an integral part of the educational preparation. By definition, a professional is autonomous in decision-making and is accountable for his or her own actions. Personal identification and commitment to the profession are strong, and individuals are unlikely to change professions. In contrast, an occupation is characterized by training that may occur on the job for varying lengths of time. The training does not incorporate, as a prominent feature, the values, beliefs, and ethics of the occupation. The workers are supervised, and ultimate accountability rests with the employer. Thus, commitment is not always strong, and individuals often changes jobs (Chitty, 1993).

Professional nursing practice involves "specialized skills essential to the performance of a unique, professional role". The two main concepts that are in the forefront of professional nursing and its services ideal are accountability and autonomy.

Accountability is the state of being responsible and answerable for one's own behavior. The sphere of a nurse's accountability is to self, the client, the employing agency, and the profession. The standards of clinical nursing practice by American Nurses Association (ANA) and standards of the various specialty nursing practices document the professional nurse's scope and limits of accountability. By virtue of these standards, society holds nurses and those under their supervision accountable for their actions.

Autonomy in nursing is the freedom and the authority to act independently. It implies control over one's practice, and it applies to both decisions and actions.

An accountability based governance system is a predominant feature of professional practice models. Responsibility and authority are established in specified processes rather than in particular individuals who, in turn, determine the placement of accountability. The nurse is central to the organization and is supported by major service components such as standards, quality assurance, continuing education, and peer process. Nursing management has no legitimate role in practice-related decisions; rather, management facilitates, integrates, and coordinates nursing operations to support the practitioner.

30.12 BASIC PRINCIPLES OF STANDARDS

1. Standards should be designed to achieve a stated purpose.
2. Standards should be based upon clear definitions of professional scope and accountability.
3. Standards should promote the fullest development of the profession in accordance with its potential social contribution.
4. Standards should be sufficiently broad and flexible to achieve their objective and at the same time permit freedom for innovation, growth and change.
5. Standards should promote universal levels of performance and encourage professional identity and mobility.
6. Standards should recognize the equality and independence of professions offering essential services.
7. Standards should be formulated according to requirements which facilitate their applicability and use by the profession.

30.13 PRINCIPLES OF NURSING PRACTICE STANDARDS

The following principles set out the requirements for practice:

1. Nurses know what specific legislation applies to their practice and follow legislated requirements.
2. Nurses collect personal and health information on a need-to-know basis.
3. Nurses ensure that clients are aware of their rights concerning their personal and health information and have consented to the collection, use and disclosure of this information.
4. Nurses share relevant personal and health information with the healthcare team.
5. Nurses explain to clients that this information will be shared and identify to them who is on the healthcare team (e.g. physicians, social workers).
6. Nurses respect clients' rights to access their own health records and to request correction of the information.
7. Nurses safeguard personal and health information learned in the context of the nurse-client relationship and disclose this information (outside of the healthcare team) only with client consent or when there is a specific ethical or legal obligation to do so.
8. Nurses have an ethical obligation to disclose in situations that involve a substantial risk of significant harm to the health or safety of the client or others. In these situations, nurses use a process of ethical decision-making before disclosing confidential information. Whenever possible, this process involves consulting with knowledgeable colleagues.
9. Nurses comply with any legal obligation to disclose confidential information that is imposed by legislation or required under a warrant, court order or subpoena.
10. In all cases where disclosure of confidential information is necessary, nurses restrict the amount of information disclosed and the number of people informed to the minimum necessary to fulfill the legal and ethical obligations.

11. Nurses access personal and health information only for purposes that are consistent with their professional responsibilities.

30.14 PROFESSIONAL STANDARDS AND NURSING PROCESS

Professional standards ensure that the highest level of quality nursing care is promoted. Excellent nursing practice is a reflection of sound ethical standards. Client care requires more than just the application of scientific knowledge. A nurse must be able to think critically, solve problems, and find the best solution for client's needs to assist clients in maintaining, regaining, or improving their health. Critical thinking requires the use of scientifically based and practice-based criteria for making clinical judgments. These criteria may be scientifically based on research findings or practice based on standards developed by clinical experts and quality improvement initiatives.

30.15 CHARACTERISTICS OF STANDARD

The characteristics of standard which undo that standard:
1. Statement must be broad enough to apply to a wide variety of settings.
2. Must be realistic, acceptable, and attainable.
3. The nursing care must be developed by members of the nursing profession preferable nurses practicing that the direct care level which consultation of experts in the domain.
4. Should be resembled in positive terms and indicate acceptable performance, i.e. good, excellence etc.
5. The nursing care must express what desirable optimal level is.
6. Must be understandable and stated in ambiguous terms.
7. Must be based on current knowledge and scientific practice.
8. Must be received and revised periodically.
9. Must be directed towards an ideal, i.e. optimum standards may only specify the minimal care that must be attained, i.e. minimum standard.
10. Standards that work are objective, acceptable, achievable and flexible.

30.16 NURSING PROFESSION AND ESSENTIAL COMPONENTS

Nursing is a helping, independent profession that provides services that contribute to the health of people. Three essential components of professional nursing are care, cure and coordination. Caring aspect is rational and requires as nurse to understand the patient's needs at a level that permits individualization of nursing therapies. To cure is to assist patients in understanding their health problems and to help them to cope. The cure aspect involves the administration of treatments and the use of clinical nursing judgment in determining, on the basis of patient outcomes, whether the plan is effective. Coordination of care involves organizing and timing the medical and other professional and technical services to meet the holistic needs of the patient. And often a patient requires many other services simultaneously in order to be well cared for. A professional nurse also supervises, teaches, and directs all of those involved in nursing care. So, there are some guidelines are essential to check how the nurses perform professionally and how they exercise the care, cure and coordination aspects of nursing. As an independent profession, nursing has increasingly set its own standards for practice. This is called standards of nursing care.

Clinical, administrative, and academic experts have developed standards of nursing practice. The most widely accepted one is American Nurses Association (ANA) 2004 within this document there are standards of professional performance and standards of practice.

30.17 RESPONSIBILITIES OF NURSE IN MAINTAINING STANDARDS

1. Maintaining general cleanliness and upkeep of the ward and its surrounding areas to provide neat and cheerful environment of the patients.
2. Coming out of the instruction of the medical officers regarding treatment of patients, observing and recording the process of treatment and generally assisting the medical officer to achieve his therapeutic aim.
3. Keeping the ward equipment in optimum state of readiness by prompt repairs and placement through condemnation boards.
4. Supervision of care and maintenance of building furniture, fitting and arranging their reports.
5. Assignment or duties for patient's care to the staff working is the ward taking into consideration the capabilities of each.
6. Ensuring that all specimens are sent to the laboratory in time and results collected when due.
7. Maintaining strict control over accounting and distribution of controlled and dangerous drugs.
8. Requisition of diet as per instruction of the medical officer and ensuring that the diets and extras are distributed to patients as per the requisition.
9. Maintenance of all registers and documents required in the ward.
10. Overall supervision of all that happens in the ward is to ensure that the patient's treatment and recovery is as smooth and pleasant as possible.

30.18 ANA-STANDARDS OF PROFESSIONAL PERFORMANCE

Table 30.2: ANA-standards of professional performance

S.N	Standards	Description	Measurements of criteria
1.	Quality of practice	The registered nurse systematically enhances the quality and effectiveness of nursing practice	1. Demonstrates quality by documenting the application of the nursing process in a responsible, accountable and ethical manner. 2. Uses quality improvement activities to initiate changes in nursing practice and healthcare delivery system. 3. Uses creativity and innovation to improve nursing care delivery. 4. Incorporates new knowledge to initiate changes in nursing practice if desired outcomes are not achieved. 5. Participates in quality improvement activities.
2.	Education	The nurse attains knowledge and competency that reflects current nursing practice	1. Participates in ongoing educational activities related to clinical knowledge and professional issues. 2. Demonstrates commitment to lifelong learning. 3. Seeks experiences to maintain clinical skills. 4. Seeks knowledge and skills appropriate to the practice setting. 5. Maintains professional records that provide evidence of competency and lifelong learning.
3.	Professional practice evaluation	The nurse evaluates one's own nursing practice in relation to professional practice standards and guide line, relevant statutes, rules and regulations	1. Engage in self-evaluation on a regular basis. 2. Seeks constructive feedback regarding one's own practice. 3. Takes action to achieve goals identified during the evaluation process. 4. Participates in systematic peer review as appropriate. 5. Practice reflects knowledge of current practice standards, laws and regulations. 6. Provides age appropriate care in culturally and ethnically sensitive manner.

Contd...

Contd...

4.	Collegiality	The nurse interacts with and contribute to the professional development of peers and other healthcare providers as colleagues	1. Shares knowledge and skills with peers and colleagues. 2. Provides peers with feedback regarding their practice. 3. Interacts with peers and colleagues. 4. To enhance ones own professional nursing practice. 5. Maintains compassionate and caring relationships with peers and colleagues. 6. Contributes to an environment that is conductive to clinical education nursing students as appropriate. 7. Contributes to a supportive and healthy work environment.
5.	Collaboration	The nurse collaborates with patient, family, and others in the conduct of nursing practice	1. Communicates with the patient, significant others, and healthcare providers regarding patient care and nursing's role in the provision of care. 2. Collaborates with patient, family and others health care providers in the formulation of overall goals and the plan of care and in the decisions related to care and delivery of services. 3. Partners with others to effect change and generate positive outcomes. 4. Document referrals, including provisions for continuity of care, as needed.
6.	Ethics	The nurse integrates ethical provisions in all areas of practice	1. Practice is guided by code of ethics for nurses with interpretive statement. 2. Maintains therapeutic and professional patient-nurse relationship. 3. Delivers care in the manner of that preserves patient autonomy, dignity, and rights. 4. Seeks available resourced in formulating ethical decisions 5. Reports illegal, incompetent or impaired practice. 6. Maintain patient confidentiality within legal and regulatory parameters.
7.	Research	The nurse integrates research findings in practice	1. Utilize best available evidence including research findings to guide practice decisions. 2. Participates in research activities as appropriate to the nurse's education and position. 3. Identifying clinical problems suitable for nursing research a. Participating in data collection b. Participating in a unit, organization, or community research committee c. Sharing research activities with others conducting research d. Critiquing research for application to practice e. Uses research findings in the development of policies, procedures, and practice guidelines for patient care f. Incorporates research as a basis for learning

Contd...

Contd...

8.	Resource utilization	The nurse considers factors related to safety effectiveness, cost, and impact on practice in the planning and delivery of nursing services	1. Evaluates factors related to safety, effectiveness, availability and cost when practice options would result in the same expected patient outcome. 2. Assists the patient and family in identifying and securing appropriate and available services to address health related needs. 3. Assigns or delegates tasks as defined by the state nurse practice acts and according to the knowledge and skills of the designated care giver. 4. Assigns or delegate tasks based on the needs and condition of the patient, the potential for harm, the stability of the patients condition, the complexity of the task, and the predictability of the outcome. 5. Assists the patient and family in becoming informed consumers about the cost, risks, and benefits of treatment and care.
9.	Leadership	The nurse provides leadership in the professional practice setting and the profession	1. Engages on team work. 2. Works to create and maintain healthy work environments. 3. Teach others to succeed through mentoring. 4. Exhibits creativity and flexibility during change. 5. Directs coordination of care across settings and care givers. 6. Serves in key roles in the work settings by participating on committees, councils, and administrative. 7. Promotes advancement of the profession. 8. Display the ability to define a clear vision, the associated goals, and a plan to implement and measure progress. 9. Demonstrates energy, excitement and a passion for quality work. 10. Willingly accepts mistakes by self and others, thereby creating a culture in which risk-taking is not only safe, but expected.

30.19 STANDARDS OF CARE

The standards of care in the ANA nursing: Scopes and Standards of practice (2004) describe a competent level of nursing care. The levels of care are demonstrated through the nursing process. The nursing process is the foundation of clinical decision-making and includes all significant actions taken by nurses in providing care to clients. Within these are the nursing responsibilities for diversity, safety, education, health promotion, treatment, self-care, and planning for the continuity of care. Standards of care are important if a legal dispute arises over whether a nurse practiced appropriately in a particular case.

Table 30.3: ANA Standards of practice

S.N	Scientific method	Description
1.	**Assessment** The nurse collects comprehensive data pertinent to the patients health or situation	1. Collects data in a systematic and ongoing process. 2. Data collection involves the patient, significant others, and health care providers, when appropriate. 3. Priorities data collection activities based on the patients immediate condition or needs determine the priority of data collection. 4. Collects pertinent data using appropriate assessment techniques. 5. Document relevant data in a retrievable form.
2.	**Diagnosis:** The nurse analyzes the assessment data to determine the diagnoses or issues	1. Derives diagnoses from the assessment data. 2. Validates the diagnoses with patient, significant others, and health care providers, when possible. 3. Documents diagnoses in a manner that facilitates the determination of expected outcomes and plan of care.
3.	**Outcomes identification:** The nurse identifies expected outcomes for a plan individualize to the patient or the situation	1. Derives outcomes from the diagnoses. 2. Formulates outcomes mutually with the patient and the health care providers, when possible. 3. Outcomes are culturally appropriate and realistic in relation to the patients present and potential capabilities. 4. Defines expected outcomes in terms of the patient, patient values, ethical considerations, environment, or situation with such consideration as associated risks, benefits, costs, current scientific evidence, and clinical expertise when formulating expecting outcomes. 5. Outcomes are attainable in relation to resources available to the person. 6. Outcomes include a time estimate for attainment for expected outcome. 7. Outcomes provide direction for continuity of care. 8. Modifies expected outcomes based on changes in the status of the patient or evaluation of the situation. 9. Documents outcomes as measurable goals.
4.	**Planning:** The nurse develops a plan that prescribes strategies and alternatives to attain expected out comes	1. The plan is individualized to the patient and patients condition or needs. 2. Develops the plan with the patient, significant others, and health care providers, when appropriate. 3. Includes strategies within the plan that address each of the identified diagnosis or issues, which may include strategies for promotion and restoration of health and prevention of illness, injury, and disease. 4. Provides for continuity within the plan. 5. Incorporates an implementation pathway or timeline within the plan. 6. Utilizes the plan to provide direction to other members of the health care team. 7. Defines the plan to reflect current status, rules, and regulations and standards. 8. Integrates current trends and research affecting care in the planning process. 9. Considers the economic impact of the plan. 10. Uses standardized language or recognized terminology to document the plan.
5.	**Implementation:** The nurse implements the identified plan of care	1. Interventions are consistent with the established plan of care. 2. Implements interventions in a safe and appropriate manner, documents interventions. 3. Utilizes evidence –based interventions and treatments specific to the diagnosis or problem. 4. Collaborates with nurse colleagues to implement the plan. 5. Utilizes community resources and systems to implement the plan.
5. A	Co-ordination of care. The registered nurse coordinates care delivery.	1. Coordinates implementation of the plan. 2. Documentation of the care.

Contd...

Contd...

B	Health teaching and health promotion	1. Provides health teaching that address such topics as healthy lifestyles, risk reducing behaviors, developmental needs, activities of daily living, and preventive self-care. 2. Uses health promotion and health teaching methods appropriate to the situation and the patient's developmental level, learning needs, readiness, ability to learn, language preference, and culture. 3. Seeks opportunities for feedback and evaluation of the effectiveness of the strategies used.
C	Consultation: the advanced practice registered nurse and the nursing role specialist provide consultation to influence the identified plan, enhance the abilities of others and effect change.	1. Synthesizes clinical data, theoretical frameworks, and evidence when providing consultation. 2. Facilitates the effectiveness of a consultation by involving the patient in decision-making and negotiating role responsibilities. 3. Communicates consultation recommendations that facilitate change.
D	Prescriptive Authority and Treatment: the advanced practice registered nurse uses prescriptive authority, procedures, referrals, treatments, and therapies in accordance with state and federal laws and regulations.	1. Prescribes evidenced-based treatments, therapies, and procedures considering the patient's comprehensive health care needs. 2. Prescribes pharmacological agents based on a current knowledge of pharmacology and physiology and based on clinical indicators, the patient's status needs, and the results of diagnostic and laboratory tests. 3. Evaluates therapeutic and potential adverse effects and potential adverse effects of pharmacological and non pharmacological treatment. 4. Provides patients with information about intended effects and potential adverse effects of proposed prescriptive therapies. 5. Provides information about costs, alternative treatments and procedures, as appropriate.
6.	Evaluation The nurse evaluates progress towards attainment of outcomes	1. Evaluation is systematic, ongoing and criterion-based. 2. Involves the patient, significant others, and the health care providers in the evaluation process, when appropriate. 3. Uses ongoing assessment data to revise diagnoses, outcomes and plan of care as needed. 4. Documents revisions in diagnoses, outcomes, and the plan of care. 5. Evaluates the effectiveness of interventions in relation to outcomes. 6. Documents the patients response to interventions.

30.20 STANDARD NURSING CARE: AN ASSET

In order to ensure quality care the nursing care needs some standards. Standards are degree of excellence. The aim of standard nursing care is to support and contribute to excellent practices. The role of nurse is constantly changing to meet the growing needs of health services.

Objectives

1. Plan
2. Holistic approach
3. Appropriate diagnosis
4. Realistic goal
5. Selecting appropriate media
6. Quality care rather than quantity
7. Economize time, material, energy.

Types of Standard Care

1. Structure -- Things we use
2. Process -- Things we do
3. Outcome -- The result

Characteristics of Standard Care

1. Dynamic
2. Reflects Changes
3. Not Static

Brief description of methods and procedure

S - Successful termination of helping relationship for client.
T - To have clear idea or conception of the distinct goal, nursing the patient and health needs of society.
A - Assertive planning.
N - Nature of client nurse interaction.
D - Directing others.
A - Analytical thinking.
R - Respect status and policies.
D - Data collection in accordance with goal.

Standard: Nursing practice requires that a conceptual model for nursing be the basis for the independent part of that practice.

Elements: Nurses are required to have clear idea or conception of the distinct goal nursing, the patient, the health needs of the society, the source of client difficulty, the focus, and modes of nursing intervention and the expected consequences of nursing activities.

Standard: Nursing practice requires the effective use of the nursing process.

Elements: Nurses are required to collect data in accordance with their conception of the goal of nursing, client, the source of client difficulty, the four and modes of intervention conceptual models for nursing.

Standard: Nursing practice requires that the helping relationship be the nature of client nurse interaction.

Elements: Nurses are required to increase the likelihood that the client will perceive the health service experience as understandable, manageable and meaningful at the outset.

Nurses are required to ensure a successful termination of the helping relationship.

Standard: Nursing practice requires nurses to fulfill professional responsibilities.

Elements: Nurses are required to respect status and policies relevant to the profession and the practice setting. Nurses are required to comply with the code of ethics of their profession. Nurses are required to function as members of a health team.

CONCLUSION

"Nursing Standards of Care" pertain to professional nursing activities that are demonstrated by the nurse through the nursing process. These involve assessment, diagnosis, outcome identification, planning implementation, and evaluation. The nursing process is the foundation of clinical decision making and encompasses all significant action taken by nurses in providing care to all consumers. While "Nursing Standards of Professional Performance" describe the roles of all professional nurses, there are many other responsibilities that are hallmarks of professional nursing. These nurses should be self-directed and purposeful in seeking necessary knowledge and skills to enhance career goals. Other activities-such as membership in professional organizations, certification in specialty or advanced practice, continuing education and further academic education, are desirable methods of enhancing the nurse's professionalism.

31 Transcultural Nursing

31.1 INTRODUCTION

Transcultural nursing is how professional nursing interacts with the concept of culture. Based in anthropology and nursing, it is supported by nursing theory, research, and practice. It is a specific cognitive specialty in nursing that focuses on global cultures and comparative cultural caring, health, and nursing phenomena. It was established in 1955 as a formal area of inquiry and practice. It is a body of knowledge that assists in providing culturally appropriate nursing care. The goals of transcultural nursing is to give culturally congruent nursing care, and to provide culture specific and universal nursing care practices for the health and well-being of people or to aid them in facing adverse human conditions, illness or death in culturally meaningful ways. Leininger (1991) notes the main goal of transcultural nursing is to provide culturally specific care. But before transcultural nursing can be adequately understood, there must be a basic knowledge of key terminology such as culture, cultural values, culturally diverse nursing care, ethnocentrism, race, and ethnography.

31.2 MEANING OF TRANSCULTURE

Transcultural nursing is an essential aspect of healthcare today. The ever-increasing multicultural population in the United States poses a significant challenge to nurses providing individualized and holistic care to their patients. This requires nurses to recognize and appreciate cultural differences in healthcare values, beliefs, and customs. Nurses must acquire the necessary knowledge and skills in cultural competency. Culturally competent nursing care helps ensure patient satisfaction and positive outcomes. This article discusses changes that are important to transcultural nursing. It identifies factors that define transcultural nursing and analyzes methods to promote culturally competent nursing care. The need for transcultural nursing will continue to be an important aspect in healthcare. Additional nursing research is needed to promote transcultural nursing.

31.3 DEFINITION

According to Medline, transcultural nursing is an area of expertise in nursing that responds to the need for developing global perspective within nursing practice in a world of interdependent nations and people. As a discipline, it centers on combining international and transcultural content into the training of nurses. It includes learning cultural differences, nursing in other countries, international health issues, and international health organizations.

31.4 CONCEPT OF TRANSCULTURE

1. Illness and wellness are shaped by a various factors including perception and coping skills, as well as the social level of the patient.

2. Cultural competence is an important component of nursing.
3. Culture influences all spheres of human life. It defines health, illness, and the search for relief from disease or distress.
4. Religious and cultural knowledge is an important ingredient in healthcare.
5. The health concepts held by many cultural groups may result in people choosing not to seek modern medical treatment procedures.
6. Healthcare provider need to be flexible in the design of programs, policies, and services to meet the needs and concerns of the culturally diverse population, groups that are likely to be encountered.
7. Most cases of lay illness have multiple causalities and may require several different approaches to diagnosis, treatment, and cure including folk and Western medical interventions.
8. The use of traditional or alternate models of healthcare delivery is widely varied and may come into conflict with Western models of healthcare practice.
9. Culture guides behavior into acceptable ways for the people in a specific group as such culture originates and develops within the social structure through interpersonal interactions.
10. For a nurse to successfully provide care for a client of a different cultural or ethnic to background, effective intercultural communication must take place.

31.5 GOALS OF TRANSCULTURAL NURSING

The goals of transcultural nursing is to give culturally congruent nursing care, and to provide culture specific and universal nursing care practices for the health and well-being of people or to aid them in facing adverse human conditions, illness or death in culturally meaningful ways According to Madeleine, the pioneer of transcultural nursing, transcultural nursing is a substantive area of study and practice that focuses on the comparative cultural values of caring, the beliefs and practices of individuals or groups of similar or different cultures. According to Medline, transcultural nursing is an area of expertise in nursing that responds to the need for developing global perspective within nursing practice in a world of interdependent nations and people. As a discipline, it centers on combining international and transcultural content into the training of nurses. It includes learning cultural differences, nursing in other countries, international health issues, and international health organizations.

31.6 APPLICATION TO NURSING

1. To develop understanding, respect and appreciation for the individuality and diversity of patients beliefs, values, spirituality and culture regarding illness, its meaning, cause, treatment, and outcome.
2. To encourage in developing and maintaining a program of physical, emotional and spiritual self-care introduce therapies, such as ayurveda and pancha karma.
3. Nurses need to be aware of and sensitive to the cultural needs of clients.
4. The practice of nursing today demands that the nurse identify and meet the cultural needs of diverse groups, understand the social and cultural reality of the client, family, and community, develop expertise to implement culturally acceptable strategies to provide nursing care, and identify and use resources acceptable to the client (Andrews and Boyle, 2002).

31.7 NURSING PROCESS AND ROLE OF NURSE

1. Determine the client's cultural heritage and language skills.
2. Determine if any of his health beliefs relate to the cause of the illness or to the problem.

3. Collect information that any home remedies the person is taking to treat the symptoms.
4. Nurses should evaluate their attitudes toward ethnic nursing care.
5. Self-evaluation helps the nurse to become more comfortable when providing care to clients from diverse backgrounds.
6. Understand the influence of culture, race and ethnicity on the development of social emotional relationship, child rearing practices and attitude toward health.
7. Collect information about the socioeconomic status of the family and its influence on their health promotion and wellness.
8. Identify the religious practices of the family and their influence on health promotion belief in families.
9. Understanding of the general characteristics of the major ethnic groups, but always individualizes care.
10. The nursing diagnosis for clients should include potential problems in their interaction with the healthcare system and problems involving the effects of culture.
11. The planning and implementation of nursing interventions should be adapted as much as possible to the client's cultural background.
12. Evaluation should include the nurse's self-evaluation of attitudes and emotions toward providing nursing care to clients from diverse sociocultural backgrounds.
13. Self-evaluation by the nurse is crucial as he or she increases skills for interaction.

31.8 CULTURAL COMPETENCE

To be culturally competent the nurse needs to understand his/her own world views and those of the patient, while avoiding stereotyping and misapplication of scientific knowledge. Cultural competence is obtaining cultural information and then applying that knowledge. This cultural awareness allows you to see the entire picture and improves the quality of care and health outcomes. Adapting to different cultural beliefs and practices requires flexibility and a respect for others view points. Cultural competence means to really listen to the patient, to find out and learn about the patient's beliefs of health and illness. To provide culturally appropriate care we need to know and to understand culturally influenced health behaviors.

Since, the perception of illness and disease and their causes varies by culture, these individual preferences affect the approaches to healthcare. Culture also influences how people seek healthcare and how they behave toward healthcare providers. How we care for patients and how patients respond to this care is greatly influenced by culture. Healthcare providers must possess the ability and knowledge to communicate and to understand health behaviors influenced by culture. Having this ability and knowledge can eliminate barriers to the delivery of healthcare. These issues show the need for healthcare organizations to develop policies, practices and procedures to deliver culturally competent care. Five essential elements that contribute to an institution's or agency's ability to become more culturally competent. These include:

1. Valuing diversity.
2. Having the capacity for cultural self-assessment.
3. Being conscious of the dynamics inherent when cultures interact.
4. Having institutionalized cultural knowledge, and
5. Having developed adaptations of service delivery reflecting an understanding of cultural diversity.

These five elements should be manifested at every level of an organization, including policy making, administration, and practice. Further, these elements should be reflected in the attitudes, structures, policies, and services of the organization.

CONCLUSION

Transcultural nursing seeks to provide care that acknowledges an individual's culture, values, beliefs and practices, the crux of which is good communication between the health professional and the patient and their family. As health professionals living in a multicultural society, it would be unusual for us not to have come across a patient that is culturally and ethnically different from ourselves. Sometimes we can cross the barrier with ease, recognizing the core values and beliefs of our patient and working with these. At other times the barrier is harder, or even impossible to cross. Communication difficulties arise - even when a translator is available, non-verbal messages may be missed by the patient, or even by the health professional.

32 Geriatric Nursing

32.1 INTRODUCTION

An elderly person needs to feel safe, remain close to other people and believe that his life continues to be meaningful. Meeting his emotional needs can help him avoid depression. Signs that he lacks sufficient support may include difficulty in sleeping, a poor appetite or an inability to concentrate, points out the American Association of Retired Persons. Emotional care for a senior should include steps designed to deal with vulnerability, loneliness, boredom and isolation.

32.2 EMOTIONAL CARE OF OLD AGE

1. **Security:** A senior citizen may feel fearful and nervous, especially if she lives alone or has mobility problems. Support a positive outlook with practical measures to guard against intruders. Arrange for the installation of additional locks or chains and a spy-hole in the door, so she can see who is calling before she opens the door. An emergency call button could reduce her fear of failing to get help should she fall or become unwell.
2. **Connection:** Help senior citizens to maintain contact with their friends and family. Encourage visits from younger family members and use the telephone to maintain regular communication. An elderly person may find Internet access helpful when family or friends are unable to offer frequent visits, but he could need help in learning to use the technology. Use photos, books and music to help him remember happy life events and involve him in important family occasions such as marriages or new babies to help him know that he continues to be an important member of the family.
3. **Community:** Maintaining links with her community can support an elderly person's feeling of connection with the world beyond her family. Arrange transport to local events, church services or shopping trips. Contact organizations in the area that may be able to offer visits or

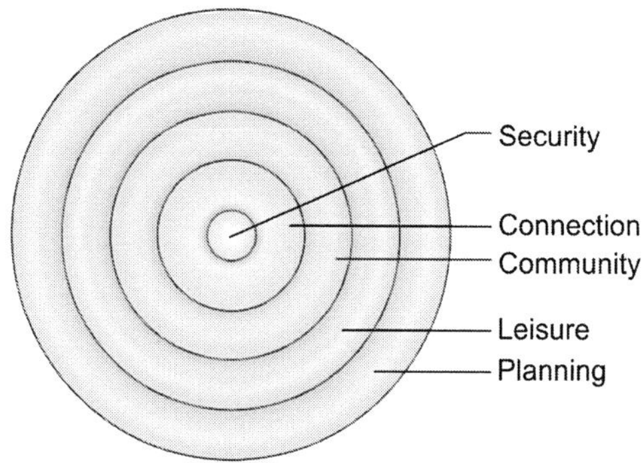

Fig. 32.1: Emotion care of old age

send newsletters that support her interests. Make sure she is able to manage the controls of her television or radio and that she knows how to access local channels so that she can continue to enjoy involvement with her neighborhood.

4. **Leisure:** Take time to listen carefully to an elderly person. Help him continue to take responsibility for himself by discussing his needs and tailoring any interventions you make to his preferences, whether he loves ball games or prefers reading. Help him overcome any obstacles to his leisure activities that aging might cause. For example, try large print books or different spectacles to overcome visual problems that prevent him from enjoying his favorite authors. Maintain his dignity, whether he lives at home or in a care facility. Ensure he has access to his own clean clothes and that any false teeth or other prosthetics fit securely so he can feel comfortable.
5. **Planning:** Look ahead to anticipate the future needs of a senior. Her circumstances will change over time and new difficulties can arise with her physical, emotional or sensory abilities. These can damage her emotional well-being. A sudden loss of the capacity to wash or dress independently needs urgent action to provide her with personal care. Watch for any deterioration in her mood and be prepared to involve health providers. Make sure she takes any medication exactly as prescribed. Sorting her tablets into the correct daily dose can help overcome a senior's fear of making mistake.

32.3 COMMON HEALTH PROBLEMS IN OLD AGE

Older adults are among the fastest growing age groups, and the first "baby boomers" (adults born between 1946 and 1964) will turn 65 in 2011. More than 37 million people in this group (60 percent) will manage more than 1 chronic condition by 2030. Older adults are at high risk for developing chronic illnesses and related disabilities. These chronic conditions include: Diabetes mellitus, arthritis, congestive heart failure, dementia.

1. **Heart disease:** In this disease, the blood to the heart is decreased due to the narrowing of the cardiac vessels which supply blood to it. This narrowing is due to atherosclerosis in which fat deposits accumulate on the walls of the blood vessels and narrowing it. The causes of this are high blood pressure, high cholesterol occurring due to high intake of animal fat, cigarette smoking, diabetes mellitus, obesity, inactivity, stress and hereditary factor.
2. **High blood pressure** is the most common ailment in almost 90% of the old people. A small rise in blood pressure (BP) also should never be neglected and lifestyle changes had to be adapted. The preventive measures are weight control, daily physical activity, treatment for diabetes, less

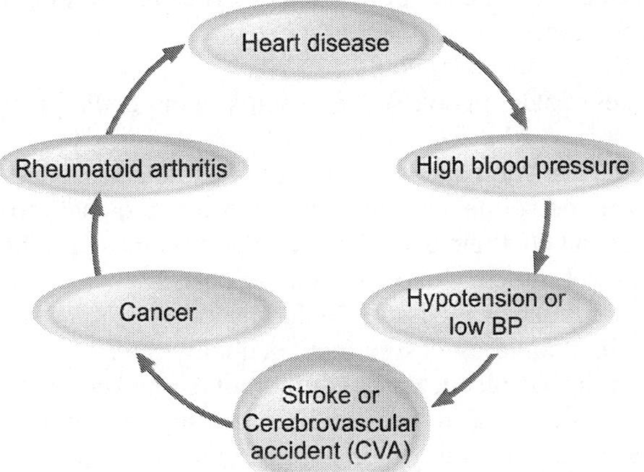

Fig. 32.2: Common health problems in old age

salt intake and saturated fat, and promoting more intake of fruits and vegetable. Fruits rich in potassium like bananas and oranges, food high in calcium are advisable.

3. **Hypotension or low BP:** This characterized by dizziness and fainting from exertion after a period of long inactivity and also it is due to anemia. This is more severe after sitting or lying down for a longer time-postural hypotension or suddenly standing after which the person loses his balance and fall to the ground. Hypotension is not in itself dangerous but can increase the risk of falls.
4. **Stroke or cerebrovascular accident (CVA):** When the heart tissue suffer from lack of nourishment due to poor blood supply, there is a disruption of blood flow to the brain tissue and death of brain cells. The impaired brain tissue circulation is called cerebrovascular disease.
5. **Cancer:** The second most common chronic disease in older people is the cancer. This greater risk of cancer in older people is due to their effects of slow acting carcinogen, prolonged development time "necessary for growth to be observable, extended pre-exposure time and failing immune capacity in old age." Certain diet and lifestyle factors may also cause cancer in old age. Diagnosing cancer in old age is often more difficult than at earlier life, because of the existence of other chronic diseases and because symptoms of cancer, such as weight loss, weakness, etc. may be thought as related to the old age.
6. **Rheumatoid arthritis** is the inflammation of the membranes lining, joints and tendons, and is characterized by pain, swelling, bone dislocation and limited range of motion, mostly effecting women and can cause severe crippling. This affects even younger people but common in older people. The symptoms are general malaise, fatigue, loss of weight, fever, joint pain, redness, swelling and stiffness affecting many joints.

32.4 GERIATRIC NURSING CARE/MANAGEMENT

1. Providing safe and effective care to older people in enhanced care settings in the community requires coordinated and competent care by a skilled work force of health care professional, working efficiently together.
2. To provide proper assessment and rehabilitation in the community settings.
3. To provide an immediate response to the care of acutely ill older.
4. To give medical support to all types of home schemes.
5. To give increased and coordinated clinical services for the people who are discharged from the hospital.
6. To coordinate the work of all healthcare people in the community.
7. To provide leadership and advice, and training for all health personnel by the concerned doctors.
8. Higher leadership is needed for health promotion designed to promote, healthier ageing, and to avoid premature dependency.
9. To provide new service for the older people.
10. To integrate all services of older people so that it helps older people who have both physical and mental problems.
11. Facilitating the development and quality assurance of enhanced services for old.
12. Teaching the healthcare personnel for more advanced and personalized care.
    This knowledge needs to help them to understand the problems of all health and social care of all professionals to a level sufficient to command their trust.
13. Basic understanding of public health issues, including local health needs knowledge of national policies for care of older people, and assessment of quality care.
14. To give proper care for the old, all necessary equipments should be available. All types of clinical staff required to support the patient care such as, nursing care, physiotherapy, occupational therapy, speech and communication therapy and mental health professionals. All types of medicines required. Proper patient records and its maintenance is required. Adequate support from social services and public health is required. Proper administration and proper assistant with good libraries also is needed.

CONCLUSION

Gerontological nursing is a specialty that focuses on enhancing the quality of life for the older person in community and institutional settings. The goal of gerontological nursing is to promote optimal health in older persons. Gerontological nursing aims to maximize independence by identifying the strengths of the older person and working with him/her to enhance or maintain these strengths. Gerontological nurses acknowledge the central role that families and friends play in the lives of older persons and their healthcare.

33 Power and Politics in Nursing

33.1 INTRODUCTION

Power is a widely used concept in both the physical and social sciences, and as a result, there are many definitions. In the physical sciences, power refers to the amount of energy transferred per unit of time. Electricians work to provide and restore this type of power as a matter of course. Mathematicians have a different notion of power in mind when they talk about a numeral to the second (or third) power. Sociologists describe power as the ability to impose one's will upon others, and savvy researchers conduct power analyses before they begin their experiments. Power means many different things to different people. For some, power is seen as corrupt. For others, the more power they have, the more successful they feel. For even others, power is of no interest at all. The five bases of power were identified by John French and Bertram Raven in the early 1960's through a study they had conducted on power in leadership roles. The study showed how different types of power affected one's leadership ability and success in leadership role.

33.2 TYPES OF POWER

I. Formal Power

1. **Coercive:** Coercive power is conveyed through fear of losing one's job, being demoted, receiving a poor performance review, having prime projects taken away, etc. This power is gotten through threatening others.
2. **Reward:** Reward power is conveyed through rewarding individuals for compliance with one's wishes. This may be done through giving bonuses, raises, a promotion, extra time off from work, etc. For example, the supervisor who provides employees comp time when they meet an objective she sets for a project.
3. **Legitimate:** Legitimate power comes from having a position of power in an organization, such as being the boss or a key member of a leadership team. This power comes when employees in the organization recognize the authority of the individual. For example, the Chief Executive Officer (CEO) who determines the overall direction of the company and the resource needs of the company.

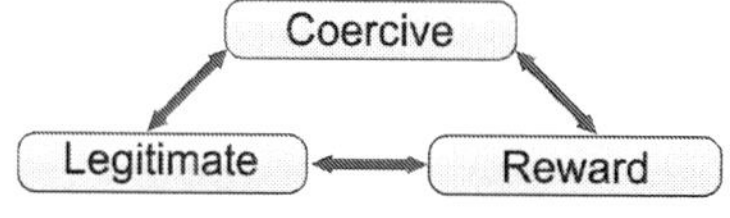

Fig. 33.1: Formal power

II. Personal Power

1. **Expert:** Expert power comes from one's experiences, skills or knowledge. As we gain experience in particular areas, and become thought leaders in those areas, we begin to gather expert power that can be utilized to get others to help us meet our goals. For example, the Project Manager who is an expert at solving particularly challenging problems to ensure a project stays on track.
2. **Referent:** Referent power comes from being trusted and respected. We can gain referent power when others trust what we do and respect us for how we handle situations. For example, the Human Resource Associate who is known for ensuring employees are treated fairly and coming to the rescue of those who are not.

33.3 CHARACTERISTICS OF NURSING POWER

The nurse leaders reflected on their own experiences and those of their nursing colleagues. They observed that the power of the nurse lies in his or her knowledge and expertise related to the technical, analytical, and interpersonal domains of nursing practice. This expertise, they observed, is uniquely interwoven into a collaborative, interdisciplinary effort focused solely on the patients and families that the nurse and care team serve and with whom they partner. The nursing profession as a whole, they said, establishes power through the practice of individual nurses who are engaged in patient care, administrative leadership, teaching, and research. The actions, behaviors, and comportment of each nurse contribute to or diminish the collective power that the profession of nursing holds in society, within a given organization, and in practice. The nurse leaders' observations regarding power underscored the power of individual nurses and highlighted how the practice of a single individual can impact patients and families, organizations, interdisciplinary colleagues, and the entire nursing profession.

Characteristics of a Powerful Professional Practice: Through our conversations with nurse leaders, we identified eight characteristics of powerful nursing practice—practice in which the nurse acts powerfully on behalf of patients and families and is recognized as powerful by others. The eight characteristics of powerful nursing practice are listed are described in more detail below.

1. **Nurses with a powerful practice acknowledge their unique role in the provision of patient centered and family centered care:** The nurse leaders observed that the nursing profession's emphasis on partnering with and caring for patients and families distinguishes nurses from other health professionals and positions them to be extremely powerful. The power of clinical nurses is significantly enhanced by the therapeutic, interpersonal relationships nurses establish with patients and families and by a nurse's expertise in relieving the burden of disease and helping patients and families cope with the continuum of health and illness. Nurses with a powerful practice, said the nurse leaders, recognize and readily acknowledge their unique contributions to patient care and realize that their relationships with patients and families put them in a position to influence the care delivery setting.
2. **Nurses with a powerful practice commit to continuous learning through education, skill development, and evidence-based practice:** All of the nurse leaders identified knowledge and expertise as an essential element of the nurse's power base and underscored the importance of continuous learning. Nurses who are powerful, they said, continuously seek new knowledge and base their practice on evidence. The educational level of nurses was also viewed as an essential element of a powerful professional practice. The nurse leaders agreed that attaining a BSN is essential, and that more education generally leads to greater power.
3. **Nurses with a powerful practice demonstrate professional comportment and recognize the critical nature of presence:** The nurse leaders noted that the professional comportment of nurses—their behaviors and how they carry themselves—is a key component of nursing power. Openness, transparency, authenticity, honesty, and integrity are some of the characteristics that the nurse leaders associated with powerful nurses.

4. **Nurses with a powerful practice value collaboration and partner effectively with colleagues in nursing and other disciplines:** Many of the nurse leaders cited the ability to collaborate with nursing colleagues and those outside of nursing as a hallmark of effective nursing leadership and a characteristic of powerful nursing practice. They noted that collaborating does not mean acquiescing or giving in. Nor does it mean competing or engaging in divisive actions and behaviors. Rather, it involves authentic, transparent discussion, debate, and deliberation and striving to reach consensus-driven outcomes. A powerful professional, said the nurse leaders, works well with others, is fair, and has opinions and perspectives that are "sought out" by others. Leading and participating on teams and partnering with others is essential to sound, expert nursing practice and is a critical element of a nurse's power base.
5. **Nurses with a powerful practice position themselves to influence decisions and resource allocation:** A number of the nurse leaders observed that powerful nurses typically position themselves to provide direction, input, and information about decisions affecting their practice, including decisions related to resource allocation. Such nurses recognize that decisions regarding staffing, technology to support practice, salaries, wages, and other factors that affect the practice environment should be in the hands of the nursing professionals who work in that environment; and if they are not, powerful nurses question whether it is because the organization does not value professional nursing practice.
6. **Nurses with a powerful practice strive to develop an impeccable character; to be inspirational, compassionate, and to have a credible, sought-after perspective:** A number of the nurse leaders observed that nurses with a powerful practice are grounded by a set of values and principles that they freely share with others and that guide their decisions and actions. The values and principles also help foster compassion, make the nurses less fearful and more open to others' ideas, and help nurses stay the course during times that may be tumultuous for patients, families, and colleagues. Nurses who are open to others and who use a values-based approach also find that others often seek out their perspective; this not only brings the nurse more power, but is the antithesis of using power as a coercive strategy.
7. **Nurses with a powerful practice recognize that the role of the nurse leader is to pave the way for nurses' voices to be heard and to help novice nurses develop into powerful professionals:** Many of the nurse leaders noted that helping novice nurses develop a voice that is based on professional credibility and expertise is a responsibility of nurse leaders at the unit, practice, program, and institutional levels. Powerful nurses, they said, recognize this and know that by fostering a nurse's professional development they promote the power of the individual nurse, enhance their own power, and strengthen the power of nursing as a profession. Powerful nurses in leadership positions also avoid using phrases such as, "My nursing staff," or "My faculty." Although, unintentional phrases like these suggest that a nurse is subservient to others and can diminish the professional stature of the individual.
8. **Nurses with a powerful practice evaluate the power of nursing and the nursing department in organizations they enter by assessing the organization's mission and values and its commitment to enhancing the power of diverse perspectives:** Many of the nurse leaders observed that nurses with a powerful practice tend to seek out and work in environments that support nurses and nursing practice, and that are led by strong nurse leaders who are themselves respected and valued by the institution. Such organizations place a high value on nurses and nursing care and, by design, uphold and contribute to the power of nurses that practice within them.

33.4 POWER AND EMPOWERMENT IN NURSING

There are compelling reasons to empower nurses. Powerless nurses are ineffective nurses. Powerless nurses are less satisfied with their jobs and more susceptible to burnout and depersonalization.

This article will begin with an examination of the concept of power; move on to a historical review of nurses' power over nursing practice; describe the kinds of power over nursing care needed for nurses to make their optimum contribution; and conclude with a discussion on the current state of nursing empowerment related to nursing care. Empowerment for nurses may consist of three components: a workplace that has the requisite structures to promote empowerment; a psychological belief in one's ability to be empowered; and acknowledgment that there is power in the relationships and caring that nurses provide. A more thorough understanding of these three components may help nurses to become empowered and use their power for better patient care. Power is necessary to be able to influence an individual or group. Nurses need power to be able to influence patients, physicians, and other healthcare professionals, as well as each other. Powerless nurses are ineffective nurses, and the consequences of nurses' lack of power has only recently come to light (Page, 2004). Powerless nurses are less satisfied with their jobs, and more susceptible to burnout and depersonalization. Lack of nursing power may also contribute to poorer patient outcomes). Studies such as these suggest that there are compelling reasons to promote power in nursing.

33.5 KINDS OF POWER OVER NURSING CARE

Kinds of Power over Nursing Care Needed for Nurses to Make Their Optimum Contribution: There are at least three types of power that nurses need to be able to make their optimum contribution. The various types of power can all be categorized as stemming from nurses' control in three domains: control over the content of practice, control over the context of practice, and control over competence. The continued lack of control over both the content and context of nursing work suggests that power remains an elusive attribute for many nurses. In this section, power will be discussed as it is manifested by nurses' control over the content, context, and competence of nursing practice.

Control over the Content of Nursing Practice: Power is an attribute that nurses must cultivate in order to practice more autonomously because it is through power that members of an occupation are able to raise their status, define their area of expertise, and achieve and maintain autonomy and influence. One of the characteristics of a profession is that professionals have power over the practice of their discipline which is often referred to as professional autonomy. Autonomy represents one kind of power nurses need, and has been defined as "the freedom to act on what one knows". Therefore, a key element of empowerment is nurses' control over their practice (Page, 2004). The ability to act according to one's knowledge and judgment is known as control over the content of nursing practice, and is often synonymous with autonomy. High levels of autonomy increased nurses' identification with the profession in one study, providing recent empirical support for this supposition.

Control over the Context of Nursing Practice: Besides control over the content of nursing practice, which represents one type of power, a related type of control is known as control over the context of practice, and represents another type of power that nurses need. Over twenty years ago it was noted that "nurses should be more meaningfully involved in the running of hospitals". Nurses' involvement in hospital affairs is one of the hallmarks of a magnet hospital environment but otherwise may not be apparent.

Control over the Competence of Nursing Practice: A necessary precursor for both autonomy and power is competence, which has its foundation in educational preparation. Power is maintained through knowledge development, which is acquired through education and expertise. The multiple entry levels into nursing practice, as well as the low educational level of nurses (relative to other healthcare professionals) may contribute to nurses' powerlessness. The statement, "Being less well-educated than other groups within the hospital puts nursing at a serious disadvantage in organizational politics", is no less true now than it was when written more than twenty years ago.

Nursing expertise is a related source of power that has a transformative effect on patients' lives. Expertise is not the same as experience, nor can expertise be acquired on nursing units with high turnover. This suggests a complex relationship between organizational factors that contribute to nursing turnover and the development of nursing expertise. Educational preparation and expertise represent two additional types of power nurses need to make their optimal contribution to patient care.

33.6 STATE NURSING EMPOWERMENT

The Current State of Nursing Empowerment Related to Nursing Care: Part of the difficulty many nurses have in being powerful may be due to their inability to develop the types of power described in the previous section. Power over the content, context, and competence of nursing practice contributes to feelings of empowerment, but control in these three domains may not be enough. An examination of the two major areas of empowerment literature in nursing, as well as a third area not yet embraced by nursing, may help inform future directions for the development of power and empowerment for nurses. Empowerment in nursing has largely been studied from two perspectives. Most nursing researchers view empowerment as either arising from the environment or developing from one's psychological state.

In conclusion, nurses' power may arise from three components: a workplace that has the requisite structures that promote empowerment; a psychological belief in one's ability to be empowered; and acknowledgment that there is power in the relationships and caring that nurses provide. Nursing research has been able to demonstrate the relationship between the first two components and empowerment; yet there remains a need for research to examine the power that exists in relationships. Nursing research from a relational theory perspective may help make nurses' power more explicit and more visible, moving our understanding of power in nursing further than has previously been possible. A more thorough understanding of these three components may help nurses to become empowered and use their power for their practice and for better patient care.

CONCLUSION

Political nursing is defined as the use of knowledge about power processes and strategies to influence the nature and direction of healthcare and professional nursing. Nurses work in organizations with varied characteristics—private or public; profit, non-profit, or charitable; large, small or medium; and in large or small cities, towns, small towns, or rural areas. In the work place, there are many issues with which nurses are involved. Power and politics may be necessary to resolve issues.

34 Cultural Diversity

34.1 INTRODUCTION

Knowledge of cultural diversity is vital at all levels of nursing practice. Ethnocentric approaches to nursing practice are ineffective in meeting health and nursing needs of diverse cultural groups of clients. Knowledge about cultures and their impact on interactions with healthcare is essential for nurses, whether they are practicing in a clinical setting, education, research or administration. Cultural diversity addresses racial and ethnic differences, however, these concepts or features of the human experience are not synonymous.

34.2 NEEDS OF CULTURAL DIVERSITY

Knowledge and skills related to cultural diversity can strengthen and broaden healthcare delivery systems. Other cultures can provide examples of a range of alternatives in services, delivery systems, conceptualization of illness, and treatment modalities. Cultural groups often utilize traditional healthcare providers, identified by and respected within the group. Concepts of illness, wellness, and treatment modalities evolve from a cultural perspective or world view. Concepts of illness, health, and wellness are part of the total cultural belief system. Culture is one of the organizing concepts upon which nursing is based and defined. Nurses need to understand:

1. How cultural groups understand life processes?
2. How cultural groups define health and illness?
3. What cultural groups do to maintain wellness?
4. What cultural groups believe to be the causes of illness?
5. How healers cure and care for members of cultural groups? and
6. How the cultural background of the nurse influences the way in which care is delivered?

34.3 NURSE ADMINISTATORS ROLE IN CULTURAL DIVERSITY

Nurse administrators need to foster policies and procedures that help ensure access to care that accommodates varying cultural beliefs. Nurse administrators need to be knowledgeable about and sensitive to the cultural diversity among providers and consumers. Nurse researchers need to utilize the cross-cultural body of knowledge in order to ask pertinent research questions. Through exploration of other cultures, nurse researchers and practitioners find that while cultures differ, there are also many similarities among groups. Nurses are in a position to influence professional policies and practice in response to cultural diversity.

34.4 CULTURAL DERVISITY IN NURSING PRACTICE

Cultural diversity in nursing practice derives its conceptual base from nursing, other cross-cultural health disciplines, and the social sciences such as anthropology, sociology and psychology. Culture is conceptualized broadly to encompass the belief systems of a variety of groups. Cultural diversity refers to the differences between people based on a shared ideology and valued set of beliefs, norms, customs, and meanings evidenced in a way of life. Culture consists of patterns of behavior acquired and transmitted symbols, constituting the distinctive achievement of human groups, including their embodiment in artifacts; the essential core of culture consists of historically derived and selected ideas and especially their attached values (Kroeber and Kluckhohn, 1952).

The impact of culture as a causative influence on the perceptions, interpretations and behaviors of persons in specific cultural groups is important. Issues such as cultural differences in defining health and in designing treatments are also important. As knowledge of specific cultures is gained, cross cultural comparison can lead to recognition of possible universal aspects as well. Ideology is comprised of the ideas of a group, their nature and source, and the doctrines, opinions or ways of thinking of a group. These are attached to an agreed upon set of beliefs or a creed. Value(s) refer to the especially favorable way of regarding the ideas, behaviors, customs, and institutions of a group as desirable, useful, estimable, important, or truthful. Ethnocentrism is the belief that one's own culture is superior to all others. This belief is common to all cultural groups, all groups regard their own culture as not only the best but also the correct, moral and only way of life. This belief is pervasive, often unconscious and is imposed on every aspect of day-to-day interaction and practices including healthcare. It is this attitude which creates problems between nurses and clients of diverse cultural groups.

34.5 ROLE OF NURSE IN CULTURAL DIVERSITY

Nurses bring their personal cultural heritage as well as the cultural and philosophical views of their education into the professional setting. Therefore, it is important for the nurse to understand that nurse-patient encounters include the interaction of three cultural systems: the culture of the nurse, the culture of the client and the culture of the setting. Access to care can be improved by providing culturally-relevant, responsive services. Individuals need choices of delivery systems in seeking healthcare. Nurses in clinical practice must use their knowledge of cultural diversity to develop and implement culturally sensitive nursing care. Nurses take pride in their role as client advocates. Recognizing cultural diversity, integrating cultural knowledge, and acting, when possible, in a culturally appropriate manner enables nurses to be more effective in initiating nursing assessments and serving as client advocates. All nursing curricula should include pertinent information about diverse healthcare beliefs, values, and practices. Such educational programs would demonstrate to nursing students that cultural beliefs and practices are as integral to the nursing process as are physical and psychosocial factors.

CONCLUSION

Diversity awareness also applies to healthcare professionals and other coworkers. Everyone belongs to one or more cultural groups. Additionally, it is important to acknowledge that diversity is ever changing, not static. Changes can occur within and between groups over time or individuals (and groups) can belong to different groups at different times. For example, beginning nursing students are challenged to learn the culture of nursing education and the nursing profession within the context of the cultural norms and expectations of a nursing student. Leininger (2002) refers to this as enculturation within the nursing profession. Similarly, a new graduate must make a transition to the new culture of the profession as a graduate nurse (and later as a registered nurse) as well as to the new organizational culture of the healthcare institution and the cultural nuances of a particular nursing unit.

35 Collective Bargaining

35.1 INTRODUCTION

Collective bargaining is the negotiation between the employer and employee to have smooth functioning of organization. It is important to have control over the demands of employees and autocratic behavior of employer and manager. Collective bargaining is the way by which employee redress their grievances and asks the employer to fulfill their needs. By this strikes can be avoided. Collective bargaining usually occurs between leaders of association or representatives of employees and the management or employer. International labour organization (ILO) has defined collective bargaining as "Negotiation about working conditions and terms of employment between an employer and a group of employees or one or more employee, organization with a view to reach an agreement wherein terms serves as a code of defining the rights and obligations of each party in their employment/industrial relations with one another".

35.2 DEFINITION

1. According to JH Richardson "Collective bargaining takes place when a number of work people enter into a negotiation as a bargaining unit with an employer or group of employer with the object of reaching an agreement on conditions of the employment of the work people. Collective bargaining is a complex process. It involves psychology, politics and power.
2. The continuous relationship between an employer and a designated labor organization representing a specific unit of employees for the purpose of negotiating written terms of employment. *–Carrell and Heavrin*
3. A process of discussion and negotiation between two parties, one or both of whom is a group of persons acting in concert... more specifically it is the procedure by which an employer or employers and a group of employees agree upon the conditions of works.
4. Tudwing Teller defines collective bargaining as an agreement between a single employer or an association of employers on the one hand and a labor union on the other, which regulate the terms and conditions of employment.

Collective bargain may, therefore, be defined as an agreement under which the organization of workers and employers collectively undertake to resolve their existing or future difference with or without the assistance of a third party.

35.3 FEATURES AND OBJECTIVES OF COLLECTIVE BARGAINING

Objectives

Collective bargaining has benefits not only for the present, but also for the future. The objectives of collective bargaining are:

1. To provide an opportunity to the workers, to voice their problems on issues related to employment.
2. To facilitate reaching a solution that is acceptable to all the parties involved.
3. To resolve all conflicts and disputes in a mutually agreeable manner.
4. To prevent any conflict/disputes in the future through mutually signed contracts.
5. To develop a conductive atmosphere to foster good organizations relations.
6. To provide stable and peaceful organization (hospital) relations.
7. To enhance the productivity of the organization by preventing strikes lock-out etc.

Collective bargaining involves discussions and negotiations between two groups as to the terms and conditions of employment. It is called 'collective' because both the employer and the employee act as a group rather than as individuals. It is known as bargaining, because the method of reaching an agreement involves proposals, counter proposals, offers and counter offers and other negotiations.

35.4 FEATURES OF COLLECTIVE BARGAINING

1. Group activity.
2. Activity in levels.
3. Flexibility.
4. Win-win situation.
5. Builds relationship.
6. An art and a science.

35.5 CHARACTERISTICS OF COLLECTIVE BARGAINING

1. It is a collective process as both employer and employee participate.
2. It is continuous process, which aims at establishing stable relationship between two parties involved.
3. It involves not only bargaining but also implementation.
4. It attempts in achieving discipline in industry.
5. It is a flexible approach, as the parties involved have to adopt a flexible attitude towards negotiations.

35.6 LEVELS OF COLLECTIVE BARGAINING

Collective bargaining operates at three levels:

1. **National level:** It is a bipartite or tripartite negotiation between union confederations, central employer associations and government agencies. It provides a floor level bargaining on terms of employment, often taken into consideration macroeconomic goals.
2. **Sectoral bargaining:** It accounts for standardization of terms of employment in one industry, includes a range of bargaining patterns.
3. **Company level:** This is a supplementary type of bargaining. It emphasizes the point that bargaining levels need not be mutually exclusive.

35.7 ADVANTAGES OF COLLECTIVE BARGAINING

1. It is flexible and mobile and not fixed or static.
2. It has fluidity or ample scope for compromise.
3. It is a complementary process not competitive.
4. It helps in achieving better planning.

5. It allows smooth functioning of organization.
6. It retents the employee in organization.
7. It encourages less strike.
8. It helps in managing conflicts.

35.8 FUNCTIONS OF COLLECTIVE BARGAINING

1. It is a rule-making or legislative process in the sense that it formulates terms and conditions under which labor and management will cooperate and work together over a certain stated period.
2. It is also a judicial process, tar in every collective agreement there is a provision or clause regarding the interpretation of the agreement and how any difference of opinion about the intention or scope of a particular clause is to be resolved. Such interpretation can be left to a joint committee of worker's and management representative or the top level management or to a third party jointly selected by the trade union and the management.
3. It is also an executive process, for both the management and the trade unions undertake to implement the agreement signed, each accepting a series of obligations under the agreement.

35.9 PRINCIPLES OF COLLECTIVE BARGAINING

For Union and Management

1. Collective bargaining should be made an education as well as a bargaining process. It should offer to trade union leaders an opportunity to present to the management the wants, desires, grievances and attitudes of its employees and make it possible for the management to explain to union leaders and through them, to its employees the economic problems which it is confronted with.
2. There must be mutual confidence and good faith, and a desire to make collective bargaining effective in practice.
3. There should be an honest, able and responsible leadership, for only this kind of leadership make collective bargaining effective and meaningful.
4. The management and trade union must look upon collective bargaining as a means of finding the best possible solution, and not as a means of acquiring as much as one can while conceding the minimum. There must be an honest attempt at solving problems.
5. Both parties to a dispute should command the respect of each other and should have enough bargaining power to enforce the terms of the agreement that they may arrive at.
6. The two parties should meticulously observe and abide by all the national and state laws which are applicable to collective bargaining.
7. Both parties must bear in mind the fact that collective bargaining is, in a sense, a form of price fixation and that the success of any collective bargaining depends, in the final analysis, on whether the management and the trade union do a good job of ensuring that the price of labor is properly adjusted to other prices.

For the Management

1. The management must develop and consistently follow a realistic labor policy, which should be accepted and carried out by its representatives.
2. The management must grant recognition to the trade union without any reservations and accept it as a constructive force in the organization.
3. The management should not wait for the trade union to bring employee grievances to its notice but should rather create the conditions in which employees can approach the management themselves, without involving the trade union.

4. The management should deal only with one trade union in the organization.
5. The management should not assume that employee goodwill will always exist. It should periodically examine the rules and regulations to determine the attitudes and degree of comfort of its employees and gain their goodwill and cooperation.
6. The management should extend fair treatment to the trade union in order to make it a responsible and conservative body.
7. While weighing the economic consequences of collective. Bargaining, the management should place greater emphasis on social considerations.

CONCLUSION

Collective bargaining generally includes negotiations between the two parties (employees' representatives and employer's representatives). Collective bargaining consists of negotiations between an employer and a group of employees that determine the conditions of employment. Often employees are represented in the bargaining by a union or other labor organization. The result of collective bargaining procedure is called the collective bargaining agreement (CBA). Collective agreements may be in the form of procedural agreements or substantive agreements. Procedural agreements deal with the relationship between workers and management and the procedures to be adopted for resolving individual or group disputes.

Collective bargaining includes not only negotiations between the employers and unions but also includes the process of resolving labor-management conflicts. Thus, collective bargaining is, essentially, a recognized way of creating a system of industrial jurisprudence. It acts as a method of introducing civil rights in the industry, that is, the management should be conducted by rules rather than arbitrary decision-making. It establishes rules which define and restrict the traditional authority exercised by the management.

36 Integration of Nursing Service and Education

36.1 INTRODUCTION

Nursing education and service are both sides of the same coin, so both are equally important, their needs something called integration which is proper blending of nursing education and practice or service in nursing curriculum. Nursing education basically involves both theoretical and practical knowledge, by theory the most advanced and valid knowledge available that can be generated and applied to many clinical situations. The nursing education to be effective, it needs a good practice, therefore best good nursing education is needed to guide for excellent nursing practice.

36.2 GOALS OF INTEGRATION

The main goals of nursing education is to equip a person with necessary skill to live effectively to provide quality nursing care. A professional nurse should be productive and humanistic, skillfully blending nursing education (science) with nursing practice (art). Further of nursing as a discrete discipline rests upon strong links between education and every sphere of practice.

Challenges in bridging the gap: The difficulties that the new graduates experiencing in making the transition from students to qualified nurses highlights the need for more bridges between education and practice. Preceptor ship is one strategy for assisting new graduates. The challenge to nursing is to discover strategies to achieve an appropriate balance between artistic and scientific components of nursing.

Role of dean in integration: Dean is a person who plays a vital role in both nursing educational institution and the nursing services. The professional task becomes precondition for ensuring that the training program is really designed to meet the population health needs. The training programs, professional profile and educational program objectives should provide basis for nursing practice in all three levels of healthcare. The advancement to adopted and develop professional skill as specialist is essential. So, that the nurses can be prepared as clinical consultants, administrators and as researcher in various fields of nursing practice in order to make both nursing education and practice identical.

36.3 OBJECTIVES OF INTEGRATION

The integration of theory and practice is perceived as a cycle, effective nursing care leading to good learning experiences, and effective education leading to effective nursing care. The paper indicates areas for further study and approaches to solving the problems. The objective of integration of nursing education and services includes the following:

1. Deliver high standards of quality care.
2. Conduct regular in-service education program based on the needed topics.
3. Organizing induction program for all the newly recruited Staff Nurse.

4. Monitor deficiencies in clinical areas through audits, feedbacks and small projects.
5. Maintain safe and happy working conditions for nurses.
6. Build resources sufficient for students learning and practice.

36.4 ROLE OF NURSE EDUCATOR

The nurse educator should choose an appropriate method to teach and practice, whatever the subjects taught in nursing. The nurse educator should make the topic meets the objectives of three domains such as cognitive, affective and psychomotor and merging of three appropriately, selection of teaching methods in a more realistic situation to the students.

36.5 ROLE OF NURSE MANAGER

Supervision of nursing practice in the clinical areas and evaluating their skills are most essential role of the nurse manager, their by the integration of nursing service and education becomes fruitful to obtain quality nursing care. Every ward should have a clinical instructor to supervise the nursing staffs and student. This is very important in nursing service where integration of education and service are practiced.

CONCLUSION

The commitment to that nursing practice based on sound, reliable knowledge is intrinsically valuable to nursing. That is to say, knowledge is desirable by its very nature. The growth and enrichment of theory and of itself is an important goal for nursing as a scholarly discipline, to pursue. Now nursing practice settings are complex, and the amount of data available to nurses are virtually endless. Nurses must analyze a tremendous amount of information about each patient and decide what to do. If a theory helps practicing nurses categorize and understand what is going on in nursing practice, if it helps them predict patients responses to nursing care, and if it is helpful in clinical decision-making, it is useful as a guide to nursing practice.

37 Women Empowerment

37.1 INTRODUCTION

Empowerment of women, also called gender empowerment, has become a significant topic of discussion in regards to development and economics. Entire nations, businesses, communities, and groups can benefit from the implementation of programs and policies that adopt the notion of women empowerment.

37.2 PROCESS OF EMPOWERMENT

The process which enables individuals/groups to fully access personal/collective power, authority and influence, and to employ that strength when engaging with other people, institutions or society. In other words, "Empowerment is not giving people power; people already have plenty of power, in the wealth of their knowledge and motivation, to do their jobs magnificently. We define empowerment as letting this power out (Blanchard, 1996)." It encourages people to gain the skills and knowledge that will allow them to overcome obstacles in life or work environment and ultimately, help them develop within themselves or in the society.

37.3 CAPABILITIES OF EMPOWERMENT

Empowerment includes the following, or similar, capabilities:

1. The ability to make decisions about personal/collective circumstances.
2. The ability to access information and resources for decision-making.
3. Ability to consider a range of options from which to choose (not just yes/no, either/or.).
4. Ability to exercise assertiveness in collective decision-making.
5. Having positive-thinking about the ability to make change.
6. Ability to learn and access skills for improving personal/collective circumstance.
7. Ability to inform others' perceptions though exchange, education and engagement.
8. Involving in the growth process and changes that is never ending and self-initiated.
9. Increasing one's positive self-image and overcoming stigma.
10. Increasing one's ability in discreet thinking to sort out right and wrong.

37.4 MODES AND METHODS OF EMPOWERMENT

1. One-way to deploy the empowerment of women is through land rights. Land rights offer a key way to economically empower women, giving them the confidence they need to tackle general inequalities.
2. Women in developing nations are legally restricted from their land on the sole basis of gender. Having a right to their land gives women a sort of bargaining power that they wouldn't normally

have, in turn; they gain the ability to assert themselves in various aspects of their life, both in and outside of the home.

3. Another way to provide women empowerment is to allocate responsibilities to them that normally belong to men. When women have economic empowerment, it is a way for others to see them as equal members of society. Through this, they achieve more self-respect and confidence by their contributions to their communities.
4. Simply including women as a part of a community can have sweeping positive effects. Not only did this drive up the efficiency of the group, but the women gained incredible self-esteem while others, including men, viewed them with more respect.
5. Participation, which can be seen and gained in a variety of ways, has been argued to be the most beneficial form of gender empowerment. Political participation, be it the ability to vote and voice opinions, or the ability to run for office with a fair chance of being elected, plays a huge role in the empowerment of peoples. It can include participation in the household, in schools, and the ability to make choices for one. It can be said that these latter participations need to be achieved before one can move onto broader political participation. When women have the agency to do what she wants, a higher equality between men and women is established.
6. Governments, organizations, and individuals have caught hold of the lure of microfinance. They hope that lending money and credit allows women to function in business and society, which in turn empowers them to do more in their communities.
7. One of the primary goals in the foundation of microfinance was women empowerment. Loans with low interest rates are given to women in developing communities in hopes that they can start a small business and provide for her family. It should be said, however, that the success and efficiency of microcredit and microloans is controversial and constantly debated.

CONCLUSION

Empowerment is a sense of having both the ability and the opportunity to act effectively. Empowerment is a process or strategy the goal of which is to change the nature and distribution of power in a specific context. It is a group activity that increases political and social consciousness, is based on the need for autonomy, and is accomplished with continuing cycles of assessment and action. Nursing organizations seek to empower nurses; nurses endeavor to empower patients to seek and adopt healthy lifestyles.

Section-8

Advanced Nursing Skills

38 Interpersonal Relationship

38.1 INTRODUCTION

The nurse is an important member of a team that must work in cooperation and harmony for the care of patients. She should be familiar with the plan of organization of the hospital and of the nursing department. The nurse must feel accountable to the organization, should be honest, dependable and willing to carry out the prescribed treatment and care for the patient. She should maintain her position and dignity. She should not accept verbal orders from the physician (medical personnel). There should be a team spirit. The nurse should have respect for the senior and concern and caring attitude towards fellow nurses, juniors and other supporting staff. She should maintain a healthy and good relationship with various departments.

38.2 ELEMENTS OF PROFESSIONAL COMMUNICATION

Professional appearance, demeanor, and behavior are important in establishing the nurse's trustworthiness and competence. A professional is expected to be clean, neat, well groomed, conservatively dressed and scent and odorfree. Professional behavior should reflect warmth, friendliness, confidence and competence. Elements which are present in the professional communication are:

1. Courtesy.
2. Use of names.
3. Privacy and confidentiality.
4. Trustworthiness.
5. Autonomy and responsibility.
6. Assertiveness.

1. **Courtesy:** Common courtesy is part of professional communication. To practice courtesy the nurse says hello and goodbye, knocks on doors before entering and uses self-introduction. The nurse also states his or her purpose, addresses people by name, says please and thank you to team members and apologizes for inadvertently making an error or causing someone distress.
2. **Use of names:** Self-introduction is important in communication. The nurse's failure to give a name, indicate status or acknowledge the client can create uncertainty about the interaction and convey an impersonal lack of commitment or caring. Addressing other by name conveys respect for human dignity and uniqueness. Avoid referring to clients by diagnosis, room number or other attribute, which is demeaning and sends the message that the nurse does not care enough to know the person as an individual.
3. **Privacy and confidentiality:** Maintaining confidentiality is an important aspect of professional behavior. It is essential that the nurse safeguard the client's right to privacy by carefully protecting information of a sensitive, private nature. Sharing personal information or gossiping

about others violates nursing ethical codes and practice standards. It sends the message that the nurse cannot be trusted and damages interpersonal relationships.

4. **Trustworthiness:** Trust is relying on someone without doubt or question. Being trustworthy means helping others without hesitation when help is needed. To foster trust, the nurse communicates warmth and demonstrates consistency, reliability, honesty and competence. Sometimes it is not easy for a client to ask for help. Trusting another person involves risk and vulnerability but it also faster's open, therapeutic communication and enhances the expression of feeling, thoughts and needs.
5. **Autonomy and responsibility:** Autonomy is the ability to be self-directed and independent in accomplishing goals and advocating for other. Professional nurses make choices and accept responsibility for the outcomes of their actions. They take initiative in problem-solving and communicate in a manner that reflects what they really need and want. Autonomy can be beneficial to the client because people who seek healthcare are often concerned about losing control of decisions that influence how they live.
6. **Assertiveness:** According to Darley, assertiveness comprises respect for others, respect for yourself, self-awareness and effective, clear, and consistent communication. Assertiveness conveys a sense of self assurance while also communicating respect for the other person. Nurses can teach assertiveness skills to others as a means for promoting personal health. Assertive people express feeling and emotions confidently, spontaneously, and honestly. They make decisions and control their lives more effectively than nonassertive individuals. Assertive responses are characterized by feelings of security, competence, power, optimism and professionalism. They are good tool for dealing with criticism, change, negative conditions in personal or professional life and conflict or stress in relationship.

38.3 PRINCIPLES OF INTERPERSONAL RELATIONSHIP (IPR)

1. Respect every one's individuality. Each member of a team is as important as the other.
2. Do not impose anything on anybody.
3. Keep emotion under control.
4. Do not be afraid to admit ignorance.
5. Do not give and take any personal favor.
6. The team leader should not make any excuse regarding his or her responsibility.
7. Develop habits of listening and focus attention on the problems.
8. Do not do or say anything that will disturb other's faith.
9. Be impartial to others and practice justice.
10. The members of team should be loyal, honest, dependable and willing to carry out the directions of the team leader.
11. There should be team spirit or we feeling among the members. The members should work for the interest of the group.
12. There should be mutual understanding between the members; they should be willing to give and take corrections.

38.4 IPR SYSTEM IN NURSING

Interpersonal relationship (IPR) is the main concept in professional field. In nursing IPR system is explained by many theorists. Imogene king explains the interpersonal relationship system in detail. Interpersonal relationship system is enhancing the nurses to promote herself and clients well-being. Interpersonal relationship system (Imogene King): King (1981) stated human being is the focus for nursing. The primary concerns of nursing are human behavior, social interaction, and social movements (1976), thus within the context of the paradigm concept of person. King (1981) included three dynamic interacting open systems:

1. Personal system.
2. Interpersonal system.
3. Social system.

The interpersonal system is composed of two, three or more individuals interacting in a given situation. King (1996) explained that, at the interpersonal system level, individuals increase consciousness and are open to interpersonal perceptions in communication and interactions with persons and things in the environment. The interpersonal system moves the focus from the individual alone to individuals interacting in dyads, triads, small groups and large groups. The major concept of the interpersonal system is interaction; sub concepts are communication, role, stress and coping.

King noted that interaction is comprehensive concept in interpersonal systems and that knowledge of interaction is essential for nurses to understand a fundamental process for gathering information about human being. King pointed out the perception, judgments, actions and reactions of the individuals cannot directly observed but must be inferred from the directly observable interaction. Elaborating, she stated, first, the informational component of interactions can be observed as communication. Second, the valuation component of interactions can be observed as transaction because one obviously values a goal, identifies means to achieve it, and takes action to attain it.

King viewed communication as the vehicle by which human relations are developed and maintained, she went to say that all behavior is communication. The general systems framework focuses on intrapersonal and interpersonal communication as well as verbal and nonverbal communication.

Communication is involved in transaction, which is defined as a process of interactions in which human being communicate with environment to achieve goals that are valued. Transactions are goal directed human behaviors. In general systems frame works, the concepts of roles was derived from the work of Bennis and Bennis, has and person. Three elements of role are interested.

1. Role is a set of behaviors expected when occupying a position in a social system.
2. Rules or procedures define rights and obligations in a position in an organization.
3. Role is a relationship with one or more individuals interacting in specific situations for a purpose.

King developed her definitions of stress from the writing of Jamis, monat and Lazarus and Selye. She stated stress is a dynamic state where by a human being interacts with the environment to maintain balance. For growth, development and performance, this involves an exchange of energy and information between the person and the environment for regulation and control of stressors. Stress is viewed as negative and positive as well as constructive and destructive. King (1981) explained that stress is reduced when transaction are made.

Interpersonal relationship system in nursing, the nurse is an important member of the health-care team that must work in cooperation and harmony for the care of the patient. This cooperation and harmony depends upon the IPR that is maintained among the members of the health team.

38.5 ESTABLISHMENT OF IPR

The head nurse is in key position for the establishment of good IPR among the personnel in her department. This will also involve communication system existing between and within the hospital departments. A warm, friendly attitude of nurses is reflected in the clients and other employees. The following points will help to establish good IPR among the personnel.

1. Every member should be kept informed about the job, any changes that are taking place from day-to-day.

2. Give personal reorganization to everyone by giving praise and showing concern whenever they deserve.
3. Known each personnel working with you and accept them with their abilities and limitations.
4. Any grievances should be dealt with promptly and appropriately.
5. Do not do or say anything that will lower the status of the members in your team.
6. Plan, organize and coordinate the activities of your team so that everything gets done in the proper time and in the correct way.
7. Remember that every member in your team is working with you and not for you or under you.
8. Try to create we feeling in your subordinates.
9. Give each person, time and opportunity to plan his work and make sure that everyone understands the work assigned to him/her.
10. Provide adequate supplies and equipment needed in the client care.
11. Except in case of emergency, avoid interrupting the personnel while they are at work.
12. Plan for frequent staff conferences.

38.6 PROBLEMS OF IMPROPER IPR

Poor organization often leads to inefficiency, misunderstanding or actual conflict among the personnel. Any conflict, however slight in the staff, is sensed by the patient and makes him feel insecure. Insecurity causes him to increase complaints, and it slows down recovery. The aim of the healthcare team is to restore the health of patient. The technical skill must be added with the warmth of human feeling and compassion. It is expedient to examine not only the behavior of the patient but also the atmosphere in which he is being treated. These problems can develop at any level of an organization and result in an inability to solve human relations problems.

I. Symptoms of organizational dysfunction frequently observed are:

1. Little personal investment by the staff in organizations' objectives and goals.
2. Policies, directives, and orders not being carried out as intended.
3. Competition between staff rather than cooperation or collaboration.
4. Failure of staff to report problems although they see anything wrong.
5. Staff blames others for problems instead to taking responsibility and seeking solutions.
6. Staff taking refuge in procedures and policies instead of searching for better alternatives.

II. Some selected causes of organizational dysfunction are as follows:

1. Tight control over decision-making with little staff participation allowed.
2. Staff judgment not being respected by administrative and Supervisory personnel.
3. Rejection of the experience of others.
4. Lack of positive feedback on good performance.
5. Lack of corrective feedback on poor performance.
6. Tradition encouraged; innovation discouraged for fear of making a mistake.
7. Inadequate mechanisms for communication up, down, and sideways in the organization.
8. Insufficient direct observation by supervisors.

III. Within the formal social system, individuals, professional and nonprofessional groups and departments compete for status, recognition, and privileges focusing on the mission of the patient care. The formal structure is often supported or subverted by the informal social relationship that emerges among personnel. These traditional groupings, norms, and goals are often informally developed in order to get the job done faster. From these nonofficial groupings emerge attitudes towards staff and toward patients that can be either detrimental to the efficiency of medical teamwork, or can help to create a positive atmosphere for achieving the formal goals of the hospital.

CONCLUSION

The ability to communicate effectively is one of the most essential skills in nursing. Broadly speaking, communication encompasses study of the patient's behavior including all observable actions, verbal and nonverbal. To be effective in communicating, the student must become astute in recognizing the effect of the patient's adaptative efforts on his or her behavior. It is also important to recognize the effect of the student's own adaptive behaviors on nurse-patient communication. Effective communication in nursing goes beyond the nurse-patient relationship and involves co-ordination and cooperation with all of the health team members.

39 Decision-Making

39.1 INTRODUCTION

Decision-making is a complex, cognitive process often defined as choosing a particular course of action. Decision-making can be regarded as the mental processes (cognitive process) resulting in the selection of a course of action among several alternatives. Every decision making process produces a final choice. The output can be an action or an opinion of choice.

39.2 CHARACTERISTICS OF DECISION-MAKING

1. Decision-making is based on rational thinking.
2. It is a process of selecting the best from amongst alternatives available.
3. It involves the evaluation of various alternatives available.
4. It is the end product because it is preceded by discussions and deliberations.
5. Decision making is aimed to achieve organizational goals.
6. It also involves certain commitment.

39.3 DECISION-MAKING PROCESS

The decision-making process goes through the various stages and the basic objectives of all these changes are to solve problem through the decision. The solution of the problem depends on how effectively the decision is made and implemented. Thus, an effective decision is one which is action oriented, goal oriented and provides efficiency in implementation. These three aspects are:

Action orientation: Decisions are action oriented and are directed towards relevant and controllable aspects of the environment and their value is dependent on the success of the actions that follow. Decisions may be treated as an intervening variable which may alternately find their utility in implementation.

Goal direction: Organizations are goal directed units and therefore any organizational process including decision making should be goal directed to enable the organization to meet its objectives. Naturally, the value of a decision is dependent on the attainment of a given goal or set of goals. Such attainment is a function of both the accuracy of the decision and its implementation.

Efficiency in implementation: An effective decision should provide the way in which it can be implemented. Therefore decision making should take into account all the possible functions, not only in terms of external context, but also in internal context. So, that a decision can be implemented properly; often the results are obtained by proper implementation of proper decision. Therefore, a brilliant decision may fall, if it is not suitable for implementation by the organization. From this point of view three characteristics of an effective decision have been identified.

1. The viability of the decision.
2. The degree of congruency between predication and reality of viability of the solution as it occurs.
3. The enthusiasm and skill with which the proposal is pursued, the alternatives of the venture.

39.4 EFFECTIVE DECISION-MAKING PROCESS

Any decision can be made effectives if decision making process is followed properly. However to make effective decision managers should take care of certain variables effecting their and its implementation. The attempt should be made a realistic decision rather than attempt at an ideal decision. This can be done by following factors are taken into consideration.

Categorical interpretation: At the very outset it may be emphasized that logical decision can be made if the real problem is interpreted and identified with in-depth study and observation. Therefore it is desirable that problem should be defined properly. It is often suggested that a problem is half solved, if it is identified properly.

Application of limiting factor: Managers can do better if they apply the principles of limiting factor. On choosing from among alternatives, the more a manager recognizes critical to the attainment of desired objectives. The more clearly and accurately, he can select the most desirable alternative. The concept of limiting may vary from one decision situation to another or for the same situation over the period of time.

Adequate information: Information is the life blood of organization because all decisions are based on this more is the quality of reliable information higher the validity of a decision. However there is a term for collecting information because of time and cost factors.

Considering other's values: While making decision it is desirable that all alternatives are considered before arriving at a decision often decision is affected by preferences and values. Moreover interpretation of many qualitative is an alternative is subject to personal judgment. Therefore, if various views or same points are taken into consideration and given adequate weight, they will contribute to the quality of decision.

Judging the effectiveness of a decision: Two major factors are relevant to the potential effectiveness of a decision. One is the objective quality of a decision and the other is the acceptability of the decision to the group who will be affected by it. Although more emphasis is usually given to quality both quality and acceptance must be present to reach most effective decision.

Quality: To determine the quality of a decision, severe factors may be considered. First what kind of imputed to the decision. A good decision cannot be made unless complete, factual, relevant, objective data are available to the decision maker. The decision make must gather and use all the available data.

The behavioral characteristics of the decision maker affect the way he/she will deal with the date and use the decision-making process. The decision maker's perception of the problem will determine what data are collected. His/her personal value system may color the way the problem is perceived. In addition, the decision maker's ability to process data will determine the manner in which he or she compiles the data devise potential solution.

Another way to gauge the quality of a decision is to ask. Is the decision defensible? A defensible decision is one that can be explained and whose every step can be recalled if necessary (bailey and clause 1975). The decision maker must be able to state how and why the decision was made, to do this, it is essential to have adequate documentation, a written report can provide valuable information, exactly after time elapse and details is forgotten documentation teaches the decision maker to be through in the use of rational processes and provide self-assurance about the decision. It serves as a concrete method for demonstrating the soundness of the decision to anyone who is interested.

Finally to determine the quality of a decision, the results of the decision must be assessed. The highest quality decision is one in which the benefits outweigh the cost. The results also refer to how well the decision met the need or solved the original problem.

Acceptability: An effective decision must be high quality but it must be acceptable to the group affected by it. If the highest quality decision is not acceptable to the group, its effectiveness will be diminished. When acceptability is included as a criterion for making the decision, a more effective decision will be made.

39.5 STEPS IN DECISION-MAKING

1. **Defining a decision:** In this phase, recognition of a problem arises and a diagnosis is made. It is of a primary importance that the manager should first determine or specify his task, i.e. the aim or purpose to be achieved.
2. **Analyzing a decision:** In this phase, we analyze the decision by asking the questions: what is the decision for, what will it change, what will it achieve, and whom will it affect.
3. **Reviewing factors:** In this phase, we review the different factors which affect a situation.
4. **Analyzing possible course of action:** During this phase, we analyze all the possible alternatives. Having examined all the relevant factors, it should become clear that there are a number of courses of action open to us.
5. **Choosing the best alternatives:** During this phase, a particular course of action is selected from among those which are available. When the mind has carried out its calculations, it offers the decision.
6. **Implementing decision:** To implement means to put into action. The process of decision is not complete until it is implemented and we have learnt to live with the consequences.
7. **Evaluating decision:** The last step is decision making is the evaluation of the decision. Sometimes, there is vigorous criticism of the decision that has been made. The manager should proposed changes and their consequences.

39.6 DECISION-MAKING MECHANISM

A rational decision has some important assumptions. For example it assumes that:
1. All the alternatives of choices are known.
2. The consequences of all the alternatives are known.
3. The decision maker has a complete utility.
4. Ordering for all possible sets of consequences.

The assumptions are seldom fulfilled in practice. Decision maker does not information about all the alternatives. Even for a single alternative he may not have all the relevant information. He makes assumptions about some aspects of the decision. In fact major decisions which are non-programmed are made under the conditions of result ignorance. Besides lack of information about the alternatives for decision making. There is a problem in anticipating the consequences of various alternatives or the objectives sought to be achieved by a decision since the outcome of a decision can be known only in future. It is virtually impossible to know the exact outcome of the decision before things actually happen. This is more pronounced in the case of non-repetitive decision.

39.7 ADVANTAGES OF DECISION-MAKING

1. It is characterized by order and direction that enables managers to determine where they are.
2. Provide a framework for data gathering which is relevant to the decision.
3. Allows application of previous knowledge and experiences that minimize errors and improve quality of patient care and work of an organization.
4. Increase manager's confidence and ability to make sound decisions.

39.8 HUMAN FACTORS IN DECISION-MAKING

A major source of limit in rationality in human factor in decision-making, personal factors affect the choice of an alternative in two ways.
1. First the choice is an ordering of a kind of personal preference and decision maker cannot eliminate his personal preference together.

2. Second choice depends on various qualitative information and its interpretation is likely to be personalized. This is the reason why major organized decisions are changed when a new chief executive with different personality features takes over the change of an organization. The major human factors which affect rationality in decision-making are the following:
   Personal value system: It is framework of personal philosophy which governs and influences the individual reaction and responses to any situation. Personal value system is viewed as a relatively permanent framework which shapes the general nature of behavior. Thus, what is good or bad as judged as the basis of personal value system. Therefore, it cannot only affect the choice of alternatives in terms of what should be best for the organization, but also in terms of perception of various situations under which an alternative is being chosen.
   Perception: Problems and their solutions are quiet abstract in nature. Then there is a likely food that individual's perception regarding the problems and their solutions are different and consequently the way of talking the problems may be different. This is so because people act according to what they seen.
   Political power and behavior: Political and power behavior in an organization also affects the extent to which a decision would be national. Since, the major choices in an organization are arrived at after a lot of consultation and involvement of various people at some stage of total decision-making process. Their interaction plays significant part in the choice process for example Mintzberg has identified three ways in which major decisions are made these are judgment, bargaining and analysis. In judgment, the choice is made in a single individual should and others do not contribute. In bargaining, choice is made by a group of decision makers with conflicting objectives. In analysis, factual data are brought to bear systematically on the evaluation process.
   Time constraints: Time factor also affects the rationality in decision-making. In many cases even though further information is needed, decisions are made only with partial data. This may be purposeful however it is often merely a reaction to the time limitation, placed on decision makers. When one makes several decisions every day. Some of major significance and others of only criteria justify making their promptly.
   Creativity and decision-making: In today's dynamic environment, creativity is vital in decision making. There are various terms which are used as synonyms to creativity, such as discover, intertion extending boundary etc. Examples of creativity in decision-making may be creation of new method, creation of new product, creation of new market and so on.

In general, creativity means a talent for unique combination or unusual association of ideas. Creativity is synthesis, thus from decision-making point of view creativity can be thought of in terms of generating ideas which are unique to the solution of the problem under consideration. John Mc has define creative thinking and the process of bringing problem before one's mind, clearly as by imagining, visualizing, supposing, contemplating or the like and then originating an idea, concept, realization or picture along a new lines.

39.9 ROLE OF CREATIVITY IN DECISION-MAKING

Creativity is vital for decision-making whether it is organizational decision or personal decision one skill that significantly differentiates good decision major from poor is creativity. The creativity to develop alternatives extracts possibilities and image consequences and role of creativity is maximum in generating alternatives which can be considered for evaluation and choice. Creativity is required specially for solving problem which is nonrepetitive and unique; such problems cannot solve by known method and past experience is not enough in this case. A fresh approach, a new twist, a novel arrangement of recognized. Parts on the addition of different materials on system are often necessary to find an acceptable solution.

For a manager, it is essential that he is thoroughly conversant with the problem at hand. For this saturation stage normally begins in thorough familiarity with a problem itself, its history, its importance, its relationship to other parts of the business and its setting. This will provide the manager a insight in identifying the real problem and he can think for suitable solution.

Preparation: Knowledge alone no matter, now complete doesn't generate creative ideas. The decision maker has to go through preparation stage at which he tries to collect information relating to the problem. He may recall his past experience and also study new materials. It should be recognized that something new does not come instantaneously or oversight. The preparation stage may last few minutes, hours; days or weeks, during this stage the person really suffer from anxiety and frustration. At this stage, creativity thinking may deliberate the problem with others deliberation usually includes three steps:

1. Analysis.
2. Building relationship and patterns.
3. Seeking useful rearrangements or combinations.

Incubation: If no solution of problem is found at the stage of preparation, creative person attempts to solve the problem and to forget about it. He may engage himself in activities totally in connected with the problem. However, he may solve the problem consciously, but it may exist in the subconscious mind. During the process of incubation, the mind will work subconsciously to create certain new ideas. This is so because a new idea is created, in the conscious mind, after certain amount of sorting and manipulating the multitude of information stored there.

Illumination: The illumination stage of creativity is characterized by a flash of insight or a sudden spontaneous solution. There are many cases where many great ideas have cone in the minds of creative thinkers, when they have not been engaged in thinking process.

Verification: This is the final stage of creative process and involves verifying, modifying or applying the ideas towards the solution of the problem under studies. During this stage, mind sets about by logical method or by experimentation to prove or disprove the solution that has been suggested. Critical thinking is used in both problem solving and decision-making.

In everyday practice, nurses make decisions about patient care. As the nurse gains experience in clinical practice, decision-making becomes somewhat automatic, but the complexity of many decisions remains. Both decision-making and problem-solving use critical thinking. Although decisions are unique to different situations, the decision-making process can be applied to each situation. The decision-making process is similar to the steps in problem-solving.

39.10 INDIVIDUAL DECISION-MAKING

There are many nonprogrammed decisions that are made by an individual in his capacity as a manager or a decision maker, but the individual decision is not generally so rational. According to Simon "it is impossible for the behavior of a single isolated individual to reach any high degree of rationality". There is consideration between certain characteristics of the decision maker such as age, intelligence, and experience in a given area, motivation, and decision accuracy confidence in the decision. There are certain impact the decision maker in decision making. They are as follows:

Information inputs: It is very important to have adequate and accurate information about the situation for decision-making.

Prejudice: Prejudice and bias are introduced by perceptual process and may cause or to make ineffective decision. First of all, the perception is highly selective which means what we want to accept and hence only such information filling down to our senses, the perception is highly subjective.

Cognitive constraints: Simon has suggested that a human brain is limited in capacity in a number of ways. Firstly our memory is short-term with a capacity of few words ideas, words and symbols. Secondly, psychologically we are always uncomfortable with decision-making and we are never sure, if our choice of the alternative was correct or optimum which makes us feel very insecure.

Attitudes, risk and uncertainty: These attitudes are developed in a person partly due to certain personal characteristics and partly due to organizational characteristics. Harrison have concluded that the risk taking attitude is influenced by:

1. Intelligence of the decision maker.
2. Expectations of the decision maker.
3. Time constraints.

Personal habits: Personal habits have great impact on organizational operations and effectiveness. Some people stick to their decisions even if these decisions are not optimal and try to shift the blame on failure on outside factors rather than their own mistakes.

Cultural and social influences: The social and group norms extent considerable influence on the style of the decision maker. Cultural upbringing and dimensions have a profound impact on the decision-making style on individual.

39.11 GROUP DECISION-MAKING

Group decisions are appropriate in nonprogrammed decisions because these decisions are complex and few individuals have all the knowledge and skills necessary to make the best decision. However, there are some factors to be considered when determining which approach to take in the process of decision-making. They are:

1. Importance of quality decision.
2. The extent to which the manager process the information and expertise to make a high quality decision.
3. The extent to which the subordinates have the necessary information to assist in generating high quality decision.
4. The extent to which the problem is structured.
5. The probability that the manager's decision will be accepted by the subordinates.
6. The extent to which the subordinates will be motivated to achieve the organizational goals.

Advantages of Group Decision-making

1. Since, the group members have different special they tend to provide more information and knowledge.
2. Implementation of the decision is more effective.
3. The input from a large numbers of people element the bases, that are generally introduced in individual decision-making.
4. It develops groundwork as a training ground for subordinates who develop the skills of objective analysis and derive conclusions.
5. The group decision-making is more democratic in nature.
6. It increases their efficiency.
7. It develops a sense of responsibility among worker.
8. Worker should make their whole heartiest efforts for the accomplishment of predetermined targets of the enterprise.

Disadvantages of Group Decision-making

1. It is highly time-consuming in assembling the right group.
2. Some members may simply agree with the others for the sake of agreement since there are social pressures to confirm not to be the odd man out.
3. The decisions made by the group may not always in accordance with goals and objectives of the organization.
4. The group members may exhibit "flows effect".

CONCLUSION

In hospital situation many problems arise. At the onset collect as many aspects as possible about the particular problem. All the factors should be thoroughly perceived and understood. All those persons concerned with the problem should be contacted and the problem should be well discussed with them. See if the past and present emotional or physical health status of any member has any connection with the problem. The problem also has to be dealt in the light of the existent rules and regulations and policies of the hospital. After having gathered all the aspects and factors of the problem. The in-charge person has to perform rather a difficult and careful task of making a decision. One should follow a routine of writing out all the facts and possible alternatives involved in the problem.

40 Supervision

40.1 INTRODUCTION

Supervision means overseeing the employees at work. It has been defined as the authoritative direction of the work of one's subordinates. It is a necessary concomitant of their hierarchical organization in which each level of subordinate to the one immediately above it and subject to its, orders. Workers at the intermediate levels of the organization supervise as well as are supervised. They supervise the work of those immediately below them and their own work is subjected to the supervision of their superior officers. At the lower level of the organization, however supervision occurs in its pure form over the first line workers who in their turn supervise on one else's work.

The nature and scope of supervision varies with the kind of the work to be supervised, the type of the people to be supervised, the extent of the supervisor's responsibility and the level of supervision. Thus, supervision of production in factories is different from the supervision of nurses' work in the hospital, or supervision of the office work.

40.2 DEFINITION

Supervision means observing the subordinates at work to see that they are working according to plans and policies of the organization and keeping the time to educate and to help them solving their work problems.

40.3 OBJECTIVES OF SUPERVISION

1. Help the staff to do their job skillfully and effectively to give maximum output with minimum resources-cost effectiveness.
2. Help the staff develop the individual capacity to the fullest extent with a view to channels the same in favor of work.
3. Guide and/or assist in meeting predetermined work objectives or targets. In nursing preventive, promotive, curative and rehabilitative care to people.
4. Help to promote effectiveness of the subordinates/staffs. Ensuring that the subordinate staff or supervise does what he/she supposed to do.
5. Help to motivate subordinates to maintain high morale, i.e. promotion of motivation and morale among all the nursing staff.
6. Help the members of the team to recognize problems, identify solutions and to take action.
7. Help to develop team spirit and promote team work for effective functioning.
8. Help to improve the attitudes of the members towards the work or programme, i.e. bridging the gap between the workers' personal goal and the organizational goal by providing guidance in the right direction.

40.4 FUNCTIONS OF SUPERVISOR

H. Nilsson gives the following list of eleven principal duties of a supervisor:

1. To understand the duties and responsibilities of his own position.
2. To plan the execution of the work.
3. To divide the work among subordinates and to direct and assist them in doing it.
4. To improve his own knowledge as technical expert and leader.
5. To improve his work methods and procedures.
6. To train the personnel.
7. To evaluate the performance of the employees.
8. To correct mistakes, solve employees' problems and develop discipline.
9. To keep subordinates informed about policies and procedures of the organization above the changes to be made.
10. To cooperate with colleagues and seek advice and assistance when needed, and
11. To deal with employee suggestions and complaints.

40.5 FACTORS INFLUENCES EFFECTIVE SUPERVISION

1. **Human relations skill:** Supervision is mainly concerned with instructing, guiding and inspiring human beings towards greater performance. For purposes of direction, the supervisor has to rely on leadership, counseling, communication and other determinants of human relations.
2. **Technical and managerial knowledge:** Guidance implies a complete understanding of all work problems, for which the supervisor should have good knowledge about technical aspect of job and also the managerial aspects.
3. **Leadership position:** The authority of supervisors must be made commensurate with their duty so as to make the job of supervision a satisfying, rewarding and challenging one. So, the supervisors are to be vested with necessary authority for enabling them to exercise leadership over the group and influence the employees.

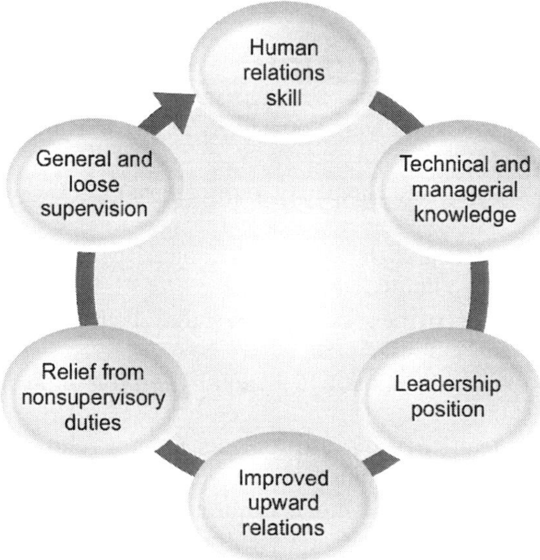

Fig. 40.1: Factor influencing effective supervision

4. **Improved upward relations:** To ensure good quality of supervision, the supervisor's upward relations must be well-established, which means to say that supervisors should be regularly allowed to present their views and suggestions to top executives in regard to the personnel and their work performance, for which, the top management must pay adequate attention and thought on supervisory jobs to ensure good quality supervisions.
5. **Relief from nonsupervisory duties:** To make the supervisory duties purposeful, the supervisors are to be relieved of many routine activities that divert their attention from the real job.
6. **General and loose supervision:** According to some experience, the general and loose supervision is more productive than close supervision. Here, the leader must allow freedom and initiative to his followers for pursuing a common course of action.

40.6 PRINCIPLES OF SUPERVISION

1. Supervision differs from one person to another.
2. It strives to make the unit good learning situation.
3. Good supervision is well-planned
4. Good supervision fosters the ability of each staff member to think and act for herself.
5. Good supervision helps the individual nurse set up objectives which are for her dynamic, reasonable and worthwhile.
6. Good supervision helps her to attain her objectives.
7. Good supervision helps the nurse to make a pattern for analysis and to analyze continuously her success in reaching her objectives.
8. Good supervision respects the personality of the nurse.
9. Good supervision stimulates the nurse's ambition to grow in effectiveness.

40.7 QUALIFICATIONS OF SUPERVISOR

1. Should be trained person—professional training and experience.
2. Should understand the training background and ability of the supervised.
3. Should have good knowledge of local practices, cultural patterns health problems in general and available resources of the community.
4. Have at least five year experience as community health nurse.
5. Be intelligent capable of learning readily and of retaining the knowledge.
6. Be able to convey knowledge to the others in an understanding and interesting way.
7. Through knowledge about administrative regulations.
8. Be able when necessary, to show authority without being too demanding and without losing the respect of subordinates.
9. Self-confidence and be able to gain the confidence of others.
10. Set the climate for cooperation between coworker and shifts for a smoothing running.

40.8 QUALITIES OF SUPERVISOR

1. Should have human approach to human problems.
2. Competent to take quick decisions.
3. Honest in dealing with subordinates.
4. Should have patience and does not lose temper.
5. Should not depend up on his formal authority too much.
6. Should be a good leader to guide the subordinates.
7. Should have sufficient technical skill to perform the jobs to be supervised.

8. Maintain interest in good nursing care.
9. Be able to promote good public relations.
10. Keep up with new trends in nursing and be able to do convey this information to others.

40.9 TECHNIQUES OF SUPERVISION

Supervision means overseeing the employees at work. It has been defined as the authoritative direction of the work of one's subordinates. Supervision is the art of overseeing, watching and directing with inspecting another's work, evaluating her or his performance and approving or correcting performance.

1. Group conference.
2. Individual conference.
3. Anecdotal records.
4. Initial conference.
5. Control of early experience.
6. Assistance with bedside care.
7. Reassurance.
8. Supervision of nursing procedure.
9. Conferences—Individual group.
10. Incidental teaching.

40.10 SUPERVISION METHODS

Supervision is a process of helping and enabling a cooperative relationship between the supervisor and the individual supervised. The primary aim of supervision is to help the individual develop his capabilities to the fullest, so that he will be able to serve most efficiently. A supervisor personally sees the performance in order to make sure that the work is done according to the rules and regulations.

Supervision strives to make the ward a platform for good learning. It should be well-planned. Good supervision helps the nurse to think and act for her, set up her own objectives and also to attain them through approval, commendation and self analysis. It helps to enhance the personality of the nurse.

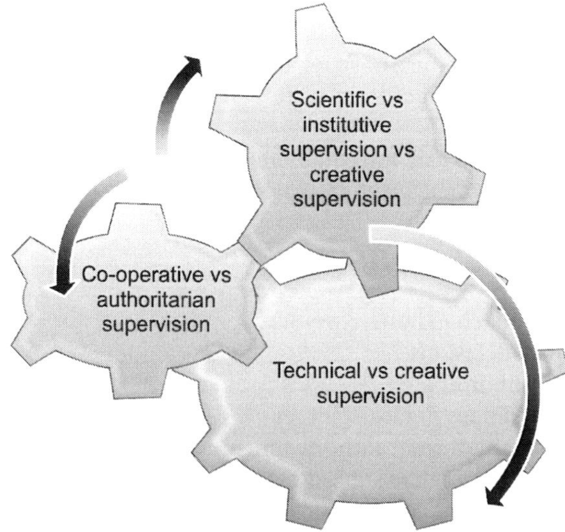

Fig. 40.2: Methods of supervision

1. **Technical vs creative supervision:** Technical methods are some of the basic supervisory skills which need to be trained. Group conferences, group discussions. For example, techniques of service study, record construction, time study etc. Creative supervision provides maximum adaptation to the situation. For example instead of a orientation period of two weeks for each new staff member, a variable plan in both contents and time according to the needs of each individual should be formulated.
2. **Cooperative vs authoritarian supervision:** In cooperative supervision there is a full participation of each member of the group in planning, action and decision whereas in authorities supervision responsibility ventures entirely on the supervisor with the staff following his/her.
3. **Scientific vs institutive supervision:** Scientific supervision relies on objective study and measurement than personal judgment or opinion. Whereas inactive supervision needs to maintain the interpersonal relationship. The supervision needs a sensitive and intuitive reaction to the emotional needs of other person.

CONCLUSION

The supervisor has to maintain thoroughness, fairness, initiation, tact, enthusiasm, emotional contact (Halsey) when dealing with his job. Prior to that, supervisor should possess personal qualifications like integrity, honesty, ability to cooperate, should be approachable ability to motivate and unite others to work, and should also have teaching ability, i.e. ability to communicate with the workers. In addition to the above, since the supervision is a process of providing constant observation, guidance and appraisal for the personnel providing nursing care, the supervisor is expected to develop certain skills like interpersonal and professional skills to acquire specific knowledge. He should have personal and professional knowledge and should be able to inculcate an attitude that will be helpful in developing leadership behavior.

41 Problem-Solving

41.1 INTRODUCTION

Problems can also be classified into two different types (ill-defined and well-defined) from which appropriate solutions are to be made. Ill-defined problems are those that do not have clear goals, solution paths, or expected solution. Well-defined problems have specific goals, clearly defined solution paths, and clear expected solutions. These problems also allow for more initial planning than ill-defined problems. Being able to solve problems sometimes involves dealing with pragmatics (logic) and semantics (interpretation of the problem). The ability to understand what the goal of the problem is and what rules could be applied represents the key to solving the problem. Sometimes the problem requires some abstract thinking and coming up with a creative solution. Problem-solving as a deliberate and serious act, involves the use of some novel methods, higher thinking and systematic scientific steps for the realization of the set goals.

41.2 DEFINITION

1. Problem-solving is a process of overcoming difficulties that appear to interfere with the attainment of a goal. It is a procedure of making adjustments in spite of interferences.
2. Problem-solving is a process and skill that you develop over time to be used when needing to solve immediate problems in order to achieve a goal.

41.3 SKILLS OF PROBLEM-SOLVING

Problem-solving requires two distinct types of mental skill, analytical and creative.

Analytical or logical thinking includes skills such as ordering, comparing, contrasting, evaluating and selecting. It provides a logical framework for problem solving and helps to select the best alternative from those available by narrowing down the range of possibilities (a convergent process). Analytical thinking often predominates in solving closed problems, where the many possible causes have to be identified and analyzed to find the real cause.

Creative thinking is a divergent process, using the imagination to create a large range of ideas for solutions. It requires us to look beyond the obvious, creating ideas which may, at first, seem unrealistic or have no logical connection with the problem. There is a large element of creative thinking in solving open problems. The creative thinking skills can be divided into several key elements:

1. **Fluency**—producing many ideas.
2. **Flexibility**—producing a broad range of ideas.
3. **Originality**—producing uncommon ideas.
4. **Elaboration**—developing ideas.

Effective problem solving requires a controlled mixture of analytical and creative thinking. Research has shown that, in general terms, each side or hemisphere of the brain is specialized to serve one of these groups of skills. The degree of specialization of each hemisphere varies from person to person, but it has given rise to the terms right-brain thinking and left-brain thinking. Left-brain thinking is more logical and analytical, and is predominantly verbal. Right-brain thinking is more holistic and is concerned with feelings and impressionistic relationships.

To be a good problem solver you need to be able to switch from one group of skills to the other and back again, although this is not always easy. Traditional education gives far greater encouragement to the development and use of left-brain thinking. This is reinforced in the way we are required to work, where emphasis is placed on rational, logical analysis of data in drawing conclusions.

Some other terms which are often used in discussions of creativity include:

1. **Intuition:** The ability to draw conclusions based on impressions and feelings rather than hard facts. It is a characteristic of right-brain thinking and some people rely on it more than others.
2. **Incubation:** The period between stopping conscious work on a problem and the time when we become aware of a solution or part solution. People struggling with problems often suddenly become aware of a solution after a period of incubation, during which the mind is occupied by other things.
3. **Invention:** The creation of new, meaningful ideas or concepts.
4. **Innovation:** Putting new ideas or concepts to a practical use, as in the development of a new product or service.

41.4 PROBLEM SOLVING CYCLE

Blood seven-step problem solving cycle: There are many different ways to solve a problem, however all ways involve a series of steps. The following is a seven-step problem solving model:

Step-1: Identify the problem: Firstly you need to identify and name the problem so that you can find an appropriate solution. You may not be clear of what the problem is or feel anxious/confused about what is getting in the way of your goals. Try talking to others, as this may help you identify the problem.

Step-2: Explore the problem: When you are clear about what the problem is you need to think about from different angles. You can ask yourself questions such as:

1. How is this problem affecting me?
2. How is it affecting others?
3. Who else experiences this problem?
4. What do they do about it?

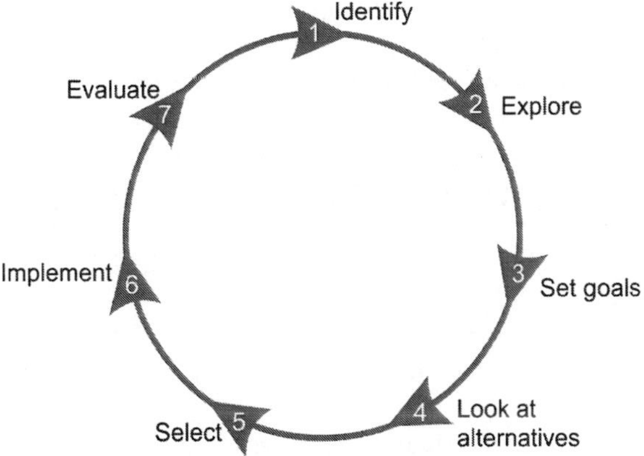

Fig. 41.1: Seven-step problem-solving cycle

Seeing the problem in different ways is likely to help you find an effective solution.

Step-3: Set goals: Once you have thought about the problem from different angles you can identify your goals. What is it that you want to achieve? Sometimes you may become frustrated by a problem and forget to think about what you want to achieve. For example, you might become ill, struggle to complete a number of assignments on time and feel so unmotivated that you let due dates pass.

1. Improve your health?
2. Increase your time management skills?
3. Complete the assignments to the best of your ability?
4. Finish the assignments as soon as possible?

If you decide your goal is to improve your health that will lead to different solutions to those linked with the goal of completing your assignments as soon as possible. One goal may lead you to a doctor and another may lead you to apply for extensions for your assignments. So working out your goals is a vital part of the problem solving process.

Step-4: Look at alternatives: When you have decided what your goal(s) is you need to look for possible solutions. The more possible solutions you find the more likely it is that you will be able to discover an effective solution. You can brain-storm for ideas. The purpose of brain-storming is to collect together a long list of possibilities. It does not matter whether the ideas are useful or practical or manageable: just write down the ideas as they come into your head. Some of the best solutions arise from creative thinking during brain-storming. You can also seek ideas about possible solutions by talking to others. The aim is to collect as many alternative solutions as possible.

Step-5: Select a possible solution: From the list of possible solutions you can sort out which are most relevant to your situation and which are realistic and manageable. You can do this by predicting the outcomes for possible solutions and also checking with other people what they think the outcomes may be. When you have explored the consequences, you can use this information to identify the solution which is most relevant to you and is likely to have the best outcomes for your situation.

Step-6: Implement a possible solution: Once you have selected a possible solution you are ready to put it into action. You will need to have energy and motivation to do this because implementing the solution may take some time and effort. You can prepare yourself to implement the solution by planning when and how you will do it, whether you talk with others about it, and what rewards you will give yourself when you have done it.

Step-7: Evaluate: Just because you have implemented the best possible solution, you may not have automatically solved your problem, so evaluating the effectiveness of your solution is very important. You can ask yourself and others:

1. How effective was that solution?
2. Did it achieve what I wanted?
3. What consequences did it have on my situation?

If the solution was successful in helping you, solve your problem and reach your goal, then you know that you have effectively solved your problem. If you feel dissatisfied with the result, then you can begin the steps again.

41.5 SCIENTIFIC METHOD OF PROBLEM SOLVING

1. Problem awareness.
2. Problem understanding.
3. Collection of relevant information.
4. Formulation of hypothesis or hunch for possible solution.
5. Selection of a proper solution.
6. Verification of the concluded solution or hypothesis.

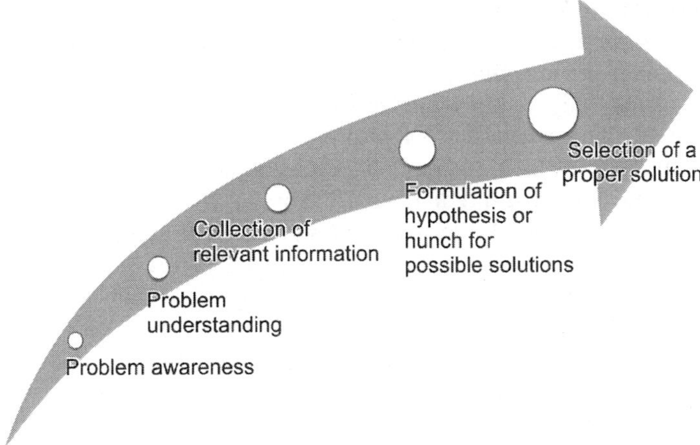

Fig. 41.2: Scientific methods of problem-solving

1. **Problem awareness:** The first step in problem solving behavior of an individual concerns his awareness of the difficulty or problem that needs a solution.
2. **Problem understanding:** The difficulty or problem experienced by the individual should be properly identified by a careful analysis. He should be clear about his problem. The problem then should be pinpointed in terms of the specific goals and objectives. Thus, all the difficulties and obstacles in the path of the solution must be properly named and identified and what is to be got through the problem-solving efforts should then be properly analyzed.
3. **Collection of relevant information:** In this step, the individual is required to collect all the relevant information about the problem through all possible sources. He may consult experienced persons, read the available literature, revive his old experiences, think of possible solutions and put in all relevant efforts for widening the scope of his knowledge concerning the problem in hand.
4. **Formulation of hypothesis or hunch for possible solutions:** In the light of the collected relevant information and nature of his problem, one may then engage in some serious cognitive activities to think of the various possibilities for the solution of one's problem. As a result, he may start with a few possible solutions for his problem.
5. **Selection of a proper solution:** In this step, all the possible solutions, thought of in the previous step, are closely analyzed and evaluated. Gates et al. (1946) have suggested the following activities in the evaluation of the assumed hypothesis or solution:
    1. One should determine the conclusion that completely satisfies the demands of the problem.
    2. One should find out whether the solution is consistent with other facts and principles which have been well-established.
    3. One should make a deliberate search for negative instances which might cast doubts on the conclusion.

The above suggestions can help the individual to consider a suitable solution for his problem out of the many possible solutions.

41.6 PROBLEM-SOLVING STRATERGY

Problem-solving strategies are the steps that one would use to find the problem(s) that are in the way to getting to one's own goal. Some would refer to this as the 'problem-solving cycle'. (Bransford and Stein, 1993) In this cycle, one will recognize the problem, define the problem, develop a strategy to fix the problem, organize the knowledge of the problem, figure-out the resources at the user's disposal, monitor one's progress, and evaluate the solution for accuracy. Although called a cycle, one does not have to do each step in order to fix the problem, in fact those who don't are usually better at problem-solving. The reason it is called a cycle is that once one is completed with a problem another usually will pop up. Blanchard-Fields (2007) looks at problem-solving from one of two facets. The first looking at those problems that only have one solution (like math problems, or fact based questions) which are grounded in psychometric intelligence. The other that is socioemotional in nature and are unpredictable with answers that are constantly changing.

The following techniques are usually called problem-solving strategies:

1. **Abstraction:** Solving the problem in a model of the system before applying it to the real system.
2. **Analogy:** Using a solution that solves an analogous problem.
3. **Brain storming:** (especially among groups of people) suggesting a large number of solutions or ideas and combining and developing them until an optimum solution is found.
4. **Divide and conquer:** Breaking down a large, complex problem into smaller, solvable problems.
5. **Hypothesis testing:** assuming a possible explanation to the problem and trying to prove (or, in some contexts, disprove) the assumption.
6. **Lateral thinking:** Approaching solutions indirectly and creatively.
7. **Means-end analysis:** Choosing an action at each step to move closer to the goal.
8. **Method of focal objects:** Synthesizing seemingly non-matching characteristics of different objects into something new.
9. **Morphological analysis:** Assessing the output and interactions of an entire system.
10. **Proof:** Try to prove that the problem cannot be solved. The point where the proof fails will be the starting point for solving it.
11. **Reduction:** Transforming the problem into another problem for which solutions exist.
12. **Research:** Employing existing ideas or adapting existing solutions to similar problems.
13. **Root-cause analysis:** Identifying the cause of a problem.
14. **Trial and error:** Testing possible solutions until the right one is found.

CONCLUSION

Problem-solving and decision-making are important skills for business and life. Problem-solving often involves decision-making, and decision-making is especially important for management and leadership. There are processes and techniques to improve decision-making and the quality of decisions. Decision-making is more natural to certain personalities, so these people should focus more on improving the quality of their decisions. People that are less natural decision-makers are often able to make quality assessments, but then need to be more decisive in acting upon the assessments made. Problem-solving and decision-making are closely linked, and each requires creativity in identifying and developing options, for which the brain storming technique is particularly useful.

42 Nursing Rounds

42.1 INTRODUCTION

There are several methods that can be used effectively in clinical teaching. Nursing rounds are conducted by the head nurse/nurse teacher for the members of her staff/students. To be successful every nurse must be prepared to participate in the discussion of nursing care.

42.2 DEFINITION

Nursing rounds are conducted by the head nurse/nurse teacher for the members of her staff/ students for a clear understanding of the disease process and the effect of nursing care for each patient.

42.3 PURPOSES OF NURSING ROUNDS

The purpose for ward rounds includes:

1. To observe the physical and the mental condition of the patients and the progress made day to day.
2. To observe the work of staff.
3. To make specific observation of the patient and to give report to doctor, e.g. wound, drainage, bleeding etc.
4. To introduce the patients to the personnel and vice versa.
5. To carry out the plan made for the care of the patients.
6. To evaluate the results of treatment and the satisfaction of the patient with his care.
7. To ensure the safety measures employed for the patient and personnel.
8. To orient the nurse/student in handing over/taking over regarding patient's treatment, care done, care yet to be completed and condition of the patient.
9. To teach the nursing students and the hospital aids regarding specific conditions.
10. To check any preventable conditions present in the patient such as bedsore, foot drop etc.
11. To cheek the emergency equipment kept near the patient and to check their safety and working order.
12. To compare the clinical manifestation of the patients having some disease so that the student understand in a better manner and gain better insight.
13. To prescribe any modification in nursing action.

42.4 IMPORTANCE OF NURSING ROUNDS

1. In nursing rounds the patient's history and the medical aspects of his care are included only as a background for the understanding of the nursing care.

2. The nurse/teacher who have been caring for the patient during the week may present the background information and tell the points in nursing care which she considers to be most essential.
3. She is then responsible for answering the questions of the class including these of the head nurse.
4. In another method of conducting rounds, the head nurse/teacher may involve any nurse in the group to tell what she knows about the patient and his nursing care; other students make addition and suggestions and help to answer the questions.
5. This method is a means of testing the student's knowledge and acquaintance with all the patients on the floor.
6. Students prepare by studying indications and actions of drug.
7. Students are told prior to rounds so that they may prepare themselves.

42.5 ROLE OF HEAD NURSE IN NURSING ROUNDS

1. In preparing for rounds the nurse selects the patients who are to be discussed in relation to the time which has been set aside for the purpose.
2. Rounds should properly not last longer than 20 minutes.
3. The head nurse needs to read the patient's progress and prognosis, their nursing care and its effectiveness.
4. She should post the time for rounds at least a week in advance and indicates the type of preparation the nurse is to make, i.e. whether she is to know thoroughly the history, care and progress of her own patients or briefly that of all patients in the ward.
5. Patient with similar diagnosis but with differing history, treatment, and prognosis may be selected or varied conditions existing in the same ward also can selected for teaching purpose.
6. Rounds for staff nurses should be held separately from those for students since the background of the two groups vary widely.
7. Rounds for students in their first clinical term may need to be held separately.

42.6 ADVANTAGES OF NURSING ROUNDS

1. This method is a means of testing the student's knowledge and acquaintance with the entire patient's on the floor.
2. The students, who are informed prior to rounds, benefit the maximum in real life teaching method.
3. No other type of rounds is a substitute for nursing rounds.
4. It is always be very valuable for the head nurse to go on regular nursing rounds with clinical instructor.
5. An intelligent nurse with creative abilities may find many other ways of successfully assisting student nurses to develop nursing skills.
6. Helps in orienting a new nurse/student to the patients.
7. An interesting strategy involving the student, teacher and the patient.
8. It offers a real life learning situation.
9. Evaluation of nursing activity, hurdles faced by nurses in implementing or success nursing care can be appraised.

42.7 DISADVANTAGES OF NURSING ROUNDS

1. The confidentiality of the patient is hampered.
2. The patient may over hear the discussion and he may not like the thought that he is being talked about if he cannot hear.

3. If the group is large the teacher may not able to speak loudly enough to be heard, in which case the attention of individuals who are on the fringes is lost.
4. Distractions are present in ward.
5. An unprepared nursing round has little teaching-learning value.
6. Quality of nursing rounds on the quality and presentation of the nurse teacher/head nurse.

CONCLUSION

Nursing care is touched on only briefly if at all. Nursing rounds are conducted by the head nurse for the members of her staff and also beneficial for students. To be successful every nurse must be prepared to participate in the discussion of nursing care.

43 Stress Management

43.1 INTRODUCTION

Stress is difficult to define precisely. The concept of stress was first introduced in the life sciences by Selye Hans in 1936. It was derived from the Latin word 'stringere'; it meant the experience of physical hardship, starvation, torture and pain. Hans Selye, 1936 defined stress as "the nonspecific response of the body to any demand placed upon it". Further, stress was defined as "any external event or internal drive which threatens to upset the organismic equilibrium" (Hans Selye, 1956). Another definition given by Stephen Robbins (1999) stress has been stated as "a dynamic condition in which an individual is confronted with an opportunity, constraint or demand related to what he/she desires and for which the outcome is perceived to be both uncertain and important."

43.2 DEFINITION

1. According to Selye (1956) stress is "any external event or internal drive which threatens to upset the organismic equilibrium".
2. Wolf and Goodell (1968) defined stress as a dynamic state within an organism in response to a demand for adaptation.
3. Cofer and Appley (1964) defined stress as a state of an organism where he perceives that his well-being is endangered and that he must direct all his energies to its protection.
4. Lazarus (1966) referred stress a state of imbalance with in an organism that is elicited by an actual/perceived disparity between environmental demands and the organism's capacity to cope with these demands; and is manifested through variety of physiological, emotional and behavioral responses.
5. McGrath (1970) defined stress as a perceived imbalance between demand and response capacity under conditions where failure to meet demand has important consequences.
6. Cox (1978) has described three classes of definitions. Stress can be variously thought of as a response, i.e. the stress response to an extreme stimulus; as a stimulus, i.e. as the stressor itself as an intervening variable.

43.3 CONCEPT OF STRESS

Stress can have physical, emotional, intellectual, social, and spiritual consequences. Usually, the effects are mixed, because stress affects the whole person. Physically, stress can threaten a person's physiologic homeostasis. Emotionally, stress can produce negative or nonconstructive feelings about self. Intellectually, stress can influence a person's perceptual and problem-solving abilities. Socially, stress can alter a person's relationships with others. Spiritually, stress can challenge one's beliefs and values. Many illness have been linked to stress.

Stress is defined in a number of ways:

1. As a stimulus.
2. As a response, and
3. As a transaction.

43.4 STRESS AS A STIMULUS

Stress may be defined as a stimulus, a life event (sometimes called a "life change") or a set of circumstances causing a disrupted response that increases the individual's vulnerability to illness.

Both positive and negative events are considered stressful. Research has shown that people who have a high level of stress are often more prone to illness and have lowered ability to cope with illness and subsequent stress.

43.5 STRESS RESPONSE

Stress is a physiological or psychological tension that threatens homeostasis or a person's psychological equilibrium. Stress is defined as a broad class of experiences in which tension occurs when demanding situations tax the resources, coping and level of adoption of individual. Stress is any characteristic of the environment which threatens a person's demands, perceived as difficult to meet or as insufficient to meet one's need.

Variations of Stress

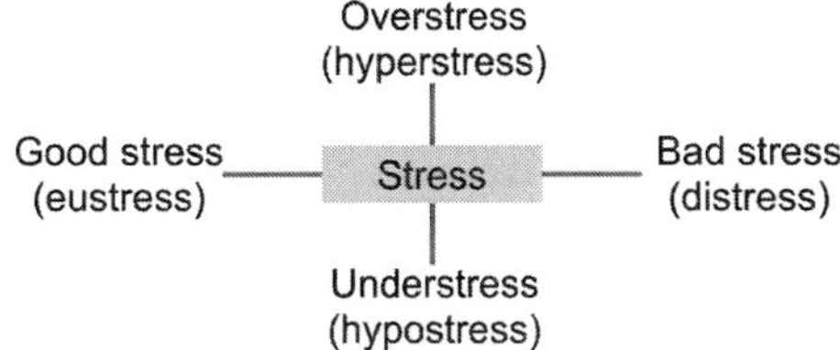

Stress is a state produced by a change in the environment that is perceived as challenging, threatening or damaging to a person's dynamic balance or equilibrium.

Stress Cycle

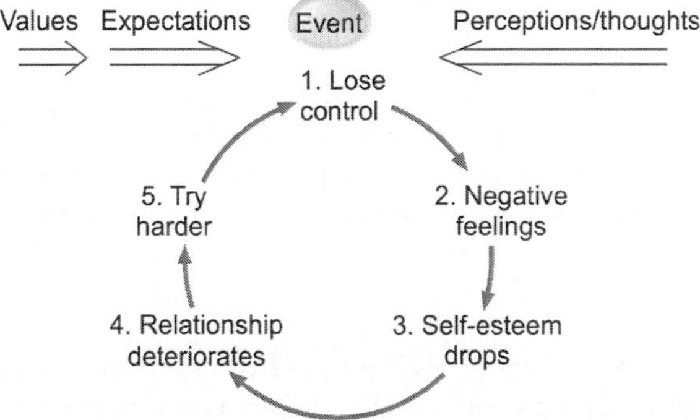

Hans Selye defined stress as "the non-specific response of the body to any kind of demand made upon it". To differentiate the cause of stress from the response of stress, Selye created the term stressor to denote any factor that produces stress and disturbs the body's equilibrium. Because stress alters the body it can be observed only by the changes it produces in the body. This response of the body, the stress syndrome or the General Adaptation Syndrome (GAS) occurs with the release of certain adaptive hormones and subsequent changes in the structure and chemical composition of the body.

In addition to adapting globally, the body can also react locally; that is, one organ or a part of the body reacts alone. This is referred to as the Local Adaptation Syndrome (LAS). One example of the LAS is inflammation.

Selye proposed that both the GAS and the LAS had three stages:

1. Alarm reaction.
2. Resistance.
3. Exhaustion.

Alarm reaction (AR): The initial reaction of the body is the alarm reaction (AR), which alerts the body's defenses against the stressor. Selye divided this stage into two parts:

1. The shock phase and
2. The counter shock phase.

During the shock phase, the autonomic nervous system reacts. The person is then ready for fight or flight. The second part of the alarm reaction is called the counter shock phase. During this time, the body changes produced during the shock phase is reversed.

Stage of resistance (SR): It is during the second stage in the GAS and the LAS syndrome that the Stage of Resistance (SR), the body's adaptation, takes place. In other words, the body attempts to cope with the stressor and to limit the stressor to the smallest area of the body that can deal with it.

Stage of exhaustion (SE): During the third stage, the stage of exhaustion (SE), the adaptation that the body made during the second stage cannot be maintained; this means that the ways used to cope with the stressor has been exhausted.

43.6 MANIFESTATIONS OF STRESS

Manifestations of the stress experience, both physiologic and psychological, may be considered coping or mechanisms. Coping is "the cognitive and behavioral effort to manage specific external and/internal demands that are appraised as taxing or exceeding the resources of the person". Coping can be adaptive o maladaptive. Adaptive coping helps the person to deal effectively with stressful events and minimizes stress. Ineffective coping results in maladaptation.

Physiologic manifestations: Physiologic manifestation may or may not occur in clients experiencing stress, depending on the way the client perceives the stressful event and on the effectiveness of the client's coping strategies. Specific physiologic manifestations are presented below:

1. Pupils dilate to increase visual perception.
2. Sweat production (diaphoresis).
3. The heart beat increases, which leads to an increased pulse rate to transport of nutrients.
4. Skin is pallid because of construction of peripheral blood vessels, and effect of nor epinephrine.
5. Blood pressure increases because of constriction of vessels in blood reservoirs.
6. The rate and depth of respirations increase because of dilation of the bronchioles, promoting hyperventilation.
7. Urinary output decreases.
8. The mouth may be dry.
9. Peristalsis of the intestines decreases, resulting in possible constipation and flatus.
10. Muscle tension increase to prepare for rapid motor activity or defense.
11. Blood sugar increases because of release of glucocorticoids and gluconeogenesis.
12. Lethargy, mental lassitude, inactivity.
13. There may be decreased physiologic functioning and loss of skeletal muscle tone (parasympathetic dominance).

Psychologic manifestations: Psychologic manifestations of stress include anxiety, fear, anger, depression, cognitive behaviors, verbal and motor responses, and unconscious ego defense mechanisms.

Cognitive manifestations: Cognitive manifestations of stress are thinking responses that include problem solving, structuring, self-control or self-discipline, suppression, fantasy, and prayer. The person assesses the situation or problem, analyses or defines it, chooses alternatives, carries out the selected alternative, and evaluates whether the solution was successful.

Verbal and motor manifestations: Verbal or motor manifestations of stress may be the first responses evident. Among these reposes are crying , verbal abuse, laughing, screaming, hitting and kicking, and holding and touching.

43.7 NURSING DIAGNOSIS

The nursing diagnoses identified by NANDA (1992), relating specifically to clients experiencing stress include the following:

1. Anxiety related to perceived threat to self-concept, health status, and socioeconomic status.
2. Ineffective individual coping related to situational crises, such as natural disasters or loss of loved ones through separation.
3. Fear related to anticipated treatment (e.g. surgery, chemotherapy) or language barrier.
4. Defensive coping.
5. Ineffective family coping: Disabling.
6. Decisional conflict related to conflict with personal values/beliefs or an ethical dilemma.

43.8 PLANNING

The nurse develops plans in collaboration with the client and significant support persons when possible, according to the client's state of health. The nurse and client set goals to change the existing client responses to the stressor or stressors. The overall client goals for persons experiencing stress-related responses are to:

1. Decrease anxiety and fear.
2. Increase the ability to manage or cope with stressful events or circumstances.

Suggested outcome criteria are: The client

1. Verbalizes a reduced level of anxiety.
2. Develops realistic goals.
3. Expresses feelings in a positive way.
4. Verbalizes feelings to another.
5. Develops effective coping mechanisms in managing stress.

43.9 IMPLEMENTATION

Although, stress accompanies every disease and illness, it is also highly individualized; a situation that to one person is a major stressor may not affect another. Some methods to help to reduce stress will be effective for one person; other methods will be appropriate for a different person. A nurse who is sensitive to client's needs and reactions can choose methods on intervention that will be most effective for each individual.

43.10 MINIMIZING ANXIETY

After clients realize that they are anxious, it is important to discuss all the possible reasons for their anxiety.

When clients can identify the cause of their anxiety, they may find it helpful to explore the cause with the objective of learning better coping strategies.

General Guidelines to Minimize the Client's Anxiety and Stress

1. Support the client and family at the time of illness: By conveying caring and understanding, the nurse can help clients reduce their stress. Feeling that someone else cares is a source of support to stressed people.
2. Orient the client to the hospital or agency: The nurse helps the client adjust to the change from independent wage earner to relatively dependent client. The nurse can help family members by giving information, for instance, about visiting hours and specific unit policies.
3. Give the client in a hospital, some way of maintaining identity: Nurses can help clients maintain identify by addressing them by the name they prefer and by assisting them to wear their own clothes in a hospital setting, when this is possible.
4. Provide information when the client has insufficient information: Fear of the unknown and incorrect information can frequently cause stress. Additional information or clarification can ally stress.
5. Repeat information when the client has difficulty in remembering: Nurses can assist clients by repeating information when it is requested/required.
6. Encourage the client to participate in the plan of care: Loss of the right to determine their own destiny can be very stressful to some people.
7. Give the client time to express feelings and thoughts: Allow time for clients to describe their feelings and worries if they wish.
8. Ensure that expectations are within the client's capabilities: Whatever the activity whether an exercise or recreation, the nurse should make sure that it is possible for the client to accomplish it.
9. Be sensitive to specific situations and experiences that increase anxiety and stress for the clients.
10. Assist a client to make a correct appraisal of a situation: Sometimes, through a lack of knowledge people draw incorrect conclusions. Having valid information might relieve the client's stress.
11. Provide an environment in which a person can function independently to some degree without assistance: By adapting eating utensils so that the clients can feed themselves, thereby nurses can lower client's stress levels.
12. Reinforce positive environmental factors and recognize negative ones to help reduce stress.
13. Arrange for other clients with similar experiences to visit the clients. For example, colostomies or similar conditions.
14. Bring the clients and their support persons into contact with people in community agencies who can help them make valid plans.
15. Communicate with competence, understanding and empathy rather than stress and anxiety.

43.11 STRESS MANAGEMENT

Management of stress involves two major changes: Change in thinking and change in behavior and life style.

I. Cognitive Approach

1. Accept death as basic existential condition.
2. Carve out a meaning of life.
3. Realize that stress is inbuilt in life. We are neither the controller of the best nor the future. Present moment is the only reality.
4. Stress inoculation is a psychological and behavioral analogue to immunization on biological level.

5. Cognitive restructuring: Modify negative self-talk to positive self-talk. Create willingness to observe own.
6. Dispute irrational beliefs.
7. Positive imagery: Self-visualization.
8. Do not ignore feelings and needs. Suppressing feelings causes frustration, irritability and stress try to gratify feelings.
9. Accept responsibility because responsibility includes the nation of authorship. Assuming the responsibility is the basic condition for change.
10. Realize we do not control world or events. Attempts to change people and events are self-defecting change attitude from other directness to self-directness.
11. Stop perfectionist attitude and set limit to ambitions and material desires.
    Do not accept mediocrity in performance but do not entangle in the knots of unrealistic ambitions and over achievement drives. Do not be obsessed with perfection and overambitious ventures.

II. Behavioral Approach

1. Planning/organizing life, set goals/objectives. Planned and organized life leads to success, goals act as a achievements.
2. Management of habits: Habits change. But do not change by sheer will power. It demands change in beliefs and attitudes. It requires a process and practice and skill management of time because time is very precious. It is not possible to save time or borrow it. It is possible to make the best and maximum out of it.
3. Time management generates inbuilt discipline in life leading to success and happiness.
4. Do not run away problems. Avoidance behavior multiplies problems.
5. Avoidance and procrastination lead to more stress. Take every crisis/situation or challenges as an opportunity for growth.
6. Be assertive: Assertion is a form of appropriate behavior develops skills of assertion.
7. Music can act like a medicine in stress and stress related disorders. Music can play an effective role in helping and live better.
8. Laughter therapy creates relaxation and reduces stress. Laughter works as an effective muscle exercise.
9. Interpersonal skills enhance self-esteem. These skills make a good communicator. These lead to a better image.
10. Physical appearance reinforces confidence. It strengthens interpersonal skills. Avoid obscene dresses.
11. Engage regularly in leisure/physical exercises. Sublimate energies. Develop and groom hobbies and interests.
12. Develop proper food and sleep habits. Take adequate sleep. Choose and take food thoughtfully.
13. Utilize support system. Supportive relationships are those marked by warmth, empathy and care. Support system helps us to manage stress at least in distinct ways. It gives emotional support.
14. Build on spiritual strength. Spirituality is an essential part of healing process in life. Thinking ourselves as an expression of higher reality. Spiritual intelligence enhances creativity, subsequently helping in setting rules amending the situations.

43.12 NURSING INTERVENTION IN STRESS REDUCTION

The first step in managing stress is to become aware of its presence. This includes identifying and expressing stressful feelings (as stated above). The role of the nurse is to facilitate and enhance the coping and adaptation. Nursing interventions depend on the severity of the stress experience and demand. The nurse's efforts are directed to life-supporting interventions and to the inclusion of approaches aimed at the reduction of additional stressors to the client. The importance of cognitive appraisal in the stress experience should prompt the nurse to assess if changes in the way the client perceives and label particular events or situations (cognitive reappraisal) are possible. So, the nurse should also consider the positive effects that result from successfully meeting, stressful demands. Greater emphasis should also be placed on the part of cultural values and beliefs enhancing or constraining various coping options.

An individual personal resource that aids in coping includes health and energy. A health-promoting lifestyle provides these resources and buffers or cushions, the impact of stressors. Lifestyle or habits that contributed to the risk of developing illness can be reduced or eliminated. Health risk appraisal is an assessment method designed to promote health by examining the individual personal habits and recommending change where health risk is identified. For example, smoking causes lung cancer and can be prevented by reducing or leaving the habit of smoking.

43.13 COPING ENHANCEMENT

Coping enhancement is a nursing intervention and defined as "assisting a patient to adapt to perceived stressors, changes, or threats which interfere with meeting life demands and roles". After completing a health risk approach, the nurse could use coping enhancement to assist the patient in an analysis of the appraisal and to explore methods to improve the person's coping abilities including appraisal of his or her own personal resources.

The activities of coping enhancement are as follows:

1. Appraise the patient's adjustment to change in body image as indicated.
2. Appraise the impact of the patient's life situations on roles and relationships.
3. Encourage the patient to identify a realistic description of change in role.
4. Approve the patient's understanding of the disease process.
5. Approve and discuss alternative responses to situation.
6. Use a calm reassuring approach.
7. Provide an atmosphere of acceptance.
8. Assist patient in developing an objective appraisal of an event.
9. Help the client to identify the information he/she made interested in obtaining.
10. Provide factual information concerning diagnosis, treatment and prognosis.
11. Provide the patient with realistic choices about certain aspects of care.
12. Encourage an attitude to realistic hope as a way of dealings with feelings of helplessness.
13. Evaluate patient's decision-making ability.
14. Seek to understand the patient's perspective of a stressful situation.
15. Discourage decision-making when patient is under severe stress.
16. Encourage gradual mastery of the situation.
17. Encourage patience in developing relationships.
18. Encourage relationships with persons who have common interests and goals.
19. Encourage social and community activities.
20. Encourage the acceptance of limitation of others.
21. Acknowledge the patient's spiritual/cultural background.
22. Encourage the use of spiritual resources if desired.
23. Explore the patient's previous achievement of success.
24. Explore patient's reason for self-criticism.
25. Confront patient's ambivalent (anger or depression) feelings.
26. Foster constructive outlets of anger and hostility.
27. Arrange situations that encourage patient's autonomy.
28. Assist patient in identifying positive responses from others.

29. Encourage the identification of specific life values.
30. Explore with the patient previous methods of dealing with life problems.
31. Introduce the patient to persons (or group) who have successfully undergone the same experience.
32. Support the use of appropriate defense mechanisms.
33. Encourage verbalization of feelings, perceptions and fears.
34. Discuss consequences not dealing with guilt and shame.
35. Encourage the patient to identify own strength and abilities.
36. Assist patient in identifying appropriate short- and long-term goals.
37. Assist the patient in breaking down complex goals into manageable steps.
38. Assist the patient in examining available resources to meet the goal.
39. Reduce stimuli in the environment that could be misinterpreted as threatening.
40. Appraise patient's needs/desires for social support.
41. Assist the patient to identify available support systems.
42. Determine the risk of the patient's inflicting self-harm.
43. Encourage family involvement as appropriate as possible.
44. Encourage the family verbalize feelings about ill family member.
45. Provide appropriate social skills training.
46. Assist the patient to solve problem in a constructive manner.
47. Instruct the patient about the use of relaxation techniques as needed.
48. Assist the patient to grieve, and work through the losses of chronic illness and/or disability if appropriate.
49. Assist the patient to clarify misconceptions. Encourage the patient to evaluate his/her own behavior.

43.14 RELAXATION TECHNIQUES

Synder (1993) and Egan (1993) identified relaxation technique as the major method used to relieve stress, included in nursing interventions. Commonly used techniques cited were progressive muscle relaxation, relaxation with guided imagery, and Senson's relaxation response. The goal of relaxation training is to produce response that counter the stress response.

Progressive muscle relaxation: It involves tensing and releasing the muscles of the body in sequence and sensing the difference in feeling. It is best if the person lies on a soft cushion on the floor, in a quiet room, breathing easily. Self-taught or instructor-directed exercise that can involve learning to contract and relax muscles in a systematic way beginning with face and ending with feet. This exercise may be combined with breathing exercises that focus on inner self.

Relaxation with guided imagery: It is the purposeful use of imagination to achieve relaxation and or direct attention away from undesirable sensations. The nurse helps the person to select a pleasant scene or experience from his or her past. This image serves as the mental device in this technique. As the person sits comfortably and quietly the nurse guides him to review the scene; trying to feel and relieve the imagery with all of the senses. A tape recording can be made for description of science of experience for the pleasant one.

Benson's relaxation response: Benson and Proctor (1984) describe the following steps for this response which include:

Step 1: Pick a brief phrase or word that reflects your basic belief systems.
Step 2: Choose a comfortable position.
Step 3: Close your eyes.
Step 4: Relax your muscle.
Step 5: Become aware of your breathing and start using your selected focus word.
Step 6: Maintain a passive attitude.

Step 7: Continue for a set period of time.
Step 8: Practice the technique twice a day.

The response combines meditation with relaxation. The other techniques of stress management will also include the following:

Thought stopping: It is a self-directed behavioral approach used to gain control of self-defeating thoughts. When these thoughts occur the individual stops the thought process and focuses on conscious relaxation.

Exercise: Regular exercise, especially, aerobic movement, results in improved circulation, increased release of endorphins on an enhanced sense of well-being.

Humor: In the forms of laughter, cartoons, funny movies, riddles, audiocassettes, comic books and joke books, humor can be used for both the nurse and patient.

Assertive behavior: Open, honest, sharing feelings, desires and opinions in a controlled way. The individual who has control over one's own life is less subject to stress.

Social support: This may take the form of organized support and self-help groups, relationships with family and friends and professional help.

In addition, meditation, breathing techniques, therapeutic touch, music therapy, and bio-feedback can be used as stress management technique.

CONCLUSION

Stress produces numerous symptoms which vary according to persons, situations, and severity. These can include physical health decline as well as depression. The process of stress management is named as one of the keys to a happy and successful life in modern society. Although life provides numerous demands that can prove difficult to handle, stress management provides a number of ways to manage anxiety and maintain overall well-being. In order to develop an effective stress management program it is first necessary to identify the factors that are central to a person controlling his/her stress, and to identify the intervention methods which effectively target these factors. Lazarus and Folkman's interpretation of stress focuses on the transaction between people and their external environment (known as the transactional model). The model contends that stress may not be a stressor if the person does not perceive the stressor as a threat but rather as positive or even challenging. Also, if the person possesses or can use adequate coping skills, then stress may not actually be a result or develop because of the stressor. The model proposes that people can be taught to manage their stress and cope with their stressors. They may learn to change their perspective of the stressor and provide them with the ability and confidence to improve their lives and handle all of types of stressors.

44 Auditing

44.1 INTRODUCTION

Audit is the instrument for quality assurance. It developed in 19th century; the nursing audit is similar to an audit performed by accounting departments. It is a process that offers the nursing personnel in a health agency. The opportunity to create and enforce standards of nursing care and to examine their own practice in systematic manner.

44.2 DEFINITION

1. **Nursing audit** is the systematic, critical analysis of the quality of clinical/community care. It is an official examination of nursing records for the purpose of evaluation verification and betterment of nursing care.
2. **Nursing audit** is a systematic formal and written appraisal by nurses of the quality of the content and process of nursing service from care record for discharged patients.

44.3 TYPES OF AUDITING

1. **Nursing management audit:** This type is more structure oriented focusing on administrative aspects of the nurse's responsibilities and nurses that the health facilities are suitably equipped to provide care.
2. **Retrospective audit:** This is the evaluation of nursing care by examining the records and charts of discharged patients.
3. **Concurrent audit:** It is the evaluation of the nursing care by the observation and retrospective method during the delivery of care. The best method of audit depends on the objective of audit.

44.4 OBJECTIVES OF NURSING AUDITING

1. Examination of the books of accounts and records with a view to test the arithmetical accuracy and correctness in recording of transactions and their reliability.
2. Verify that the balance sheet and profit and loss account are drawn in conformity with the accounts and records.
3. Ascertain that proper accounting principles and procedures and management policies are followed.
4. Ensures that book of accounts and records as required by law are kept.
5. Report on the balance sheet as to whether it reflects the true and fair. State-of affairs of the institution and that the profit or loss of the institution.
6. Inspect all the documents, records and books of accounts of the institution and express opinion on matters required by the statistics.

44.5 AUDIT CYCLE

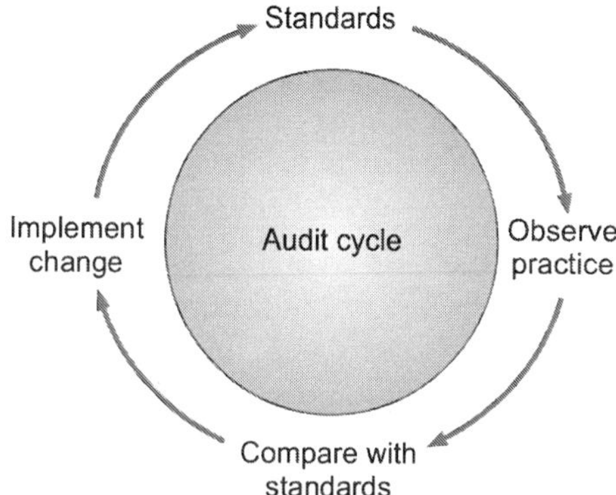

Fig. 44.1: Audit cycle

44.6 CHARACTERISTICS OF AUDITING

1. Audit looks at the entire process of care including administration and not just at clinical management.
2. Compares the care which actually is given. Standard procedures are agreed to decide which care should be given.
3. Concentrates on finding solutions for the problems identified.

44.7 BENEFITS OF AUDIT

1. **Patient:** The fundamental principle behind nursing care audit to everyone involved in care.
2. **Nursing staff:** For nurses, nursing care audit offers the opportunity to concentrate on areas of care where their skills and efforts can have positive outcomes, greater senses of achievement, autonomy, responsibility and provides a means for self-improvement.
3. **Community:** The new purchases provides environment in the hospital requires practitioners to quantity the work they do. Nursing care audit allows nurses to measure the mole intangible aspects of their work, in particular the quality care and so demonstrate the contribution.

44.8 NURSING AUDIT

Nursing audit is an evaluation of nursing service. Before 1955 very little was known about the concept. It was introduced by the industrial concern and the year 1981 was the beginning of medical unit. George Groword, pronounced the term physician for the first time medical audit. Ten years later Thomas R Pondon MD established a method of medical audit based on procedures used by financial account. He evaluated the medical care by reviewing the medical records. First report of nursing audit of the hospital published in 1955. For the next 15 years, nursing audit is reported from study (or) record on the last decade. The program is reviewed from record nursing plan nurses notes, patient condition, nursing care.

44.9 NURSING AUDITOR

1. **Internal auditor**: The nursing experts from within the hospital are deputed for internal audit and the auditing is done within the agency or hospital.

2. **External auditor**: Nursing and the medical administrations from the ministry other agencies of professional association like TNAI undertake the nursing audit in the desired agency or hospital.

44.10 METHODS OF AUDIT

S.N	Types	Description
1	Continuous audit	Continuous audit is on in which the audit staff is engaged in checking of the accounts during the whole year.
2	Final audit	Final audit is otherwise known as complete audit. It is commonly understood as an audit which is carried out after the close of the accounting year.
3	Periodical audit	Periodical audit refers to the audit at periodical intervals. During each visits the auditor completes his work up to the period of next visit.
4	Balance sheet audit	This audit consists mainly of the verification of each of the items in the balance sheet. Naturally, the verification of each item in the balance sheet leads to complete examination of the different items of expenditure and their allocation into capital and revenue.
5	Interior audit	Interior audit is one where the auditor conducts the audit for apart of the accounting year.

44.11 QUALITIES OF NURSING AUDITOR

1. **Knowledge:** Knowledge of accountancy and commercial law, the auditor has to cheek the books of accounts and satisfy that they reveal the true and fair view of the state of affairs of the business.
2. **Honesty and integrity:** An auditor certificates are taken as true and the profession is recognized for its morale and honesty.
3. **Skill and tact:** An auditor often has to act with care and skill to elicit information from his clients and the accounting staff of the business and to satisfy about the truthfulness of the transaction.
4. **Patience and perseverance:** An auditor must have utmost patience in carrying out his duties. He must hear his clients fully. He should have firm conviction of his actions.
5. **Ability to work hard:** An auditor should be witching to undertake hard work and evidence interest in his work.
6. **Ability to maintain secrets:** Auditor while dealing with the books of accounts of his clients may come across information which needs to be maintained secret.
7. **Report writing:** The observations and findings of the auditor are to be written in the form of a report and sent to the client for information. The report is to be written in a concise form and in an understandable language, free from ambiguity and contradictions.
8. **Common sense:** Above all these qualities, an auditor must possess common sense. He must have practical wisdom and act with presence of mind.

44.12 ADVANTAGES OF NURSING AUDIT

1. Can be used as a method of measurement in all areas of nursing.
2. Functions are easily understood.
3. Scoring system is fairly simple.
4. Results easily understood.
5. Assesses the work of all those involved in recording care.
6. May be useful tool as part of a quality assurance program in areas where accurate records of care are kept.

44.13 DISADVANTAGES OF NURSING AUDIT

1. Appraises the outcomes of the nursing process, so it is not so useful in areas where the nursing process has not been implemented.
2. Many of the components overlap making analysis difficult.
3. It is time consuming.
4. Requires a team of trained auditors.
5. Deals with a large amount of information.
6. Only evaluates record keeping. It only serves to improve documentation not nursing care.

CONCLUSION

A profession concerns for the quality of its service constitutes the heart of its responsibility to the public. An audit helps to ensure that the quality of nursing care desired and feasible is achieved. This concept is often referred to as quality assurance. An audit is a systematic and official examination of a record, process or account to evaluate performance. Auditing in health care organization provide managers with a means of applying control process to determine the quality of service rendered. Nursing audit is the process of analyzing data about the nursing process of patient outcomes to evaluate the effectiveness of nursing interventions. The audits most frequently used in quality control include outcome, process and structure audits.

Section-9

Quality Nursing Care

45 Quality Nursing Care

45.1 INTRODUCTION

The head nurse's conception of the patient determines to a large extent the quality of care the patient receives. Hopefully the head nurse sees the patient as a person with the basic needs shared by all human beings, yet with additional needs because she/he is ill and hospitalized. If she sees the patient in this way the care and attention she gives will be different than if she merely sees him as a sick individual in need of nursing care.

45.2 DEFINITION

1. Quality is defined primarily as the "degree of conformity with pre standards" and is focused on patient care as oppose medical or healthcare.
2. Nursing process and quality assured nursing care: Nursing process is a means by which good quality care is given to the patients. For good quality patient care there should be adequate facilities, proper management of man money material but what the patent got that is important. Some institutions have more buildings, sophisticated facilities.

45.3 STANDARDS OF NURSING CARE

The quality of nursing care is broad, but quality can be interpreted and applied to nursing through, the quality is caring, which is the heart of nursing. It is relative, which is in the eye of the beholder. It is dynamic and every changing, which is a sign of our times. It is satisfaction, which is achievement of professional standards. It is control, which is essential in a competitive environment, which is difficult to measure, but quality is a challenge, which is being accepted and pursued by nursing.

Standards of Nursing

1. Improving the quality of nursing care.
2. Evaluation of nursing care.
3. Provision of scientific and rationalized care with a definite direction.
4. Supervision and performance appraisals.
5. Attaining distinct position by drawing a demarcating line as to how nursing is different and unique from other professions.
6. Justifying demands in resource allocation.
7. Time conservation and time management.
8. Proper utilization of available resources.
9. Avoiding duplication of work (as healthcare involves multidisciplinary team).

45.4 PRINCIPLES OF QUALITY NURSING CARE

The nurse managers who have implemented quality assurance programs have identified certain principles.

1. The physicians and nurse contribute to patient care outcomes neither physicians nor nurses should unilaterally carry responsibility for quality care.
2. In planning, a comprehensive quality care program of a health institution coordination is needed to ensure that objective and activities of health profession.
3. Care should be taken to ensure that resource expenditure for quality assurance activities is appropriate in amount.
4. In order to ensure that resources expended for quality assurance yield significant findings or results, investigators should focus their attention on monitoring only critical performance factors.
5. The key to ensuring quality in patient care in accurate evaluation of care and they key successful auditing of care in adequate documentation of care.
6. The ability to achieve nursing objectives depends on optimal functioning of the entire process and effective monitoring of nursing system.
7. Evaluation of care will not by itself improve practice; feedback to practitioners is required both to perpetuate good practice and to replace unsatisfactory interventions with more effective methods.
8. Once quality of care has been assessed and needed improvements have been identified, peer pressure can provide the impetus required to effect prescribed changes practice.

The quality of nursing care which is significance of quality assurance in nursing, status of quality nursing care principles at international and national level, the need for preparing local and national standards which are more feasible and implement in various aspects and inculcating the concept and culture of quality among nursing professionals

45.5 ADMINISTRATING NURSING CARE TO THE PATIENT

Quality care to the patient is to provide physical and social environment which will contribute in speedy recovery of patient from illness and maintain all physical and mental functions of the individual and restore lost functions.

1. **Environment:** Management of environment is the responsibility of the head nurse, provision of physically safe and comfortable environment helps in speedy recovery of the patient which includes regulation of atmospheric temperature, humidity and ventilation.
2. **Cleanliness:** Provision of clean equipment, clean linen, clean floors and walls free from pathogenic organisms. Unclean, contaminated equipment can transmit infection from one person to another. Safety of patients and personnel depends upon the degree of cleanliness.
3. **Orderliness:** Cleanliness and orderliness go side by side, things in the ward should not only be clean but also in order. Nothing should be thrown on the floor or on the bed or furniture. The beds, furniture, trolleys, cupboards should be kept in neat and orderly manner. The whole surrounding should give the appearance of restful, relaxed atmosphere.
4. **Adequate lighting and ventilation:** Proper ventilation is required for comfort and health of the patients. Ventilation includes maintenance of temperature, exchange of air and humidity of air. Number of visitors should be restricted, since the number of people in a room or ward effect the temperature and humidity.
5. **Prevention of noise:** A sick person is very sensitive to noise, a little noise may disturb, it increases the nervous tension and pain in patient. The head nurse should maintain peaceful environment by speaking in low tone, walking quality and handling equipment without producing minimum choice.
6. **Well-functioning equipment:** The head nurse and her staff and responsible for the maintenance of proper functioning of equipment and keep where it is easily available.

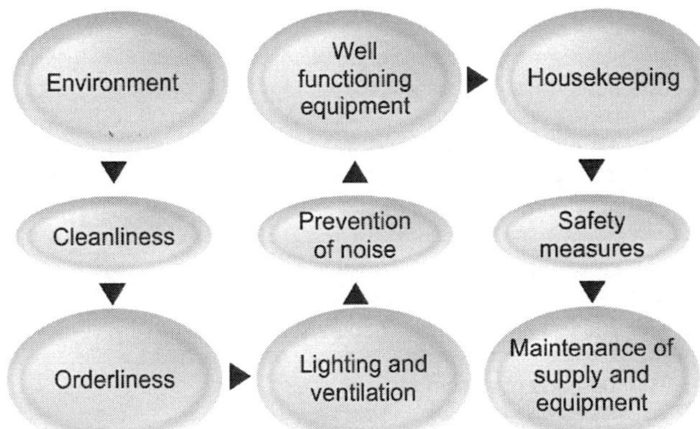

Fig. 45.1: Administrating nursing care

7. **Housekeeping:** Supervision of housekeeping of her unit is the responsibility of the head nurse. The head nurse should observe the principles of good housekeeping and must attend to the details of environment. The head nurse should see that hand washing, scrubbing, drying equipment are available in her unit.
8. **Safety measures:** Safety of the patient is the concern of every member of the staff and nursing sister. Every measure should be taken to product patient from mechanical, thermal, chemical and bacteriological injuries.
9. **Maintenance of supply and equipment:** Well functioning and adequate supply of equipment is must for providing optimum patient care. The head nurse must maintain adequate supply of material and keep in mind the principles of material management.

45.6 FACTORS INFLUENCING QUALITY OF PATIENT CARE

Good nursing care is impossible without good nurses, but they alone are no assurance that patients will be nursed. Other factors enter into the situation, namely, the amount of nursing care provided, the stability of the service, the quality of ward teaching and supervision and the quality of ward management.

1. **The type of service:** Medical, surgical, maternity, pediatric, communicable disease, psychiatric etc. more nurses are needed to care for children than for adult.
2. **The acuteness of the service** and the rate of turnover in patients. The degree of illness affects the amount of nursing care needed.
3. **The experience of the nurse** who are to give the patient care, graduate nurses are usually more mature in judgment, more skilled and are able to work more rapidly than students.
4. **The number of nurse's aids** and other nonprofessional workers, the quality of their work, their stability in service.
5. **The amount and quality of teaching** which precedes the assignment of personnel to the service as well as that given as in-service preparation.
6. **The amount and quality of supervision:** Individuals who are well-taught and supervised learn to use their time to good advantage so that fewer nurses are needed if they are well-prepared.
7. **The methods of appointment** of the medical staff.
8. **Affiliation of the hospital with medical school:** This arrangement may well over-balance the increase in nursing load due to an open staff.
9. **The plan of the ward:** In an open ward all patients are in full view of the nurses. It is easier to recognize patient's needs for attention, to local doctors and nurses for messages, and to

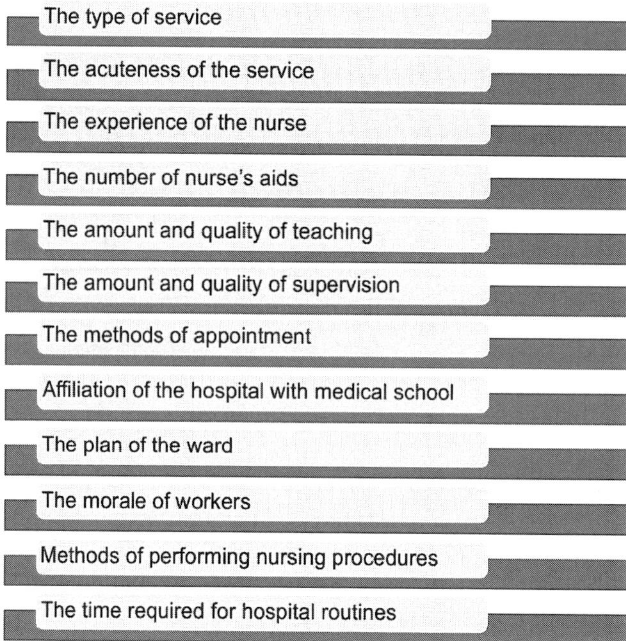

know what is happening than when patients are housed in small units behind walls and doors, desirable as the later may be.

10. Physical facilities.
11. The amount, type and location of equipments and supplies.
12. The number of hours in the working week of nurses and other personnel and the flexibility in hours.
13. **The morale of workers:** Morale determines to a large extent the interest consciousness of all personnel. It is depended upon good personnel practices.
14. **Methods of performing nursing procedures**.
15. **The time required for hospital routines**: The more complex the system of record keeping and reporting the more nursing time is consumed in desk work.

45.7 METHODS OF PATIENT CARE

Five methods have been in vogue, although in many situations a combination of one with the other will generally be observed.

1. **Care method:** The nurse provides all nursing functions for the patient. A one-to-one relationship of 'my patient my nurse' exists resulting in more individual care and greater work satisfaction.
2. **Group assignment method:** One nurse is assigned to a group of patient to provide total nursing care. This can be considered an enlargement of the case method described above.
3. **Functional assignment method:** Nurses are assigned to functions, e.g. TPR taking, medication, sponging, maintenance, duty and so on. Here, the nursing care becomes fragmented among many nurses, and impersonal. This method has some advantages which make those accustomed to it hesitant to change it. In this method, more can be accomplished in a given period of time. However, this gives the patient a service which is to some extent unsatisfactory and unsatisfying-unsatisfactory because responsibility for the attention given to patient is arbitrarily divided between several people, unsatisfying because the attention itself is apt to be impersonal.

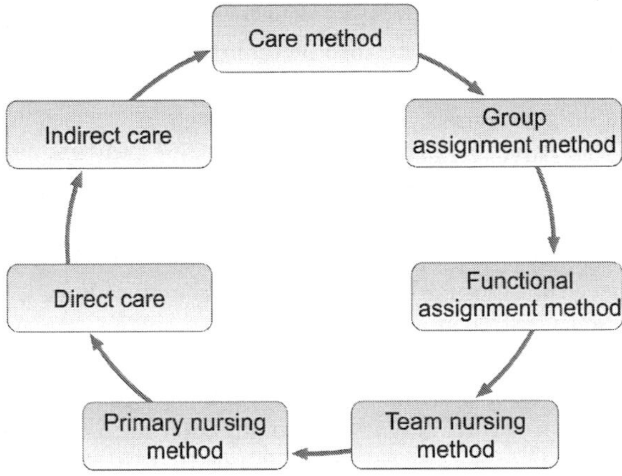

Fig. 45.2: Methods of patient care

4. **Team nursing method:** Assignment of a group of the patients to a team of the nursing (2 to more) staff headed by a staff nurse. This method has resulted due to shortage of staff to give total care. Other nurses and nurse aides are incorporated in the team to take care of the load, as many parts of care do not require the technical ability of a highly skilled professional nurse. The assignment of duties is based upon analysis of functions to be performed, competencies available and supervision required. This approach is quite effective if properly organized and supervised. However, here too nursing care is fragmented and nonpersonalized. The concept is based on the philosophy that a group of nursing personnel with graded competencies working together in a coordinated, cooperative way can meet all needs of patients more economically.
5. **Primary nursing method:** Primary nursing method is akin to the case method. The primary nurse assumes 24-hour accountability for the care, planning and evaluation. When on duty on a shift, the primary nurse herself assumes responsibility for providing total care. Other functions of primary nurse are the coordination of nursing activities with physician and other health professionals. In determining the number of nurses required for a service in the hospital, it has to be understood that nurses have to carry out two types of actions in relation to patient care. They are as follows:
6. **Direct care:** These are defined as those that are performed in the presence of the patient for the purpose of meeting his or her physical, emotional and social care needs.
7. **Indirect care:** They are those actions that are not necessarily performed in the presence of the patient but are essential to effective nursing care. Such actions include the process of carrying out nursing assessment, formulating and writing nursing plans, and evaluating the effectiveness of each.

45.8 ROLE AND FUNCTIONS OF A NURSE

Nurses assume a number of roles when they provide care to patients. Nurses often carry out these roles concurrently not exclusively of one another. For example, the nurse may act as a counselor while providing physical care and teaching aspects of the care.

1. **Caregiver:** The caregiver role traditionally included those activities that assist the patient physically and psychologically while preserving the patient's dignity. Care giving encompasses the physical, psychological, developmental, cultural and spiritual levels.
2. **Communicator:** In the role of communicator, nurses identify patient's problems and then communicate these verbally or in writing to other members of the health team. The nurse must be able to communicate clearly and accurately in order for a client's healthcare needs to be met.

3. **Teacher:** As a teacher, the nurse helps the client learn about their health and the healthcare procedures they need to perform to restore or maintain their health. The nurse assesses the client's learning needs and readiness to learn, sets specific learning goals in conjunction with the client, enacts teaching strategies, and measures learning.
4. **Client advocate:** A client advocate acts to protect the client. In this role the nurse may represent the client's needs and wishes to other health professionals, such as relaying the client's wishes for information to the physician.
5. **Counselor:** The nurse counsel's primarily healthy individual with normal adjustments difficulties and focuses on helping the person develop new attitudes, feelings and behaviors by encouraging the client to look at alternative behaviors, recognize the choices, and develop a sense of control.
6. **Change agent:** The nurse acts as a change agent when assisting others that is clients, to make modifications in their own behavior. Nurses also often act to make changes in a system, such as clinical care, if it is not helping a client return to health. Nurses are continually dealing with change in the healthcare system.
7. **Leader:** The leader role can be employed at different levels individual client, family, groups of clients, colleagues or the community.
8. **Manager:** The nurse manager also delegates nursing activities to ancillary workers and other nurses, and supervises and evaluates their performance.
9. **Case manager:** Nurse case managers work with the multidisciplinary healthcare team to measure the effectiveness of the case management plan and to monitor outcomes. Each agency or unit specifies the role of the nurse case manager.
10. **Research consumer:** Nurses often use research to improve client care. In a clinical area, nurses need to (a) have some awareness of the process and language of research, (b) be sensitive to issues related to protecting the rights of human subjects, (c) participate in the identification of significant researchable problems, and (d) be a discriminating consumer of research findings.

45.9 MANAGEMENT OF PATIENT CARE

Table 45.1: Patient care activities

S.N	Activities	Description
1.	Admission and orientation of the client	There are definite procedures prescribed by the hospital policies regarding the admission of the client. Nurses should remember that for a client and his relatives the hospital is strange place and they need orientation by the nurses.
2.	Assessment of clients needs and planning for the client care	Maslows hierarchy needs can be a guide for priority to meet the client's needs. The nurse makes use of every opportunity to collect necessary data for making diagnosis and nursing interventions. After collecting the data, she makes a plan for the care of the client. The plan is made known to all the members of her team to provide continuity care.
3.	Progressive client care	This is organizing client care units according to client's needs for medical and nursing care instead of segregating clients, according to services-medical, surgical, gynecological, orthopedics etc. Clients are nursed in different units according to the degree of illness suffered by them. a. **Intensive care units:** The critically ill clients, such as those suffering from coronary thrombosis, cardio-respiratory failures, cerebro-vascular accidents, clients who are undergoing major surgery and other clients who are need constant attention are admitted to the intensive care units. b. **Immediate care units:** When clients no longer need closed attention by the nurses they are transferred to the immediate care units. c. **Self care units:** Most of the clients are in the self care units are ambulatory, the work load in these units is very less compared to other units.

Contd...

Contd...

4.	Priority nursing care	The saving of a life depend on promptness of action, every moment is precious. When a client is brought to the hospital. Maslow's hierarchy of needs is helpful in determining priorities. Abraham Maslow described a hierarchy or pyramid of needs with primary or physiological needs at the base and secondary or nonphysiological needs at the higher levels.
5.	Assignments of personnel for the client's care	When the nurse has made the plan of care, she needs the right personnel for the implementation of her plan. **a. The functional method:** In functional method, the work is divided among the personnel, and each person is concerned with a particular task. For example one nurse may take temperature, gives all the injections and medications and does all the charting. Another nurse may serve the diets and maintains the intake and output of the all the clients.
		b. The client method of assignment: The head nurse assign the total care of a group of clients to each personnel's in the ward. Each personnel are responsible for the complete care of each client assigned to her, regardless of her abilities and experiences. **c. The nursing team method of assignment:** It has advantages over both functional and the client methods of assignments. The team method of assignment developed from a need to utilize the knowledge and skills of the staff nurse to better advantage and ensure the supervision of auxiliary nursing personnel. The concept of nursing team is based on the philosophy that a group of nursing personnel working together in a coordinated, cooperative way can carry out the full functions of nurse in giving the individualized care. **d. Nurse-client ratio:** The generally accepted staffing pattern ideal for an intensive care unit is 1:1 per shift, in intermediate care unit the staffing strengths varies with shift. In morning shift, it may be one nurse for 3 to 5 clients, in the evening shift it may be one nurse for seven clients, and in night shifts there can be one nurse for 11 clients.
6.	Planning the time schedules and work schedules	Time schedules and work schedules are useful administrative devices for the orderly regulation of activities for avoiding omissions. The work schedule outlines the basic duties of the various grades of personnel's.
7.	Ward rounds	The head nurse makes two types of ward rounds, the ward rounds made with the physician and the ward rounds made by herself or with her nursing staff. When a doctor's round is expected, the head nurse collects all the available information relevant to each client. She see that all charts are made up-date, the latest reports and X-rays are kept ready for inspection. Immediately after rounds the head nurse should be prompt to carry out the doctor's orders.
8.	Reports and records	Complete and concise report is vital for good management and administration. No team can function effectively without this method of communication. Report can be oral or written; giving a good report is an art. A well prepared report will help to communicate all information's to the persons concerned. Every report should be given promptly at the proper time. The important report that are written in the ward situations are 24 hours report, census report, the anecdotal reports and accidental reports.
9.	Management of emergencies	The nurses should keep the unit ready at all times with equipments, supplies and drugs for immediate resuscitation of the client, so that no time is lost to initiate the treatment. The nurses may follow the standing orders and the policies of the hospital to resuscitate the client while waiting for the doctor's arrival.
10.	Teaching clients	Every client has the right to know the nature of his illness, its progress, its treatment, and its preventive, promotive and rehabilitative aspects. The client teaching should start with the admission of the client and it should be encouraged throughout his stay in the hospital and even after his discharge from the hospital.
11	Appraisal of nursing services	Periodical evaluation of the nursing service is indispensable to maintain high quality of nursing care. The focus of evaluation should be: **1. Structural:** Physical facilities, equipments and supplies, staffing. **2. Process:** Nursing techniques, nursing procedures, quantitative and qualitative care, adequacy and appropriateness of care. **3. Outcome:** Client's satisfaction, satisfaction of personnel engaged in the client care, lower accident and complication rates and promptness in the performance of the task.

45.10 PATIENT SAFETY IN THE HOSPITAL

Medical errors may occur in different healthcare settings, and those that happen in hospitals can have serious consequences. The Agency for Healthcare Research and Quality, which has sponsored hundreds of patient safety research and implementation projects, offers these 10 evidence-based tips to prevent adverse events from occurring in the hospital.

1. **Prevent central line-associated blood stream infections:** Be vigilant preventing central line-associated blood stream infections by taking five steps every time a central venous catheter is inserted: wash your hands, use full-barrier precautions, clean the skin with chlorhexidine, avoid femoral lines, and remove unnecessary lines. Taking these steps consistently reduced this type of deadly healthcare-associated infection to zero in a study at more than 100 large and small hospitals.
2. **Re-engineer hospital discharges:** Reduce potentially preventable readmissions by assigning a staff member to work closely with patients and other staff to reconcile medications and schedule necessary follow-up medical appointments. Create a simple, easy-to-understand discharge plan for each patient that contains a medication schedule, a record of all upcoming medical appointments, and names and phone numbers of whom to call if a problem arises.
3. **Prevent venous thromboembolism:** Eliminate hospital-acquired venous thromboembolism (VTE), the most common cause of preventable hospital deaths, by using an evidence-based guide to create a VTE protocol. This free guide explains how to take essential first steps, layout the evidence and identify best practices, analyze care delivery, track performance with metrics, layer interventions, and continue to improve.
4. **Educate patients about using blood thinners safely:** Patients who have had surgery often leave the hospital with a new prescription for a blood thinner, such as warfarin brand name: Coumadin®), to keep them from developing dangerous blood clots. However, if used incorrectly, blood thinners can cause uncontrollable bleeding and are among the top causes of adverse drug events. A free 10-minute patient education video and companion 24-page booklet, both in English and Spanish, help patients understand what to expect when taking these medicines.
5. **Limit shift durations for medical residents and other hospital staff if possible:** Evidence shows that acute and chronically fatigued medical residents are more likely to make mistakes. Ensure that residents get ample sleep and adhere to 80-hour workweek limits. Residents who work 30-hour shifts should only treat patients for up to 16 hours and should have a 5-hour protected sleep period between 10 pm and 8 am.
6. **Consider working with a Patient Safety Organization:** Report and share patient safety information with Patient Safety Organizations (PSOs) to help others avoid preventable errors. By providing both privilege and confidentiality, PSOs create a secure environment where clinicians and healthcare organizations can use common formats to collect, aggregate, and analyze data that can improve quality by identifying and reducing the risks and hazards associated with patient care.
7. **Use good hospital design principles:** Follow evidence-based principles for hospital design to improve patient safety and quality. Prevent patient falls by providing well-designed patient rooms and bathrooms and creating decentralized nurses' stations that allow easy access to patients. Reduce infections by offering single bed rooms, improving air filtration systems, and providing multiple convenient locations for hand washing. Prevent medication errors by offering pharmacists well-lit, quiet, private spaces so they can fill prescriptions without distractions.
8. **Measure hospital's patient safety culture:** Survey hospital staff to assess your facility's patient safety culture. AHRQ's free *Hospital Survey on Patient Safety Culture* and related materials are designed to provide tools for improving the patient safety culture, evaluating the impact of interventions, and tracking changes over time. If the health system includes nursing homes or ambulatory care medical groups, share culture surveys customized for those settings.

9. **Build better teams and rapid response systems:** Train hospital staff to communicate effectively as a team. A free, customizable toolkit called Team STEPPS™, which stands for Team Strategies and Tools to Enhance Performance and Patient Safety, provides evidence-based techniques for promoting effective communication and other teamwork skills among staff in various units or as part of rapid response teams. Materials can be tailored to any healthcare setting, from emergency departments to ambulatory clinics.

CONCLUSION

The quality of nursing care is broad, but quality can be interpreted and applied to nursing through, the quality is caring, which is the heart of nursing. It is relative, which is in the eye of the beholder. It is dynamic and every changing, which is a sign of our times. It is satisfaction, which is achievement of professional standards. It is control, which is essential in a competitive environment, which is difficult to measure, but quality is a challenge, which is being accepted and pursued by nursing.

46 Nursing Service Department

46.1 INTRODUCTION

The role and responsibilities of today's nurse administrator are more complex than those of counterparts a century or even a decade ago. The current healthcare system is characterized by sicker patients, specialized personnel, expensive technology, increasing regulation and shorter lengths of hospital stay. In a climate of uncertainity, rapid change and a national shortage of nurse, the challenge to the nurse administrators to ensure the delivery of quality care is greater than ever. Nursing service department is responsible for providing comprehensive and continuing care to the patients in collaboration with members of the other healthcare services. Good nursing care is the result of ideal coordination between administrative and clinical planning. The nursing service administration unit is responsible for establishing and maintaining standards and for supervising the work of the nursing care personnel.

46.2 PHILOSOPHY OF NURSING SERVICE

Leddy and Pepper (2003) defined philosophy of nursing as the intellectual and affective outcomes of the professional nurses' efforts to understand the ultimate relationship among humans. environment, and health; to approach nursing as a scientific discipline; to integrate a sense of values into practice; to appreciate esthetic elements that contribute to health and well-being; and to articulate a personal belief system about human beings, environment, health and nursing. Hubert H Humphrey Comprehensive Health Center our nursing philosophy is providing an atmosphere of comfort while delivering care to the public we serve, it is our belief that the dignity and worth of individual must be respected and preserved. We further believe that the nursing care must be consistent with and specifically designed to meet the needs of the patient, and his family and the community in which he lives.

Our mission statement is "To provide quality healthcare in a culturally sensitive manner" (2000). The American Nursing Association is the professional organization for nurses in the United States. It major purposes are to promote high standards of nursing care to improve the quality and availability of healthcare, and to foster the professional development of nurses. Nurses are responsible for promoting excellence in nursing practice, patient advocacy, and for protecting the practice of nursing in all clinical settings. In keeping job philosophy and mission in mind I believed that I have developed a philosophy that reflects the values of caring, human life and dignity, the environment, health, professional nursing, cultural diversity, and educational achievement.

Caring is an essential component of nursing which involves the therapeutic use of self within the context of nursing practice. Caring requires a personal, social, moral and spiritual engagement of the nurse. The nurse is committed to self and others. Caring involves the protection.

46.3 MEANING OF NURSING SERVICE

Nursing service provides safe, effective and well-planned nursing care for patients as a result of development of nursing as a science, it has become a highly complex function the demands much training and skill. This department has constant contract with patients and naturally ir requires the coordination of all other services for best patient care. Control and coordination will be possible only when there is proper organizational structure and adequate supervision. Activities to perform led and personnel needed must be grouped in such a way as to achieve smooth functioning lines of authority should be clearly marked and above all everyone should know for what, to whom and for whom the nurse in responsible.

46.4 DEFINITION

1. **WHO expert committee** on nursing defines the nursing services as the part of the total health organization which aims to satisfy major objective of the nursing services is to provide prevention of disease and promotion of health.
2. **Nursing services:** Nursing service is the part of the total health organization which aims at satisfying the nursing needs of the patients/community. In nursing services, the nurse works with the members of allied disciples such as dietetics, medical social service, pharmacy etc. in supplying a comprehensive program of patient care in the hospital.

46.5 NURSING SERVICE DEPARTMENT

The nursing department is the largest department in the hospital. The head of department is the director of nursing (the nursing administrator, matron, nursing officer). She is responsible directly to the hospital administrator for the efficient management of the department. She have at least on assistant for each period of the day since the nursing department serves 24 hours. The director of nursing delegates the management of two or more nursing units within the hospital to a nurse supervisor who in turn delegates the management of the nursing unit to the first line nurse manager (Head nurse). The first-line nurse manager (Head nurse "RN"), in turn delegates the care of the patients to the unit staff.

46.6 GOALS OF NURSING SERVICE DEPARTMENT

1. To recognize the needs of the patient.
2. To assess the patients level of readiness to learn in relation to their illness.
3. To provide "an effective patient care".
4. To provide favorable atmosphere to the patients.
5. To upgrade nursing standards by evaluating the employees performance in the nursing department.
6. To work in coordination with all the nursing units within the hospital.

46.7 OBJECTIVES OF NURSING SERVICE DEPARTMENT

1. To provide highest possible quality of nursing care in terms of total patient needs.
2. To assist the doctor in the medical care of the patient and to carry out therapy as he prescribes.
3. To promote programmes of nursing education and to provide facilities for the development of all categories of nursing service personnel.
4. To promote and encourage nursing research studies.

5. To assess the quality of the nursing service.
6. To promote participation in health programmes and supportive community activities.

46.8 ESSENTIALS OF NURSING SERVICE

The outcome of our journey is the achievement of the eight essentials of a Magnet Designated facility; fundamentals to create an environment that:

1. Embraces patient care as the priority.
2. Promotes interdisciplinary collaboration.
3. Encourages professional development.
4. Supports evidence-based autonomous practice.
5. Provides adequate staffing.
6. Recruits and retains qualified and competent staff.
7. Shares control for professional practice.
8. Provides excellent leadership and management.
9. Through our nursing vision, values, and philosophy it is our passion to promote excellence in nursing practice and support the health system's mission to improve the health of the communities we serve with quality and compassion by providing extraordinary nursing care.

Together with professional care, warmth, friendliness and the sharing of joys and sorrows help to make each hospital and hospice a place where hearts can be lightened, work enjoyed, happiness shared and health restored. The care provided by the nurse and other staff and the ethos of the hospital are formed and shaped by the traditions, principles. The values on which their clinical care is based include a profound respect for human life and for each individual person irrespective of color, race, creed, gender, and sexual orientation, physical or mental disabilities.

46.9 CLASSIFICATION OF NURSING PRACTICE PERSONNEL

The department consists of two main classifications:

a. **Professional nursing personnel:** They are director, assistants, supervisors, first-line managers (RN) and staff nurses.
b. **Nonprofessional nursing personnel:** They are practical nurses (assistant nurses), nurse aides, orderlies and clerks.

46.10 FUNCTIONS OF NURSING SERVICE DEPARTMENT

1. To plan, provide and evaluate nursing care for patient and families.
2. To define and implement the philosophy, objectives and standards for nursing care of the patients.
3. To provide and implement a departmental plan of administrative authority which delineates responsibilities and duties of each category of nursing personnel.
4. To coordinate the functions of the department with the functions of all other departments.
5. To estimate the requirements of the department.
6. To interpret hospital and nursing practice objectives to the patients and community.
7. To participate in the formulation of personnel policies, to implement established policies and evaluate their effectiveness.
8. To develop an effective system of nursing records and reports.
9. To estimate needs for facilities, supplies and equipment.
10. To participate in financial planning.
11. To participate in studies and research projects for the improvement of patient care and hospital services.

12. To provide and implement continuing education program for all nursing personnel.
13. To participate in and or facilitate all educational programs of students in the healthcare field.

Specific Functions of Nursing Unit

1. Provide and maintain the highest quality patient care with the lowest possible cost.
2. Furnish the most desirable environment (safe, comfortable and pleasant) for patients and health service personnel, i.e. medical and nursing staff as well as the other hospital personnel.
3. Consider needs of patients families and significant others.
4. Provide adequate space to facilitate the carrying out of all the activities needed, i.e. using different types of equipment with minimum waste of personnel time, i.e. wide doors and corridors, wheel chair with IV stand, patient movement in their beds with attached apparatus—improves quality care.
5. Promote job satisfaction of the health personnel.

46.11 FACTORS INFLUENCING NURSING SERVICE

Organization of nursing service unit involves the design of nursing departmental framework. It included activities to be undertaken, organizational authority delegated, as well as an understanding of authority and informational relationships with other positions; the more adequately the individual responsible can contribute towards accomplishing enterprise organizational objectives. First and middle-level managers generally have their greatest influence on the organizing phase of the management process at the unit or department level. Here the managers organize how work is to be done, shape the organizational climate and determine how patient care delivery is organized, and resources necessary for selected care delivery system to he effective. The nursing service unit manager/leader determines how best to plan work activities so that organizational goals are met effectively and efficiently. This involves using resources wisely and to co-ordinate activities with other departments. How activities are organized can facilitate communication flexibility and job satisfaction.

Nursing personnel composed of professional nurses, nurses as practitioners and nursing assistants constitute the largest single body personnel in the nursing department / unit of the hospital. Nursing care refers to the care of the clients with specific regard to nursing. While the nursing service refers to coordinating responsibility of the nurse, Who in addition to giving nursing care also works with members of allied disciplines such as dietetics, medical service, social service. Pharmacy and various others in supplying a comprehensive program of hospital care. Nursing considers the whole patient body, mind and spirit and recognizes him as an individual.

Nursing services must be maintained throughout the day. Good nursing care needs good nurses, but they alone are no assurance of that patients will be well nursed. Other factors enter into the situation, like the amount of care provided, the stability of the service and the quality of the work management, many variable factors influence the number of nurses needed in a ward to render a high quality nursing care.

These factors include:

1. The type of service to be provided, i.e. medical, surgical, obstetrics, gynecology, pediatrics, psychiatric etc. The acuteness of the service.
2. The experience of the nurses who are to give the patient care.
3. The number of non-nurses who involve in patient care, their quality and stability of service.
4. The amount of quality of teaching given in-service preparation.
5. The physical facilities available.
6. The amount, type, location of equipment and supplies.
7. The number of working hours of nurses and the flexibility in hours.
8. The morale of the workers.
9. The method of assignment.

For organizing functions to be productive and facilitate meeting the organizations needs, the leader must know the organization and its members well.

Roles and Functions of the Leader/Manager in Organizing Groups

Leadership roles associated with organizing patient care

1. Periodically evaluates the effectiveness of the organizational structure for the delivery of patient care.
2. Determines if adequate resources and support exist before making any changes in the organization of patient care.
3. Examines the human element in work redesign and supports personnel during adjustment to change.
4. Inspires the work group toward a team effort.
5. Inspires subordinates to achieve higher levels of education, clinical expertise, competency, and experience in differentiated practice.
6. Ensures that chosen nursing care delivery models advance the practice of professional nursing.

Management functions associated with organizing patient care

1. Examines the unit philosophy to ensure that it supports any change in the patient care delivery system.
2. Selects a patient care delivery system that is most appropriate to the needs of the patients being served.
3. Uses scientific research and current literature to analyze proposed changes in nursing care delivery models.
4. Uses a patient care delivery system that maximizes human and physical resources as well as time.
5. Ensures that non professional staff are appropriately trained and supervised in the provision of care.
6. Organizes work activities to attain organizational goals.
7. Groups activities in a manner that facilitates communication and coordination within and between departments.
8. Organizes work so that it is cost-effective as possible.
9. Makes changes in work design to facilitate meeting organizational goals.
10. Clearly delineates criteria to be used for differentiated practice roles.
11. Nursing service management is one of the prerequisite for good nursing care.
12. Management of work, management of personnel and maintenance of records and reports are important in ward management.

Management of work: To manage the work the manager/leader should have the knowledge of all the duties and activities to be performed in unit or ward.

Knowledge of ward routines and its planning: Each days work is to be planned to save time and use available time for nursing the clients. Ward routines must be established/planned to delegate the duties/responsibilities which include writing and giving reports, handling orders, checking medicine cards and administering medicines, summarizing charts, handling telephone calls, checking and ordering supplies, keeping cupboards. Stocked, distributing linen, collecting specimens and providing individualized nursing, supervision and teaching.

Providing equipment linen and supplies: There should be provision for proper supplies and equipment for efficient work. All the materials should be adequate, functional, and accessible according to their use to deliver healthcare services. Without equipment and suppliers, health personnel cannot work effectively, they feel frustrated and society, community lacks confidence in health services. Supplies are expendable items which are used up and it must be recorded such as soaps. Detergents, paper towels, stationary etc. Equipment include permanent articles may be classified as fixed and movable. Fixed equipment is attached to walls or floor such as sinks, movable equipment includes furniture, instruments syringes etc. In planning for equipment, linen and supplies. There should be provision of supplies and equipment to meet the requirements of extra patients.

1. A cot for every patient or failing that, a mattress or thick quilt for every floor patient.
2. An almost 100% replacement of sheets yearly.
3. Provision of linen in accordance with type of ward.

Providing safe environment: Safe and restful environment is necessary to the patient's welfare and comfort. Cleanliness and orderliness improve morale and makes workers careful and neat in their habits, maintenance of building and equipment is economical as well as safe and efficient.

46.12 COMMON NURSING SERVICE ACTIVITIES

Hygiene, nutrition, medications, fluid management, skin and wound care, respiratory care, circulatory care, elimination, mobility, special diagnostic and treatment procedures, health teaching and daily activities of living. After care descriptors have been selected, the levels of care, intensity is defined for each descriptor. The level is differentiated by the amount of nursing time and frequency of each care measure.

1. **The factor system** is referred to as objective because specifying particular indicators or factors associated with patient care helps to ensure objectivity by the rater.
2. **Prototype evaluation system:** This is considered subjective and uses broad descriptive categories to describe the patient and needs. Characteristics are listed for a typical patient in each of the categories.

Type-I: Patients with acute, episodic disease or disability who will return to their pre-illness level to functioning and for whom the goal is to relieve existing health problem.

Type- II: Patients with chronic disease with acute episode of illness but has potential to return to pre-episodic level of functioning where the chronic health problem can be managed by self or the family.

Type-III: Patients with chronic disease where return to pre-illness level of functioning but potential to increase level of functioning with care goal is rehabilitation to a maximum level of functioning with agency support.

Type-IV: Patients with chronic disease who cannot be maintained at home without ongoing agency support.

Type-V: Patient with end stage of illness. However, the most effective patient classification system is one that is specifically tailored to the clinical situation where it will be used.

46.13 ROLES AND RESPONSIBILITIES

There are six main roles and functions of the nurse manager listed by American Organization of Nurse Executives (AONE):

1. The nurse manager is accountable for excellence in the clinical practice of nursing and the delivery of patient care on a selected unit or area within the healthcare institutions.
2. The nurse manager is accountable for managing human, fiscal and other resources needed to manage clinical nursing practice and patient care.
3. The nurse manager is accountable for facilitating development of licensed and unlicensed nursing and healthcare personnel.
4. The nurse manager is accountable for ensuring institutional compliance with professional, regulatory, and government standards of care.
5. The nurse manager is accountable for planning as it relates to the units or areas, department, and organization as a whole.
6. The nurse manager is accountable for facilitating cooperative and collaborative relationship among disciplines/departments to ensure effective delivery of quality care.

CONCLUSION

Nursing service department is responsible for providing comprehensive and continuing care to the patients in collaboration with members of the other health care services. Good nursing care is the result of ideal coordination between administrative and clinical planning. The nursing service administration unit is responsible for establishing and maintaining standards and for supervising the work of the nursing care personnel. The nursing department is the largest department in the hospital. The head of department is the director of nursing (the nursing administrator, matron, nursing officer). She is responsible directly to the hospital administrator for the efficient management of the department. She/he have at least on assistant for each period of the day since the nursing department serves 24 hours.

47 Nursing Process

47.1 INTRODUCTION

The nursing process is a problem-solving approach used by nurses to meet the needs of the patient. It is a deliberative method that relies on the use of cognitive, interpersonal and psychomotor skills. The nursing process is the systematic, rational method of planning and providing nursing care. Its goal is to identify a client's health status, actual or potential healthcare problems, to establish plans to meet the individual needs and to deliver specific nursing interventions to meet those needs. The nursing process is cyclical, that is the component of the nursing process follows a logical sequence, but more that one component may be involved at any given time. The nursing process provides a framework for accountability in nursing.

47.2 DEFINITION

1. The nursing process is cyclical, that is the component of the nursing process follows a logical sequence, but more than one component may be involved at any given time. The nursing process provides a framework for accountability in nursing.
2. The nursing process can be defined as an orderly, systematic way of identifying the clients (patient) problems, making plans to solve them, initiating the plans or assigning others to implement it and evaluating the extent to which the plan was effective in resolving the problems identified.
3. Nursing Process: An evolving procedure consisting of five components by which a person's health status and needs are identified (assessment and diagnosis), plans are developed (planning), care is delivered (implementation), and outcomes are evaluated (evaluation) as the physical, social, and emotional problems of the person are resolved and/or new problems are identified.

47.3 STEPS AND APPLICATION IN NURSING PROCESS

The nursing process consists of five steps or components. These five steps of the nursing process are assessment, nursing diagnosis, planning, implementation and evaluation. The scientific nursing activities and responsibilities are associated with each steps of the nursing process.

Assignment: It is collecting, verifying and organizing data about the client's health status. Data about physical, emotional, developmental, social, cultural, intellectual and spiritual aspects of the client's are obtained from a variety of sources and are the basis for actions and decisions taken at a subsequent phases.

Nursing diagnosis: It is a process of making a clinical judgment about a client's potential or actual health problem. Nursing diagnosis is the statement of the judgment. In this phase, the nurse sorts, clusters the data and analyses, what are the actual and potential health problems for which the client needs nursing assistance and what may be the contributing factors to this problem.

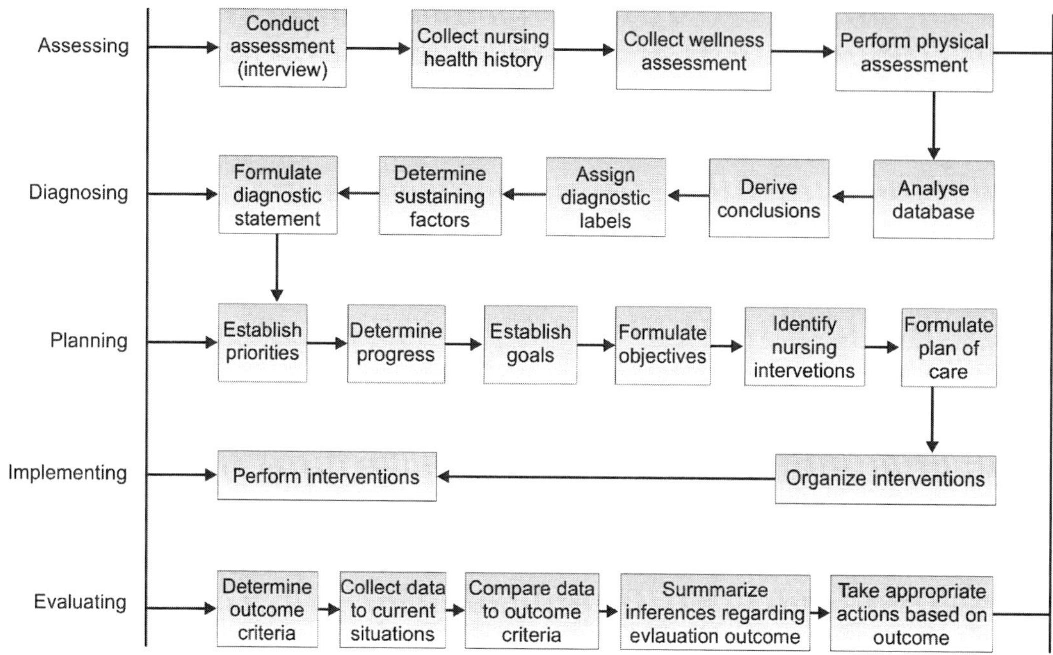

Fig. 47.1: Nursing practice application

Steps and Application of Nursing Process Model

Planning: It involves a series of steps in which the nurse and client set priorities, formulate goals or expected outcomes and establish a written care plan for nursing interventions. The plan to resolve or minimize the identified problems of the client and to coordinate the care provided by all the health team members.

Implementation: It is putting the nursing care plan into action. During the implementation phase, the nurse continues to collect data and carries out the prescribed nursing activities or delegates the care to an appropriate person who validates the nursing care plan.

Evaluation: It is assessing the client's response to nursing interventions and then comparing the response to predetermined standards. These standards are often referred to as 'outcome criteria.'

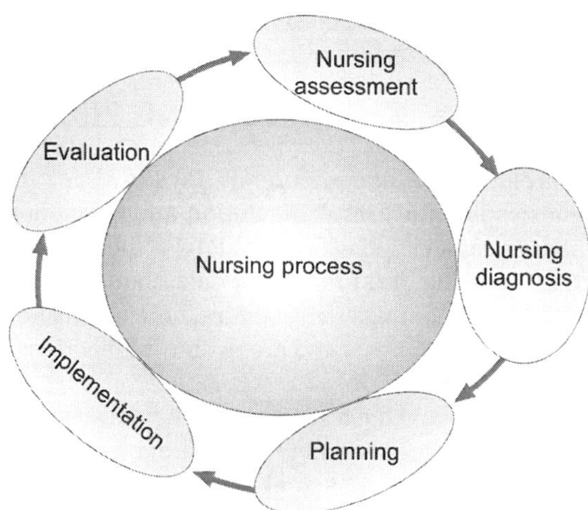

Fig. 47.2: Steps of nursing process

The nurse determines the extent to which the goals are predetermined and the outcomes of care that have been achieved, partially achieved or not met.

47.4 BENEFITS OF NURSING PROCESS

Benefits for the Client

1. **Quality clients care:** The nursing care is planned to meet the unique needs of the individual, family or community. Continuous evaluation and reassessment of the client's changing needs ensure an appropriate level of care.
2. **Continuity of care:** The written care plan is accessible to all the persons involved in the client's care and it prevents the client from repeating information and preferences to each caretaker.
3. **Participation by the client in their healthcare's:** The process can help the clients to develop skills related to their healthcare and to become more committed to the goals of care.

Benefits for the Nurse

1. **Consistent and systematic nursing education:** The agency which accredits nursing education programmes requires all graduates to be competent in using the nursing process.
2. **Job satisfaction:** Well written care plans, has given the nurses to be confident about that nursing interventions which are based on correct identification of the clients problems, thus preventing the uncoordinated, trail- and- error nursing.
3. **For professional growth:** By elevating the effectiveness of the nursing interventions, the nurse learns which interventions are most effective and which ones can be adapted to meet the needs of other clients.
4. **Meet professional standards:** Learning and implementing the nursing process while providing client care is a basic requirement for professional nursing competence.

A Framework for Accountability

1. Accountability is the condition of being answerable and responsible to someone for specific behaviors that are part of the nurse's professional role.
2. The nursing process provides a framework for accountability and responsibility in nursing and maximizes accountability and responsibility for standards of care.
3. Nurses are accountable to the client (public), to their professional statuary nursing body, to colleagues, to the employing agency and to themselves.
4. The nursing process provides a framework for accountability in all areas. A professional nurse is accountable for activities in all five phases of the nursing process.

47.5 ADVANTAGES OF NURSING PROCESS

When used effectively, the nursing process offers many advantages:

1. It's patient-centered, helping to ensure that your patient's health problems and his response to them are the focus of care.
2. It enables you to individualize care for each patient.
3. It promotes the patient's participation in their care, encourages independence and concordance and gives the patient a greater sense of control—important factors in a positive health outcome.
4. It improves communication by providing you and other nurses with a summary of the patient's recognized problems or needs.
5. It promotes accountability for nursing activities, which in turn promotes quality assurance.
6. It promotes critical thinking, decision-making and problem-solving.
7. It's outcome-focused and encourages the evaluation of results.
8. It minimizes errors and omissions in care planning.

CONCLUSION

The nursing process is a problem-solving approach used by nurses to meet the needs of the patient. It is a deliberative method that relies on the use of cognitive, interpersonal and psychomotor skills. The nursing process is the systematic, rational method of planning and providing nursing care. Its goal is to identify a client's health status, actual or potential healthcare problems, to establish plans to meet the individual needs and to deliver specific nursing interventions to meet those needs. The nursing process is cyclical, that is the component of the nursing process follows a logical sequence, but more than one component may be involved at any given time. The nursing process provides a framework for accountability in nursing.

48 Nursing Assessment

48.1 INTRODUCTION

The first step of nursing process is assessment. Assessment is the collection of data about the client from a variety of sources. Assessment is the continuous process carried out during all phases of the nursing process. It may be used during the diagnosis phase to validate a diagnosis. A "systematic, dynamic process by which the nurse, through interaction with the client, significant others, and healthcare providers, collects and analyzes data about the client. Assessment is broader than observing and data gathering. It includes the application of processes such as critical thinking and professional judgments used in prioritizing, identifying immediate and anticipated need, analyzing medical and nursing interventions aimed at appropriate outcomes, and providing for holistic continuum of care" (ANA, Nursing Scope and Standards of Practice).

48.2 PREREQUISITES TO ASSESSMENT

1. **Beliefs:** The nurse's belief encompasses a caring philosophy about the client's, responsibilities and health and illness and the role of nursing in healthcare. These philosophies do not blossom overnight but are molded during the course of nursing education by nurses, other students, instructors and clients.
2. **Knowledge:** The knowledge base for nurses is extensive and nurses are required to use information from sciences such as nursing, anatomy, physiology, microbiology, pharmacology, chemistry and nutrition using all of these sciences is guidelines, the nurse can analyze data collected about the client.

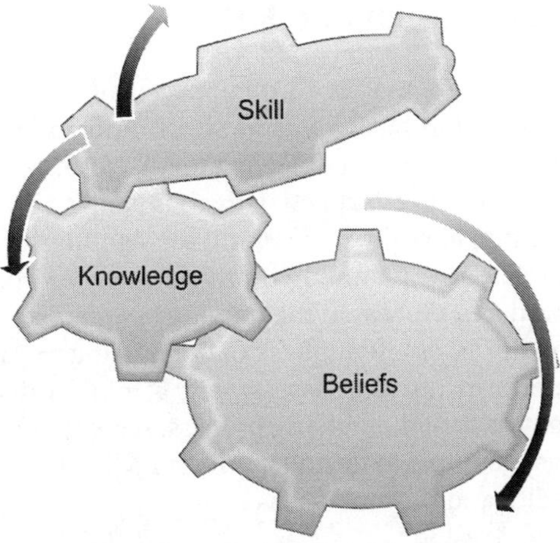

Fig. 48.1: Prerequisites to assessment

3. **Skill:** A variety of skills are required to perform a complete assessment of the client. They include psychomotor and interpersonal.

Psychomotor skills are the technical skills required in many phases and nursing process. During the assessment phase, the most common skills are those of physical assessment such as inspection, palpation and auscultation.

Interpersonal skills are important in all phases of nursing process but are a critical component of the assessment phase. The term therapeutic relationship is often used to describe the communication techniques that allow the client and family to share views and telling openly.

48.3 DATA COLLECTION

Data collected from a patient includes both objective and subjective data. Objective data are detectable by an observer. Examples of objective data are blood pressure recording, checking body temperature, detecting cyanosis in a patient. Subjective data are apparent only to the patient concerned. Examples of subjective data are feeling of pain, inching, etc.

Sources of Data

1. **Client:** The chief source of data is usually the client unless the client is too ill, young or confused to communicate clearly. The client can provide subjective data that no one else can offer.
2. **Significant others:** Significant others are supporting person who knows the client well and often provide data. They might convey information about the stress the client was experiencing before the illness, family attitudes to illness and health and the client's home environment.
3. **Health personnel:** Health personnel are often the sources of information about a client's health. Nurses, physicians, social workers and physiotherapist. Physician who knows the client's home setting may provide valuable data about the family and the environmental stress.
4. **Medical records:** Medical records are often a source of a client's present and past health and illness patterns. This record can provide nurses with information about a client's coping behaviors, health practices, previous illness and allergies.
5. **Other records and reports:** Other records and reports can also provide information pertinent to health, laboratory, and tests are frequently ordered as part of the physician's initial examination to aid in a medical diagnosis.
6. **Literature:** The review of nursing and related literature, such as professional journals and reference texts, can provide additional information for the database.

48.4 METHODS OF DATA COLLECTION

1. **Observation:** The nurse observes mainly through sight, all of the senses are engaged during careful observations. Observation has two aspects: (a) noticing the stimuli and (b) selecting organizing and interpreting the data, i.e. perceiving them. Observation is a conscious, deliberate skill that is developed only through effort and with an organized approach.
2. **Interviewing:** The nurse interviews the patient and his significant others obtain data by asking relevant questions. Interview is a planned communication or conversation with a purpose. Interviewing can be viewed as a process in the nursing health history, which is the primary tool for data collection during the assessment phase of the nursing process.
3. **Examination:** Nurses perform physical assessment to obtain the objective data needed to complete the assessment phase of the nursing process. A complete database of both subjective and objective data allows the nurse to formulate nursing diagnosis, to develop client goals and intervene to promote health and prevent disease.

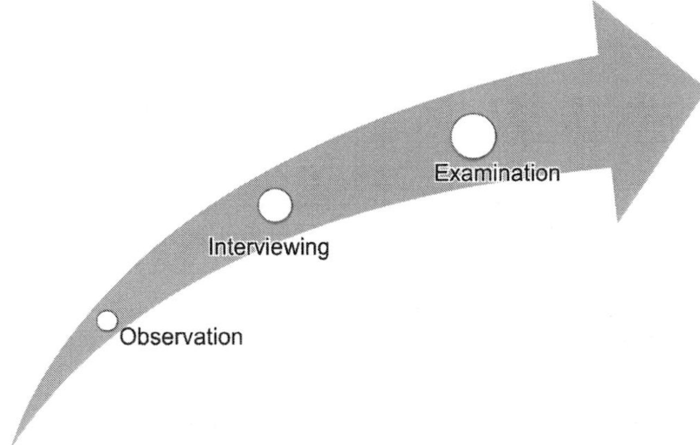

Fig. 48.2: Methods of data collection

Guidelines for Data Collection

1. **The initial history:** The data collected in this step usually include the historical data (pat illness), current data (the current complaint) and demographic data (date of birth, address). It is helpful to address the client's chief complaint early in the interview process.
2. **Symptom analysis:** When a client expresses a problem the nurse conducts a complete analysis of a symptom. This process begins with symptoms analysis which is the collection of subjective data about the problem. Symptoms analysis requires the client to identify the location of the symptoms, describe the symptoms, severity of the pain, and timing of the symptoms. (Including onset, duration and frequency).
   Aggravating and relieving symptoms and any associated symptoms. It is crucial that the nurse be able to perform a complete symptoms analysis. The data obtained can guide the nurse in detecting what the problem is and what degree of priority is should be given.
3. **Approaches to history taking:** There are various approaches that can be used to provide a systematic guide to assessment. Gordon has devised functional health patterns and the North American Nursing Diagnosis Association (NANDA) has devised human response patterns based on patterns of unitary persons.
4. **Physical examination:** Physical examination of the client is the second portion of assessment. Examination allows the nurse to gain objective data through the use of inspection, percussion, palpation and auscultation. These data further define the client's response to the disorder, provide a baseline of data for further comparison, and elaborate on the subjective data provided in the client's history.

48.5 PHYSICAL EXAMINATION

Assessment of physical findings should confirm data obtained in nursing history. Baseline information is obtained on admission. The proper examination proceeds logically from head to be starting with general appearance, blood pressure, pulse, hands, head and neck, heart, lungs, abdomen, feet and legs.

Definition: Physical examination is defined as a complete assessment of patient's physical and mental status.

Purpose

1. To understand the physical and mental well-being of the patient.
2. To detect disease in its early stage.
3. To determine the cause and the extent of disease.
4. To understand any changes in the condition of diseases, any improvement or regression.
5. To determine the nature of the treatment or nursing care needed for the patient.
6. To safeguard the patient and his family by noting the early signs especially in case of a communicable disease.
7. To contribute to the medical research.
8. To find out whether the person is medically fit or not for a particular task.

48.6 METHODS OF PHYSICAL EXAMINATION

Inspection: Visual examination of the body is called inspection. It is the observation with the naked eyes to determine the structure and functions of the body. It means looking with eyes. It reveals any rash, scar, color, size, shape, contour or symmetry of body parts. The quality of inspection depends on the time spent by the nurse to be thorough and systematic. In a hurry we may overlook significant findings and make an incorrect conclusion. The following principles should be kept in mind for making accurate inspections:

1. Good lighting and exposure are essential.
2. Inspect each area for size, shape, color, symmetry and proposition and find out any deviations from normal.
3. Use additional lights for examining body cavities, e.g. oral.
4. Use sense of olfaction along with visual to detect abnormalities, e.g. bad breath indicates unhygienic mouth conditions. Acidotic smell is significant of diabetic acidosis.

Palpation: It is the feeling of the body or a part with the hands to note the size and positions of the organs. In palpation, the finger pads and not the finger tips are used. Palpation is an assessment technique in which the examiner feels with his/her fingers and one or both hands. Skill and gentleness are important. The degree of pressure applied during palpation varies, depending on, e.g. tenderness of the area and the depth of palpation required. It reveals any swelling, coldness, hotness, stiffness, hardness, smoothness, roughness, pain, vibration, firmness and flaccidity.

The following points are to be kept in mind while doing palpation:

1. The client should be relaxed and comfortable. Observe nonverbal signs of discomfort during palpation.

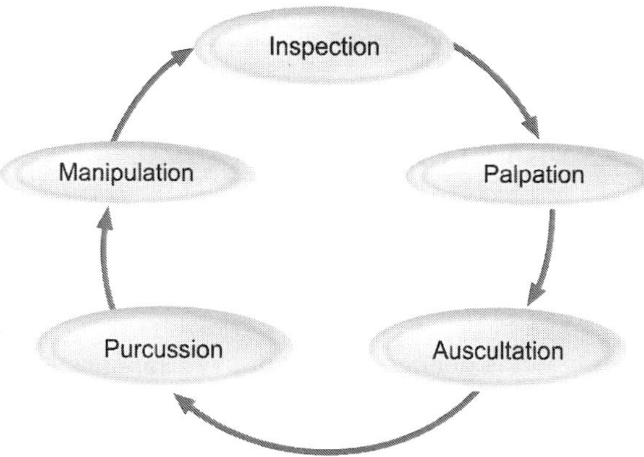

Fig. 48.3A: Methods of physical examination

2. Palpation to be done with warm hands, short fingernails and a gentle approach.
3. Palpation to be done slowly, and gently.
4. For light palpation the hand is depressed about 1 cm (1/2 inch) and for deeper palpation it should be approximately 2.5 cms (1 inch).
5. Use appropriate parts of the hands for doing various palpations.

Percussion: It is the examination by tapping with the fingers on the body to determine the condition of the internal organs by the sounds that are produced. It is done by placing a finger of the left hand firmly against a part to be examined and tapping with the finger tips of the right hand. It means striking/tapping with fingers. It elicits sounds, which indicate whether the underlying tissues are solid or filled with air or fluid. The sounds may be:

1. **Resonance:** A low pitched and loud sound heard over the normal lung tissues.
2. **Hyper resonance:** Very loud, very low pitch sound longer than resonance and is of booming quality signifies emphysema.
3. **Tympany:** A drum-like sound heard over the air-filled tissues such as gastric air bubble.
4. **Dull:** A medium-pitched sound with a medium duration without resonance heard over solid tissues such as heart and liver.
5. **Flat:** A high-pitched sound with a short duration without resonance heard over complete solid tissues such as hand and thigh.

Methods of percussion: The percussion can be done by two methods. These are:

1. **Direct percussion:** Striking the body surface directly with one or two fingers, e.g. ascitic thrill.
2. **Indirect percussion:** Placing the middle finger of the nondominant hand firmly against the body surface and striking the distal joint of no dominant finger with the middle fingers of the dominant hand.

Auscultation: It means listening with stethoscope/placing ear against the body. It reveals sounds produced within the body and the blood vessels such as heart beats, bowel sounds, while auscultation frequency loudness, quality and duration of the sound to be noted.

Manipulations: It is the moving of a part of the body to note its flexibility. Limitation of movements is discovered by this method.

Testing of reflexes: The response of the tissues to external stimuli is tested by means of percussion hammer, safety pin, wisp of cotton, hot and cold water, etc.

48.7 HEAD TO TOE EXAMINATION

The examination is carried out in an orderly manner focusing upon one area of the body at a time. The observation of the patient starts as the patient walks into the examination room, e.g. a limp may be noted as the patient walks in. The following observations are made:

General Appearance

1. Nourishment: Well-nourished or under-nourished.
2. Body build: Thin or obese.
3. Health: Healthy or unhealthy.
4. Activity: Active or dull (tired).

Mental Status

1. Consciousness: Conscious, unconscious, delirious, talking incoherently.
2. Look: Anxious or worried, depressed, etc.

Posture

1. Body curves: Lordosis, kyphosis, and scoliosis.
2. Movement: Any limp.
3. Height and weight.

Skin Conditions

1. Color: Pallor, jaundice, cyanosis, flushing, etc.
2. Texture: Dryness, flaking, wrinkling or excessive moisture.
3. Temperature: Warm, cold, and clammy.
4. Lesions: Macules, papules, vesicles, wounds, etc.

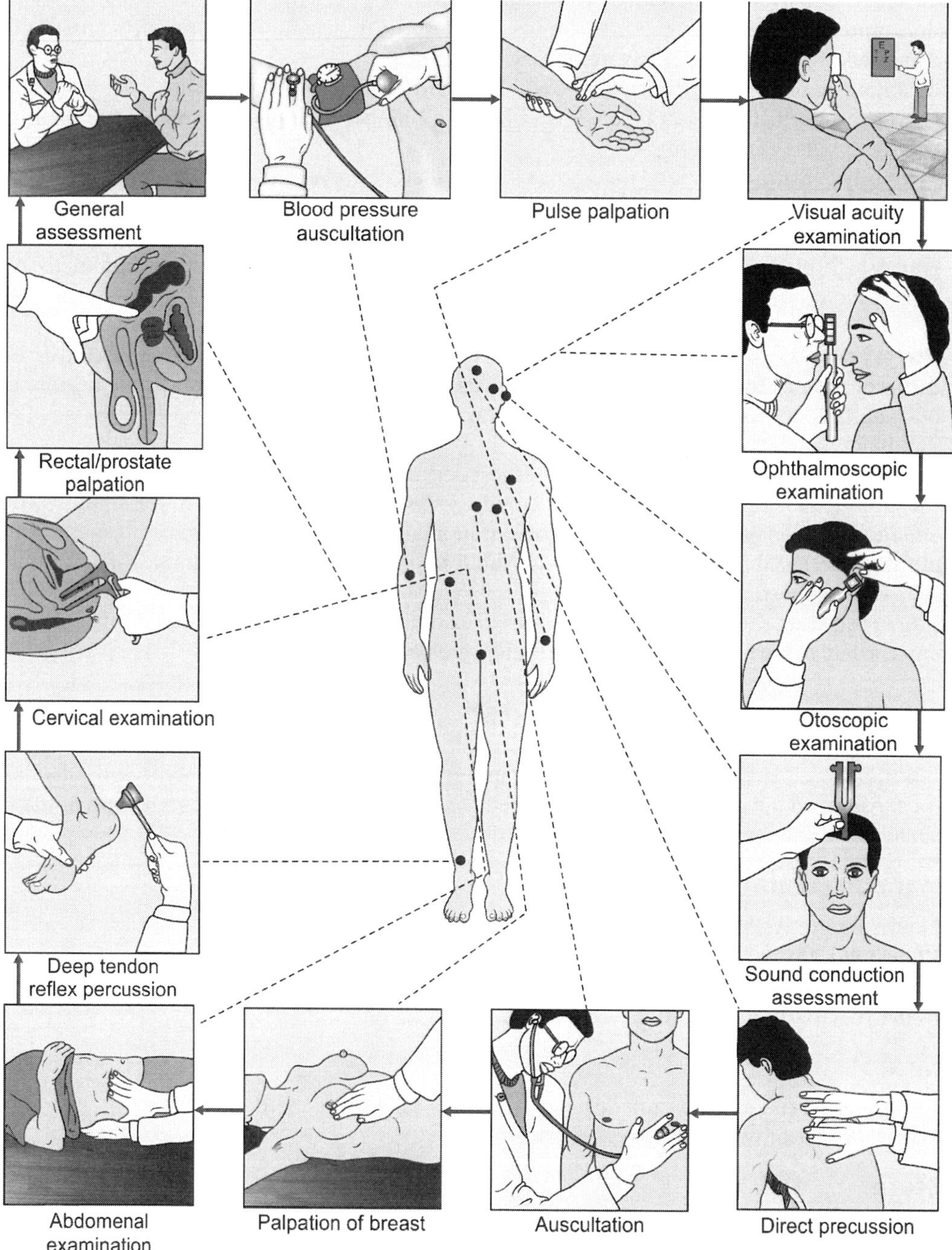

Fig. 48.3B: Methods of physical examination

Head and Face

1. Shape of the skull and fontanel.
2. Skull circumference.
3. Scalp: Cleanliness, condition of the hair, drandruff, pediculi, infections like ringworm.
4. Face: Pale, flushed, puffiness, fatigue, pain, fear, anxiety, enlargement of parotid glands, etc.

Eye

1. Eye brows: Normal or absent.
2. Eyelashes: Infection, sty.
3. Eye lids: Edema, lesions, ectropion, entropion.
4. Eye-balls: Sunken or protruded.
5. Conjunctiva: Pale, red, purulent.
6. Sclera: Jaundiced.
7. Cornea and iris: Irregularities and abrasions.
8. Pupils: Dilated, constricted reaction to light.
9. Lens: Opaque or transparent.
10. Fundus: Congestion, hemorrhagic spots.
11. Eye muscles: Strabismus (squint).
12. Vision: Normal, myopia, hypermetropia.

Articles Appropriate for Specific Examination

1. **Eye:** Torch, ophthalmoscope, snellens chart, wisp of cotton.
2. **Ear:** Head mirror, light bulb fixed on the wall or a table lamp and a torch, a tuning fork.
3. **Nose:** Nasal speculum, forceps, a head mirror and a light bulb.
4. **Throat:** Tongue depressor, a laryngeal mirror, a kidney tray, a paper bag, throat swabs in a container. Torch gauze pieces in a bowl.
5. **Chest and Abdomen:** Stethoscope, tape measure.
6. **Vaginal:** Sterile vaginal speculum, gloves, a kidney tray, a bowl with swabs (sterile), and an antiseptic lotion.
7. **Rectal:** Proctoscope, gloves, finger cots, a kidney tray, water-soluble jelly.
8. **Neurological:** A percussion hammer, safety pins, a wisp of cotton, hot or cold water.

Ears

1. External ear-discharges, cerumen obstructing the ear passage.
2. Tympanic membrane: Perforations, lesions, bulging.
3. Hearing: Hearing acuity.

Nose

1. External nares: Crusts or discharges.
2. Nostrils: Inflammation of the mucus membrane, septal deviations.

Mouth and Pharynx

1. Lips: Redness, swelling, crusts, cyanosis, angular stomatitis.
2. Odor of the mouth: Foul smelling.
3. Teeth: Discoloration and dental caries.
4. Mucus membrane and gums: Ulceration and bleeding, swelling, pus formation.
5. Tongue: Pale, dry, lesions, sords, furrows, tongue tie, etc.
6. Throat and pharynx: Enlarged tonsils, redness and pus.

Neck

1. Lymph nodes: Enlarged, palpable.
2. Thyroid gland: Enlarged.
3. Range of motion: Flexion, extension and rotation.

Chest

1. Thorax: Shape, symmetry of expansion, posture.
2. Breathe sounds: Sigh, swish, rustle, wheezing, rales, crepitations, pleural rub, etc.
3. Heart: Size and location, cardiac murmurs.
4. Breasts: Enlarged lymph nodes.

Abdomen

1. Observation: Skin rashes, scars, hernia, ascites distension, pregnancy, etc.
2. Auscultation: Bowel sounds, fetal heart sounds.
3. Palpation: Liver margin, palpable spleen, tenderness at the urea of appendix, inguinal hernias.
4. Percussion: Presence of gas, fluid or masses.

Extremities: Movement of joints, tremors, clumbing of fingers, ankle edema, varicose veins, reflexes, etc.

Back: Spina bifida curves.

Genital and Rectum

1. Inguinal lymph glands: Enlarged, palpable.
2. Patency of urinary meatus and rectum (in infants).
3. Descent of the testes.
4. Vaginal discharges.
5. Presence of sexually transmitted diseases.
6. Hemorrhoids.
7. Enlargement of the prostate gland.
8. Pelvic masses.

Neurological Tests

1. Coordination tests.
2. Reflexes.
3. Equilibrium tests.
4. Tests for sensations.
5. Role of the nurse in the physical examination.

48.8 PREPARATION OF THE ENVIRONMENT

1. Maintenance of privacy.
2. A separate examination room is needed.
3. Keep the doors closed. The relatives are not allowed.
4. Drape the patient according to the parts that are exposed.
5. Lighting: As far as possible natural light should be available in the examination room, because if a patient is jaundiced, it may not be detected in the artificial light. There should be adequate lighting.
6. Comfortable bed or examination table: The patient should be placed comfortably throughout the examination. There should be provision for the maintenance of a suitable position, e.g. a

lithotomy position may be maintained when examining the genitalia. To maintain this position, a special examination table with stirrup rods is needed.

7. The room should be warm and without draughts.

48.9 PREPARATION OF THE EQUIPMENT

All the articles needed for the physical examination are kept ready for the examination at hand.

1. Sphygmomanometer
2. Stethoscope
3. Foetoscope
4. TPR Tray
5. Tongue depressor
6. Pharyngeal retractor
7. Laryngoscope
8. Tape measure
9. Flash light
10. Weighing machine
11. Ophthalmoscope
12. Otoscope

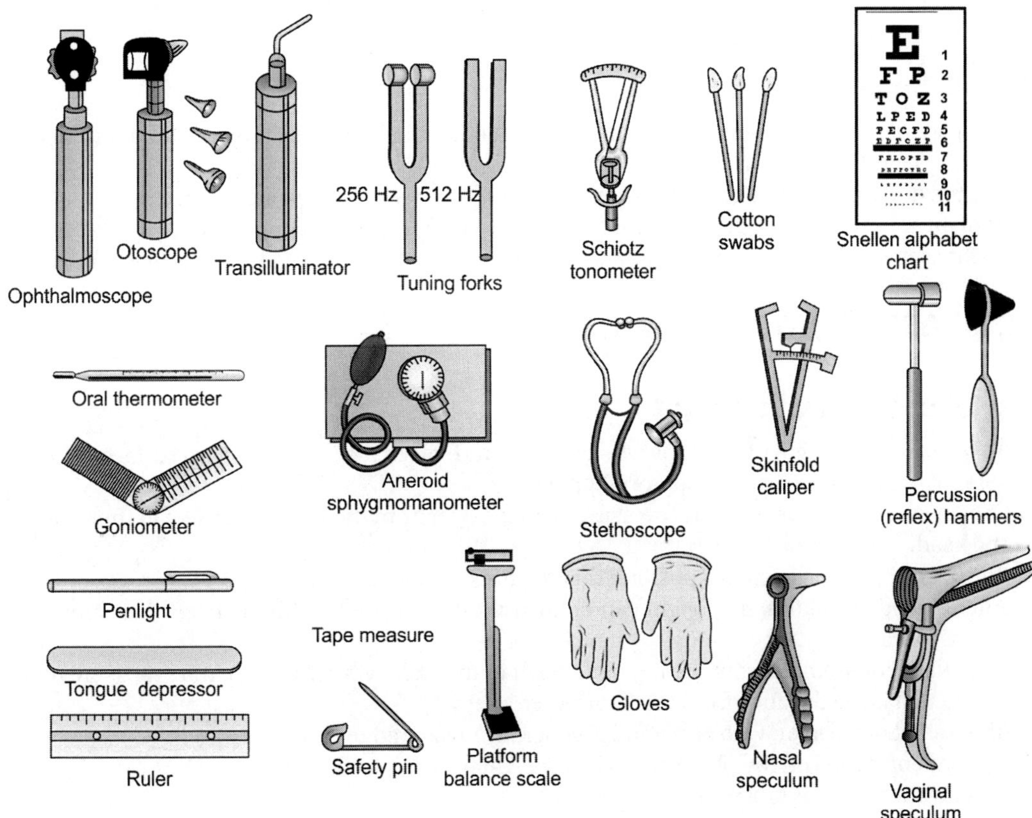

Fig. 48.4: Equipments for physical examination

13. Tuning fork
14. Nasal speculum
15. Percussion hammer, safety pins
16. Cotton wool, cold and hot water
17. Test tubes
18. Vaginal speculum
19. Protoscope
20. Gloves
21. Sterile specimen bottles, slides
22. Cotton applicators.

48.10 PREPARATION OF THE PATIENT

Physical Preparation

1. Keep the patient clean.
2. Shave the part if necessary.
3. Keep the patient in a comfortable position which is convenient for the doctor to examine the patient.
4. Empty the bladder prior to the examination. Empty the bowels by an enema if required.
5. Loosen the garments and change into the hospital dress, if it is the custom.
6. Drape the patient with extra sheets and expose only the need areas.
7. Avoid unnecessary exposure.

Mental Preparation

1. The patient may be quite new to the hospital situation and he may be anxious about his illness.
2. He may have false ideas about the medical examination.
3. It is the duty of the nurse to allay his anxieties and fears by proper explanations.
4. Explain the sequence of the procedure to gain his confidence and cooperation.
5. As far as possible a nurse should remain with a female patient during the physical examination.

48.11 ASSISTING IN EXAMINATION

I. To Take Height and Weight

1. To measure the length of the baby who cannot stand, place the baby on a hard surface, with the soles of the feet supported in an upright position.
2. The knees are extended and the measurement is taken from the soles of the feet to the vertex of the head.
3. The head should be in such a position that the eyes are facing the ceiling.
4. After a child can stand, the height can be measured, if the child with the heels back and head against a wall.
5. A small flat board held from the top of he head to the wall, will give an accurate measure of the height that is the distance from the floor to the board.
6. The weight of a person who can stand is generally measured by a standing scale.
7. The patient stands on the platform and the weight is noted on the dial.
8. Usually the weight is taken without shoes.
9. To take the weight of the baby, a baby weighing scale is used, in which there is a container, where the baby can be laid.

10. It is important to weigh a baby unclothed. If the body is weighed with the cloth then weigh the clothes separately and subtract this weight.

II. To Measure the Skull Circumference

The skull is measured at its greatest diameter from above the eyes to the occipital protuberance.

III. Examination of the Eyes

1. The examination is done in a lying or sitting position.
2. The examiner frequently uses a head mirror that reflects light to the patient's face.
3. The first examination is one of inspection to determine the movements of the eyes, reaction to light, accommodation to near and far objects.
4. For detailed examination of the internal parts of the eye an ophthalmoscope is used.

IV. Examination of the Ears

1. The patient may be placed either in a lying or sitting position with the ear to be examined turned towards the examiner.
2. Articles used for the examination are a head mirror, ear speculum of various sizes, cotton tipped applicators and autoscope.
3. Tuning fork is used to test the hearing.
4. A child needs to be carefully restrained.
5. Young children sit on their mother's lap with their legs restrained between the mother's knees and their arms held against their back.
6. The mother then holds the child's head against the chest.
7. Very small infants can be laid on the examination table.

V. Examination of the Nose, Throat and Mouth

1. The patient is usually seated with the head resting against the back of the chair.
2. For the examination of the throat, a tongue depressor and a good light are needed.
3. For examination of the nose, a nasal speculum and a head mirror are used. Sometimes the autoscope is also used.

VI. Examination of the Neck

The neck needs to be palpated for lymph nodes. In order to assess the thyroid glands, the patient is asked to swallow saliva.

VII. Examination of the Chest

1. While examining the anterior chest, the patient is placed in a horizontal recumbent position.
2. The chest is examined in several ways.
3. It is percussed to determine the presence of fluid or congested areas.
4. The physician listens to the sound within the chest by means of a stethoscope.
5. To examine the posterior chest, the patient is placed in a sitting position.
6. The heart and lungs are examined by percussion and auscultation.
7. The breasts are examined by palpation for the presence of lumps or growths.
8. The axilla are palpated for enlarged lymph nodes.
9. During the examination, the patient's face is turned away from the doctor.

VIII. Examination of the Abdomen

1. Extremities are inspected, palpated and moved.
2. A fine tremor suggestive of hyperthyroidism can be observed, if the patient is asked to hold the arms out in front of him for a few minutes.

Care of after examination

1. Assist him to dress and help him to remain in a comfortable position in the bed.
2. After-care of equipment: Wash the equipment with soap and water, rinse, dry and sterilize, as needed.
3. Replace the equipments in their usual places.
4. Label specimens properly and send them to the laboratory immediately.

Nurse's Responsibilities During Physical Examination

1. A separate examination room is needed. Keep the doors closed, screen the patient and provide privacy if he is not in a separate room. Relatives are not allowed.
2. Drape the patient according to the parts that are to be examined. Natural light should be available in the examination room.
3. There should be adequate lighting in the room. The patient should be comfortable throughout the examination.
4. There must be provision for the maintenance of a suitable position, e.g. Lithotomy position. The room should be warm.
5. The nurse must stay in the room at all times while the doctor examines a female patient.
6. During the examination of a male patient's genitals, the nurse must leave the room. Take the patient's temperature, pulse, respiration and blood pressure, if recent readings are not available.
7. Give health teaching to the patient as need arises.

CONCLUSION

Nursing assessment is the continuous, systematic, critical, orderly and precise method of collecting, validating, analyzing and interpreting information about physical, psychological and social needs of an individual nature of self-care deficits and other factors influencing conditions. Assessment is a primary skill in nursing. Almost from the very moment you learn a patient's name, you begin your assessment. Honing your assessment skills is an ongoing process. In the exciting and challenging field of nursing, you will learn something new every day.

49 Nursing Diagnosis

49.1 INTRODUCTION

The second step of the nursing process is often referred to as analysis, as well as need (or problem) identification or nursing diagnosis. Although, all these terms may be used interchangeably, the purpose of this step of the nursing process is to draw conclusions regarding a client's specific needs or human responses of concern so that effective care can be planned and delivered.

Today, the use of the nursing process and nursing diagnoses is rapidly becoming an integral part of an effective system of nursing practice. It is a system that can be used within existing conceptual frameworks, because it is a generic approach adaptable to all academic and clinical settings. In addition, -organizing schemata of nursing problems other than North America Nursing Diagnosis Association (NANDA) are used within the profession.

49.2 DEFINITION

1. The nursing diagnosis is a conclusion drawn from the data collected about a client that serves as a means of describing a health need amenable to treatment by nurses. A uniform or standardized way of identifying, focusing on, and labeling specific phenomena allows the nurse to deal effectively with individual client responses.
2. Nursing diagnosis is defined as "a clinical judgment about individual, family, or community experiences/responses to actual or potential health problems/life processes. A nursing diagnosis provides the basis for selection of nursing interventions to achieve outcomes for which the nurse has accountability."
3. The process of assessing potential or actual health problems, including those pertaining to an individual patient, a family or community, that fall within the scope of nursing practice; a judgment or conclusion reached as a result of such assessment or derived from assessment data.
4. A nursing diagnosis is a standardized statement about to the health of a client (individual, family, or community) for the purpose of providing nursing care. One organization for defining standard diagnoses is the North American Nursing Diagnosis Association now known as NANDA-International.

49.3 CONCEPT OF NURSING DIAGNOSIS

1. Nursing diagnosis is actual or potential problems that are amenable to resolution by nursing actions.
2. The five national conferences on the classification of nursing diagnosis held in 1970's and the early 1980's have provided an impetus for the identification and classification of nursing diagnosis according to symptomatology.

3. When developing the nursing diagnosis for a particular patient, the nurse must first identify the commonalities among the assessment data collected. These common features lead to the categorization of related data that reveal the existence of a problem and the need for nursing intervention. The patient's nursing problem is then defined as the nursing diagnosis.
4. It must be remembered that nursing diagnosis are not medical diagnosis, they are not medical treatments prescribed by the physician; they are not diagnostic studies; they are not the equipment utilized to implement medical therapy.
5. They are not the patient's actual or potential health problems that are amenable to resolution by nursing actions. Nursing diagnoses that are succinctly stated in terms of the specific problems of the patient will guide the nurse in the development of the nursing care plan.

49.4 MEANING OF NURSING DIAGNOSIS

Nursing diagnosis is a statement of a health problem or of a potential problem in the client's health status that a nurse is licensed and competent to treat. Four steps are required in the formulation of a nursing diagnosis. A database is established by collecting information from all available sources, including interviews with the client and the client's family, a review of any existing records of the client's health, observation of the client's response to any alterations in health status, a physical assessment, and a conference or consultation with others concerned in the client's care. The database is continually updated. The second step includes analysis of the client's responses to the problems, healthy or unhealthy, and classification of those responses as psychologic, physiologic, spiritual, or sociologic. The third step is the organization of the data so that a tentative diagnostic statement can be made that summarizes the pattern of problems discovered. The last step is confirmation of the sufficiency and accuracy of the database by evaluation of the appropriateness of the diagnosis to nursing intervention and by the assurance that, given the same information, most other qualified practitioners would arrive at the same nursing diagnosis. In use, each diagnostic category has three parts: the term that concisely describes the problem, the probable cause of the problem, and the defining characteristics of the problem. A number of nursing diagnoses have been identified and are listed as accepted by the NANDA, and they are updated and refined at periodic meetings of the group.

49.5 NURSING DIAGNOSIS CLASSIFICATION

The NANDA-I system of nursing diagnosis provides for four categories.

1. **Actual diagnosis:** A clinical judgment about human experience/responses to health conditions/life processes that exist in an individual, family, or community". An example of an actual nursing diagnosis is: Sleep deprivation.

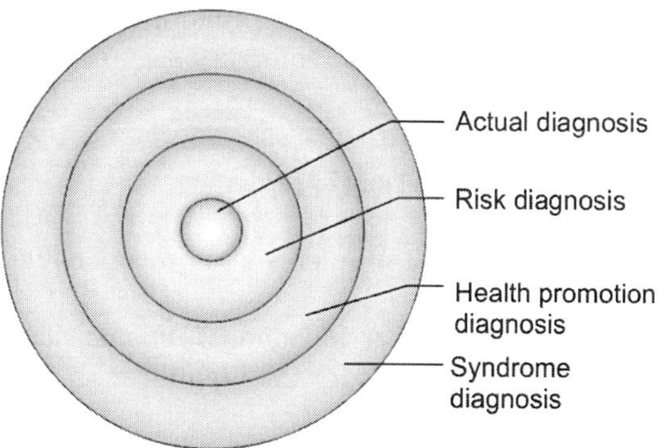

Fig. 49.1: Classification of nursing diagnosis

2. **Risk diagnosis:** Describes human responses to health conditions/life processes that may develop in a vulnerable individual/family/community. It is supported by risk factors that contribute to increased vulnerability. An example of a risk diagnosis is: Risk for shock.
3. **Health promotion diagnosis:** A clinical judgment about a person's, family's or community's motivation and desire to increase well-being and actualize human health potential as expressed in the readiness to enhance specific health behaviors, and can be used in any health state. An example of a health promotion diagnosis is: Readiness for enhanced nutrition."
4. **Syndrome diagnosis:** A clinical judgment describing a specific cluster of nursing diagnoses that occur together, and are best addressed together and through similar interventions." An example of a syndrome diagnosis is: Relocation stress syndrome.

49.6 STRUCTURE OF DIAGNOSIS

There are five types of nursing diagnoses in the NANDA system.

1. **An actual diagnosis** is a statement about a health problem that the client has, and could benefit from nursing care. An example of an actual nursing diagnosis is: Ineffective airway clearance related to decreased energy and manifested by an ineffective cough.
2. **A risk diagnosis** is a statement about a health problem that the client doesn't have yet, but is at a higher than normal risk of developing in the near future. An example of a risk diagnosis is: Risk for injury related to altered mobility and disorientation.
3. **A possible diagnosis** is a statement about a health problem that the client might have now, but the nurse doesn't yet have enough information to make an actual diagnosis. An example of a possible diagnosis is: Possible fluid volume deficit related to frequent vomiting for three days and manifested by increased pulse rate.
4. **A syndrome diagnosis** is used when a cluster of nursing diagnoses are often seen together. An example of a syndrome diagnosis is: Rape-trauma syndrome related to anxiety about potential health problems and as manifested by anger, genitourinary discomfort, and sleep pattern disturbance.
5. **A wellness diagnosis** is used to describe an aspect of the client which is at a high level of wellness. An example of a wellness diagnosis is: Potential for enhanced organized infant behavior, related to prematurity and as manifested by response to visual and auditory stimuli.

49.7 DIAGNOSTIC REASONING

1. **Classification:** The initial step of data analysis is classification of the date. Data need to be organized in order to be clearly analyzed and the most logical means to organize data is to classify them. The body systems approach functional health pattern approaches are two convenient methods of classification. When these methods are used for taking a history and performing a physical examination, the data are already classified.
2. **Validation:** The next step of data analysis is validation. In this step, the nurse verifies the diagnosis by speaking to the client. The nurse can validate finding with the family, especially if the client is unable to communicate. For example, the nurse could ask about scars or wounds and therefore, expand the data base on the client. The nurse can also validate the diagnosis by comparing it to textbook material or by talking to other nurses.
3. **Inductive versus deductive reasoning:** The nurse may use inductive or deductive reasoning to interpret data. Inductive reasoning begins with a set of facts from which a conclusion is drawn. Inductive reasoning is the use of cues to draw a conclusion.

   Deductive reasoning begins with the facts that the client is on bed rest and taking narcotics and concludes (deduces) that the client is at an increased risk.

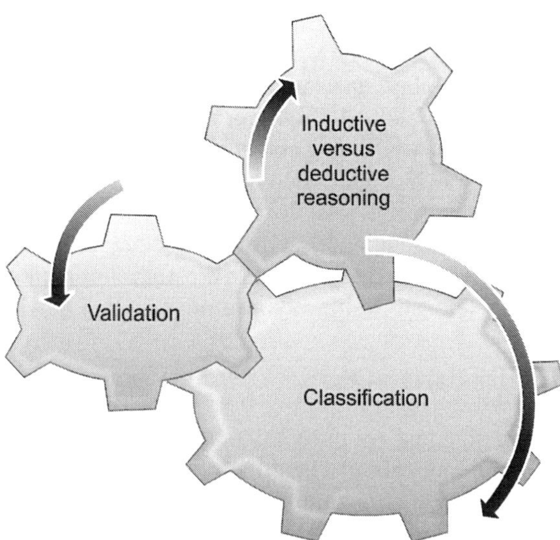

Fig. 49.2: Diagnostic reasoning

49.8 ERRORS IN DIAGNOSIS

1. **Incomplete data:** Common cause of incomplete data occurs during the interview phase of assessment. Some clients withhold information intentionally because some they feel embarrassed or are unsure how the nurse would react to the information.
2. **Inaccurate interpretation:** Data from the client can be misinterpreted in several ways. The problem can be diagnosed in several ways. The problem can be diagnosed before the data are completely collected. Sometimes, the nurse can have a personal prejudice about the client.
3. **Lack of knowledge or experience:** The clinical experience and knowledge may result in inaccurate data processing. Failure to recognize a problem is a common experience for most nurses. The inexperienced nurse may overlook important data or fail to realize the significance of the data.

49.9 IMPORTANCE OF NURSING DIAGNOSIS

1. The diagnosis is anything abnormal or that concerns the client, or strengthens of the client. Diagnoses within the realm of nursing are the response of the client to a state of health or illness and include physical, psychological, spiritual and educational areas.
2. These nursing diagnosis and their treatment are within the legal scope of nursing practice. The actual conditions that nurses are educated to handle and licensed to treat are called nursing diagnosis.
3. The role of the nurses can vary greatly between settings; there has always been difficulty in describing the work in nursing. NANDA has provided national leadership in the development of standardized statements or nursing diagnosis, to describe human response to actual or potential health problems which nurses treat.

49.10 WRITING NURSING DIAGNOSIS

A nursing diagnosis should be written in three parts indicating the human response, related factors and defining characteristics.

1. **Human response:** The human response is the client's problem attached as a nursing diagnosis. Most nurses use NANDA nursing diagnosis as the human response statement, but other form of problem statements are possible.
   The human response should always be stated as a response to care rather than as a need for care. Needs for care such as needs to be fed or needs to be turned every 2 hours, describe a nursing intervention rather than a client problem?
2. **The related factors:** The related factors are the possible causes or etiology of the problem. This section of the statement describes the factors associated with the problem. These factors may be environmental, psychological, physiological, sociocultural or spiritual.
   Because these factors direct nursing actions aimed at resolving, preventing or reducing the problem, the related factor should be directed at an aspect of the client response on which the nurse have an impact.
3. **The defining characteristics** are the data indicating the problem is present. When the client is at risk of developing a problem, the risk factors are identified rather than defining characteristics.

49.11 TEN RULES OF WRITING NURSING DIAGNOSIS

1. Write the diagnosis in terms of the client's response rather than nursing need.
2. Use "related to" "rather than" "due to" "or" "caused by" to connect the first two parts of the statement.
3. Write the diagnosis in legally advisable terms.
4. Write the diagnosis without value judgments.
5. Avoid reversing the parts of the statement.
6. Avoid using single clues as the first part of the statement.
7. The two parts of the statement should not mean the same thing.
8. Express the related factor in terms that can be changed.
9. Do not include the medical diagnosis in the nursing diagnosis.
10. State the diagnosis clearly and concisely.

49.12 COLLABORATIVE PROBLEMS

1. As nurses have continued to work with nursing diagnosis, shortcomings of the system have been identified.
2. Carpenito defines collaborative problems as the psychological complications that have resulted or may result from the pathophysiologic and treatment-related conditions, and from other situations.
3. Nurses monitor to detect the onset and status of complications and collaborate with physicians in treatment.

CONCLUSION

Nursing diagnosis is defined as "the statement that describes the client's actual and potential response to health problem that the nurse competent to treat. ANA supported nursing diagnosis in nursing. A social policy statement which defined nursing as "the diagnosis and treatment of human responses to actual or potential health problems". It is a process of making a clinical judgment about a client's potential or actual health problem. Nursing diagnosis is the statement of the judgment. In this phase, the nurse sorts, clusters the data and analyzes, what are the actual and potential health problems for which the client needs nursing assistance and what may be the contributing factors to this problem.

50 Nursing Planning

50.1 INTRODUCTION

The next step in the nursing process is planning activities to promote healthy client responses or prevent, correct or reduce unhealthy client responses.

Planning and setting expected outcomes begins by determining the priority of human response. (in five-step nursing process) a category of nursing behavior in which a strategy is designed to achieve the goals of care for an individual patient, as established in assessing and analyzing. Planning includes developing and modifying a care plan for the patient, cooperating with other personnel, and recording relevant information. To develop the plan the nurse anticipates the patient's needs according to established priorities; involves the patient and the patient's family and significant others in designing the plan; uses all information necessary for managing the patient's care, including recorded information from other health professionals and the age, sex, culture, ethnicity, and religion; plans for the patient's comfort, activity, and function; and chooses nursing measures that are necessary to deliver care as planned. With the cooperation of other health personnel the nurse coordinates care for the benefit of the patient and identifies resources in the healthcare facility or community for social or health assistance as needed by the client or the patient's family. All information relevant to the management of the patient's care plan is recorded. Planning follows analyzing and precedes implementing in the five-step nursing process.

50.2 PHASES OF PLANNING

1. The assessment of priorities to nursing diagnosis.
2. The specification of short-term, intermediate and long-term goals of nursing action.
3. The identification of specific nursing interventions appropriate for attaining the goals.
4. The documentation of the nursing diagnosis, goals nursing interventions and expected outcomes in the nursing care plan.

50.3 STEPS IN PRIORITIES

1. The assignment of priorities to the nursing diagnosis should be a joint effort by the nurse and the patient or his family members.
2. Consideration must be given to the urgency of the problems. The most critical receiving the highest priorities.
3. Maslow's hierarchy of needs provides a useful framework for the determination of priority problems. The use of this hierarchy requires that high priorities be given to physical needs.

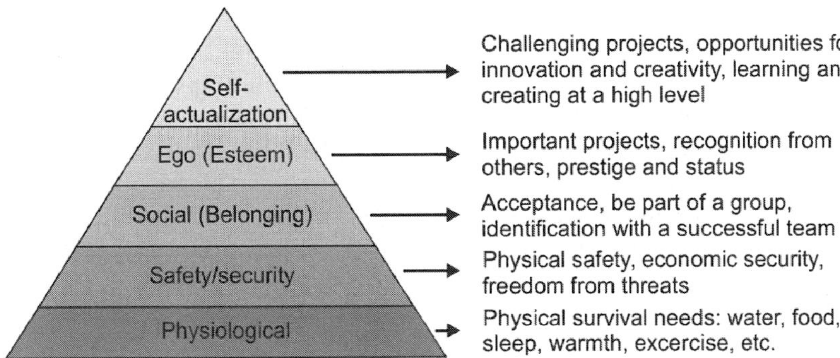

Maslow's hierarchy of needs is shown above the pyramid illustrates the five levels of human needs. The most basic are physiological and safety/security, shown at the base of the pyramid. As one moves to higher levels of the pyramid, the needs become more complex.

50.4 ESTABLISHING GOALS FOR NURSING

1. After the priorities of the nursing diagnoses have been establish, the short-term goals and the nursing actions appropriate for attainment of the goals are identified.
2. The patient and his family should be included in the establishment of the short-term intermediate and long-term goals of the nursing actions.
3. Short-term goals are those that are of immediate concern and that can be reached in a short period of time.
4. The critical time periods provide a time for determining the effectiveness of the nursing interventions and the existence of a need for additional or altered nursing care.

50.5 TEAM NURSING

1. Ideally, the accomplishment of all aspects of the planning phase of the nursing process is a group effort.
2. The nurse collaborates with other members of the nursing team, with the patient and his family and with appropriate resource persons from the healthcare agency and community agencies.
3. It is also important to remember that the patient is part of a family. The family members have need that arises from the patient's illness.
4. Another aspect of care planning takes into the account is the fact that the patient comes from the community. Community agencies have an interest in the patient and are involved in planning.

50.6 FORMULATING NURSING CARE PLAN

The nursing care plan serves to communicate the following information to all members of the nursing team:

1. Nursing diagnosis and their priorities.
2. The goals of the nursing interventions.
3. The nursing interventions which are expressed in the form of nursing orders.
4. The outcomes criteria, which identify the expected behavioral outcomes for the patient.
5. The critical time period within which each outcome must be met.

CONCLUSION

The third step of the nursing process includes the formulation of guidelines that establish the proposed course of nursing action in the resolution of nursing diagnoses and the development of the client's plan of care. It involves a series of steps in which the nurse and client set priorities, formulate goals or expected outcomes and establish a written care plan for nursing interventions. The plan to resolve or minimize the identified problems of the client and to coordinate the care provided by all the health team members.

51 Nursing Implementation/Intervention

51.1 INTRODUCTION

Implementation as a phase of the nursing process involves putting the plan of care into effect. The nurse coordinates her activities with those of others responsible for contributing to patient care and delegates responsibility to other professional and technical caregivers as appropriate. During implementation, the care plan is tested for effectiveness. Nursing interventions may not have had the desired effect, or a change in the patient's condition may present more critical problems that have a higher priority, thus requiring revision of the plan and different interventions. Nursing interventions are the actual implementation of the care plan. Nursing interventions are designed to promote, maintain or restore the client's health.

51.2 DEFINITION

1. Nursing intervention an action for which nurses are responsible that is intended to benefit a patient or client.
2. Nursing interventions are actions undertaken by a nurse to further the course of treatment for a patient. In several nations, professional nursing organizations have created complex classification systems for such interventions, creating a standardized system that can be used by all nurses to provide a high level of care. The goal is to improve the health and comfort of the patient.

51.3 MEANING OF INTERVENTION

Nurses carry out nursing interventions during the implementation phase of the nursing process. Some examples of nursing interventions would be: administer pain medication as needed, turn and reposition every two hours or perform range-of-motion exercises. An order may be required of certain nursing interventions before they can be carried out. A standing order would be an example of this. Standing orders are made by doctors in case certain situations arise, such as giving a medication when the patient shows signs of agitation or insomnia. Some interventions are actually carried out by other licensed healthcare professionals, for example a physical or respiratory therapist. The nurse records all interventions performed as well as the patient's response and outcome. This information is also relayed at the end of the shift to the nurse who will be caring for the patient next during the oncoming shift.

Nursing intervention is an act by a nurse that implements the nursing care plan or any specific objective of that plan, such as turning a comatose patient to avoid the development of decubitus ulcers or teaching insulin injection technique to a patient with diabetes before discharge from the hospital. The patient may require intervention in the form of support, limitation, medication, or treatment for the current condition or to prevent the development of further stress. As stress increases, the need to adapt and the need for nursing intervention increase.

51.4 CHARACTERISTICS OF NURSING INTERVENTION

Nursing interventions have following seven characteristics:

1. Be congruent with the overall plan of care.
2. Be based on scientific principles.
3. Be individualized to the client.
4. Be designed to provide a safe and therapeutic environment.
5. Consider the need for teaching and learning.
6. Use resources appropriately.
7. Be clearly communicated.

51.5 STAGE OF NURSING INTERVENTION

There are four stages to nursing interventions. The first is the assessment, in which the nurse determines what the problem is, as for instance in the case of someone with a nail in his or her foot. After the assessment, the nurse formulates an appropriate intervention plan, which in the case of this fictional patient would involve removal of the nail, irrigation of the wound, the administration of prophylactic antibiotics, and a tetanus shot. After planning, the nurse implements the treatment he or she has formulated, and then evaluates the patient to determine the outcome of the interventions, and to decide if additional interventions need to be undertaken.

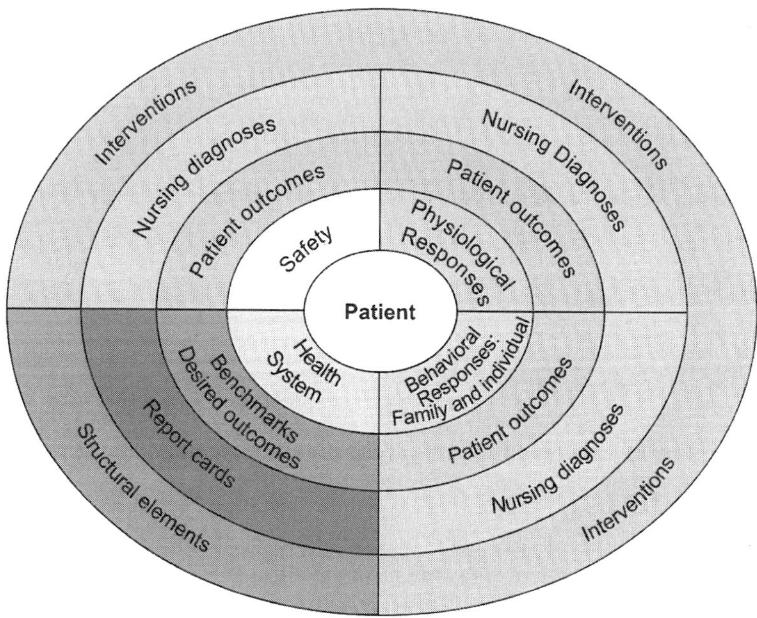

Fig. 51.1: Nursing intervention stages

51.6 PROVING SELF-CARE

The nurse should identify what skills are required for providing the intervention. It is important to remember that when a skill is delegated to another healthcare team member, the registered nurse remains legally responsible for the client's outcome.

Nurses can work alone or as part of patient care teams and interventions work in the same way in both cases. When a patient is admitted to the hospital, for example, he or she may have medical orders from a doctor, such as a standing order for medication, but the nurses also formulate a plan, which may include things like regularly checking patient vitals, monitoring fluid output, and educating the patient and his or her family about the situation.

Another aspect of providing self-care is continuous monitoring for complication. There are many complications that can allow surgery, medication administration and disease states. While the care is being given, the nurse continues to assess the client and evaluate his or her response to the care. The nurse also needs to consider which of the interventions could be modified, if the client shows no progress toward the desired outcome.

51.7 RATIONALE

At times, the scientific rationale for an intervention is required on a student care plan or listed within a standardized plan of care. It is important that the care given has its basis in scientific study, not in habit or old wives tales. The use of rationale assists in identifying the professional nurse from other providers of healthcare.

51.8 NURSING ROLES

Providing care teller into seven categories, according to Benner:

Helper role, teaching coaching, diagnostic and patient monitoring, management of rapidly changing conditions, administering and monitoring therapeutic regimens, monitoring and ensuring quality of health care practices and organizational and work role competencies. Nursing interventions can include things like counseling, referrals, patient advocacy, the administration of medication, and the performance of minor medical procedures. As in all medical care, the primary concern is keeping the patient stable enough to receive treatment, while the secondary concern is evaluating all patient needs and deciding on a course of action. When a patient comes in with an obstructed airway and a broken leg, for instance, the airway must be secured before the broken leg can be treated. Nurses are also unafraid to call in support from other medical professionals when they need it.

In nursing schools, students are usually taken through a number of theoretical cases in which they are presented with a hypothetical assessment, and asked to come up with a nursing plan which includes specific interventions. Nursing students also discuss routine interventions that are used on a regular basis, and learn about how to assess patients, how to work with other medical staff to achieve a treatment plan, and how to interact with patients and their families to ensure that everyone stays informed, comfortable, and happy.

CONCLUSION

Nursing implementation consists of doing and documenting the activities that are the specific nursing actions needed to carry out the interventions or nursing orders. It is putting the nursing care plan into action. During the implementation phase, the nurse continues to collect data and carries out the prescribed nursing activities or delegates the care to an appropriate person who validates the nursing care plan.

52 Nursing Evaluation

52.1 INTRODUCTION

The last step in the process is evaluation. Evaluation examines the degree of goal attainment and basically asks, "Did the client achieve the goal he or she was supposed to?" and if not why not? Evaluation begins with collecting data about the client's health status, closely re-examining the outcome criteria. The degree of outcome attainment is determined and a revised plan of care is established, if needed.

52.2 MEANING OF EVALUATION

During the evaluation phase of the nursing process, the nurse assesses whether the patient's goals have been achieved, and to what degree. Some goals are met partially or not at all and in these cases the nurse must determine what nursing actions should be implemented to bring about full achievement of goals. Goals that are met fully must be assessed to determine whether the implementation of nursing actions is necessary to continue or not. The evaluation is also documented. Evaluation is continuously done and depends upon all other phases of the process.

Evaluation will answer the following questions

1. Were the nursing diagnoses accurate?
2. Did the patient meet the outcome criteria?
3. Did the patient meet the criteria within the critical time periods?
4. Have the patient's nursing problems been resolved?
5. Have the patient's nursing needs been met?
6. Should the nursing interventions be retained, altered or discontinued?
7. Have new problems evolved for which nursing interventions have not been planned or implemented?
8. What factors influenced the achievement or lack of achievement of the goals?
9. Do priorities need to be reassigned?
10. Should changes be made in the goals and outcome criteria?

52.3 FORMAL EVALUATION MODELS

This type of evaluation can be viewed as informal. There is also a formal method of evaluation through a system called quality assurance.

1. Quality assurance is the planned and systematic evaluation of care given to group of clients. The organization most actively involved in formal quality assurance is the joint commission for accreditation of healthcare organizations.
2. Quality assurance programs in nursing are viewed as evaluation system composed of three dimensions — structure, process and outcome.

3. The structural dimension: Focuses on the organization within which nursing care is provided.
4. The process dimension: Focuses on patient welfare and end results of the care provided to the patient.

52.4 OUTCOME CRITERIA

Goals for accountability and quality assurance in nursing are being realized. The American Nurses Association has developed basic standards that provide a general model for nursing practice by which the quality of nursing practice may be evaluated. Record-keeping has been revised to provide a problem-oriented approach to documentation of data. The use of outcome criteria as validations of the nursing process has become an accepted trend. The nursing audit has become an accepted method for comparing results of the actual nursing performance with the established criteria.

CONCLUSION

Evaluation is an ongoing process that determines the extent to which the goals of care have been achieved. The nurses assess the progress of the patient/client, institute corrective measures if required and revise the nursing care plan. Evaluating is, in part, appraising by an authority. The nurse may be viewed as the authority in a given situation because of theory base, past experience and assessment skill. The client, however, is the authority on his or her particular strengths and needs. Therefore, implicit in this interpretation of evaluating is the collaboration of the nurse and client, each using his or her particular authority to decide together on future directions of care. The very essence of nursing requires the nurses to evaluate constantly the patient's nursing needs as well ass her own activities in meeting these needs guiding the patient in his own evaluating of his own health needs, determining how well he is meeting them and planning with him to maintain an optimal level of health.

53 Quality Assurance

53.1 INTRODUCTION

The Joint Commission on the Accreditation of Health Care Organizations (JCAH) advocates that each hospital is required to conduct a comprehensive integrated Quality Assurance Program to ensure continuing control of quality care for patients. The need for nursing quality assurance active is spelt out in the nursing standards of JCAH Manual. It states that "the Nursing Service Department" has a planned and systematic process for the monitoring and evaluation of the quality and appropriateness of patient care and for resolving identified problems. Nursing manager's understanding of the concept of quality assurance will enhance their role in implementing and evaluating standards of care.

53.2 DEFINITION

1. Quality assurance (QA) is the process of establishing a target degree of excellence for nursing intervention and taking action to ensure that each patient receives the agreed upon-level of care.
2. Quality assurance is a judgment concerning the process of care based on the extent to which that cares contributes to valued outcomes. *–Donabedian 1982*
3. Quality assurance is the measurement of provision against expectations with declared intention and ability to correct any demonstrated weakness. *–Shaw*
4. Quality assurance is a management system designed to give maximum guarantee and ensure confidence that the service provided is up to the given accepted level of quality, the standards prescribed for that service which is being achieved with a minimum of total expenditure. *–British Standards Institute*

53.3 CONCEPT OF QUALITY ASSURANCE

Quality assurance is a dynamic process through which nurses in both academic and clinical practice assume accountability for quality of care they provide (George, Veigas and Isaac, 1984). It is a guarantee to the society that members of the nursing profession are regulating services provided by nurses. Kozier et al. (2004) define quality assurance as the defining of nursing practice through well written nursing standards and the use of those standards as a basis for evaluation on improvement of client care.

53.4 OBJECTIVES OF QUALITY ASSURANCE

Quality assurance whether in health or education had two main objectives:

1. To provide technical assistance in designing and implementing effective strategies for monitoring quality and correcting systemic deficiencies and

2. To refine existing methods for ensuring optimal quality healthcare through an applied research programme (Decker, 1985 and Schroeder, 1984).

53.5 APPROACHES TO QUALITY ASSURANCE

There are three approaches from which nursing care can be evaluated to assure quality nursing practice:

1. Structure,
2. Process, and
3. Outcome.

Since, each of these interaction elements contributes to the quality of nursing care delivered, an improvement in any of the three tends to produce favorable change in the other two.

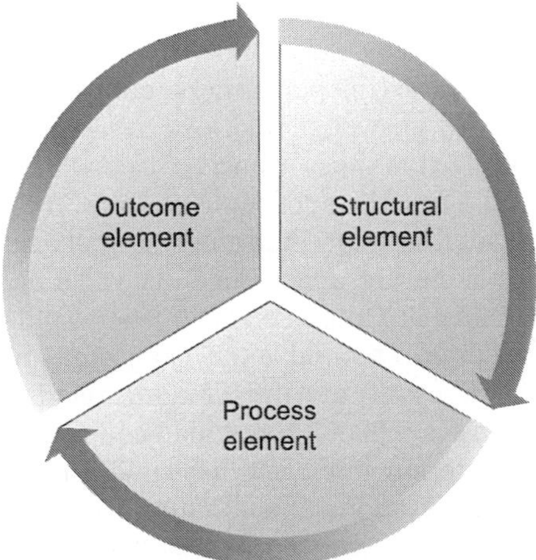

Fig. 53.1: Approaches to quality assurance

Structural element: It includes the physical setting, instrumentality and conditions through which nursing care is administered, such as philosophy, objectives, policies, procedures, records, organizational structures, financial resources, equipment and expectations and attitudes of patients and employees.

Process element: It includes steps of the nursing process itself—assessment, diagnosing, planning, implementation and evaluation and all subsystems within the nursing process, such as taking a health history, performing a physical examination, making a nursing diagnosis, determining nursing care goals, writing a nursing care plan, performing each care, cure and coordination of tasks prescribed by the care plan, measuring patient care outcome and recording and reporting patient's response to treatment. It is the criteria for measuring nursing care to determine if nursing standards of practice are being met, so they are task oriented.

Outcome element: It includes changes in patient health systems that result from nursing interventions. For example, modification in signs and symptoms, knowledge, attitudes satisfaction, skill level and compliance with treatment regimen, and established patient outcome criteria.

53.6 STEPS OF QUALITY ASSURANCE

Quality assurance is the systematic process of evaluating the quality of care given in a particular unit or institution. It involves the following steps:

1. **Setting standards:** A standards is a desired quantity, quality or level of performance with reference to a criterion against which performance is to be measured. The nursing profession through the American Nurses Association (ANA) itself has designated generic standards of nursing practice. In addition, each patient care unit must designated standards specific to the patient population served. These standards are the foundation upon which all other measures of QA are based.
   For example: "Every patient will instruments are developed and selected to collect evidence that indicates standards are being met. There are three basic forms of nursing audits: structure, process and outcome. Standards define nursing care customers as well as nursing activities of structural resources needed. They are used for planning nursing care as well as for evaluating it.
2. **Assign responsibility:** Assign responsibility to individual or committee.
3. **Delineate scope of care:** Develop an inventory including the type of patients served, the conditions and diagnoses treated, the treatment or activities performed, the type of practitioners providing care, the site where care is provided. This will provide bases for subsequent steps in the evaluation process.
4. **Identify important aspects of care:** Unit personnel should ask themselves "which of the things we do are most important?" the answer should lead to identifying important aspects of care (criteria). Priority should be given to those aspects of care which occur frequently, affect large number of patients involves risk or serious consequences or will deprive patient from substantial benefit if the care is not provided correctly or problematic behavior.
5. **Determining criteria:** Criteria must be determined that will indicate if the standards are being met and to what degree they are met. Criteria must be general and specific to the individual unit. A criterion is the value-free name of a variable that is known to be reliable indicator of quality. For example: a criterion to demonstrate that the standard regarding care plan for every patient is being met would be: "A nursing care plan is developed and written by a registered nurse within 12 hours of admission." This criterion provides a measurable indicator to evaluate performance.
6. **Data collection:** Sufficient observations and random samples are necessary for producing reliable and valid information. A useful rule is that 10 percent of the institutional patient population per month should be sampled.
   Data collection methods include:
   - Patients' Observations and interviews.
   - Nurses Observations and interviews.
   - Review of Charts.
7. **Evaluating performance**
   The methods include:
   - Reviewing documented records.
   - Observing activities as they take place.
   - Examining patients.
   - Interviewing patients, families and staff.

   Records are most commonly uses source for evaluation but they are not as reliable as direct observations. It is quite possible to write in the patient's chart activities that were not done or to not record these things that were done. Also, the chart indicates the care provided but it does not demonstrate the quality of that care.
   For the stated criteria example: This step will be: Records would be examined to determine if care plans were written on each patient within 12 hours of admission and, if so, that standards had been met.
   Another example: To measure quality of the care plan: Every care plan will include patient education appropriate to the patient's medical diagnosis, nursing diagnosis, interventions planned and discharge planning.

8. **Problem identification:** Analysis and reporting of the data gathered from the evaluation process will lead to problem identification and isolation and the evidence is gathered through round, observation and records. The nurse manager's responsibility is to look for patterns or trends of deviation from normal, further data collection and analysis could be done for the identified problems.
9. **Problem solution:** Once problem has been defined and isolated, plans are made to solve them on a priority bases. Those that are critical, which involves safety and welfare of the patient take first priority. Other factors use in determining priority will include severity, frequency, benefit, cost, and liability.
   The first step is that the nursing unit must determine how much deviation from the standard is acceptable before changes are made. In the example of developing, a written nursing care plan for every patient as a standard, the unit should decide if 45 out of 50 patients admitted have a care plan recorded within 12 hours of admission and the other 5 have recorded care plans within the next 6 hours, is this deviation acceptable? If not, then how should this be corrected?
   - Is the unit short-staffed?
   - Have there been an unusually large numbers of admissions recently?
   - Are a number of new graduates being oriented on the unit?

   After collecting all pertinent information about the possible causes, the nurse manager after consultation with staff and/or supervisor should make plans for correcting deficiencies in performance.
   - What needs change? Structural element?
   - Process element?
   - Outcome element?
10. **Monitoring and feedback:** Follow-up on how effective changes have been in improving performance is very necessary step in the QA process.

If in the example prescribed, the nurse manager found that the next 50 patients had care plans recorded within 12 hours, then the performance had improved relative to that standard. If it had not improved, then another approach would need to be taken, or possibly, the criterion should be evaluated for appropriateness for that unit.

53.7 QUALITY ASSURANCE METHODS

The purpose of a nursing QA program is to measure and improve the quality of patient care delivered in the organization. Therefore, a variety of QA methods have been used. These include:

Nursing audit: It is a method for evaluating quality of nursing care through the appraisal of the nursing process or customers of care as it is reflected in the patient care records. There are two types of audits: 1. Concurrent and 2. Retrospective audit.

Peer review: It is a process by which nurses evaluate one another's job performance against accepted standards.

Patient care profiles analysis: The analysis of longitudinal or cross-sectional complications of data about patients with a particular diagnosis or problem.

Quality circles: A quality circle is a small group of 5 to 15 employees who perform similar work and meet for one hour each week to solve problems related to their work.

Patient satisfaction (Client feedback): Patient satisfaction is used as one of several indicators of quality.

53.8 QUALITY ASSURANCE CYCLE

In practice, QA is a cyclical, iterative process that must be applied flexibly to meet the needs of a specific program. The process may begin with a comprehensive effort to define standards and norms as described in Steps 1-3, or it may start with small-scale quality improvement activities (Steps 5-10). Alternatively, the process may begin with monitoring (Step 4). Some teams may even choose to simultaneously begin in two places. For instance, comprehensive monitoring and focused problem solving may start as a coordinated, parallel effort. The ten steps in the QA process are discussed in the following section.

1. **Planning for quality assurance:** This first step prepares an organization to carry out QA activities. Planning begins with a review of the organizations scope of care to determine which services should be addressed.
2. **Setting standards and specifications:** To provide consistently high-quality services, an organization must translate its programmatic goals and objectives into operational procedures. In its widest sense, a standard is a statement of the quality that is expected. Under the broad rubric of standards there are practice guidelines or clinical protocols, administrative procedures or standard operating procedures, product specifications, and performance standards. For some programs, setting standards and specifications involves a simple review of current guidelines and standard operating procedures to ensure that they are up-to-date.
3. **Communicating guidelines and standards:** Once practice guidelines, standard operating procedures, and performance standards have been defined, it is essential that staff members communicate and promote their use. This will ensure that each health worker, supervisor, manager, and support person understands what is expected of him or her. This is particularly important if ongoing training and supervision have been weak or if guidelines and procedures have recently changed. Assessing quality before communicating expectations can lead to erroneously blaming individuals for poor performance when fault actually lies with systemic deficiencies. Additionally, QA efforts that begin with a surprise examination are likely to cause suspicion rather than support.
4. **Monitoring quality:** Monitoring is the routine collection and review of data that helps to assess whether program norms are being followed or whether outcomes are improved. By monitoring key indicators, managers and supervisors can determine whether the services delivered follow the prescribed practices and achieve the desired results.

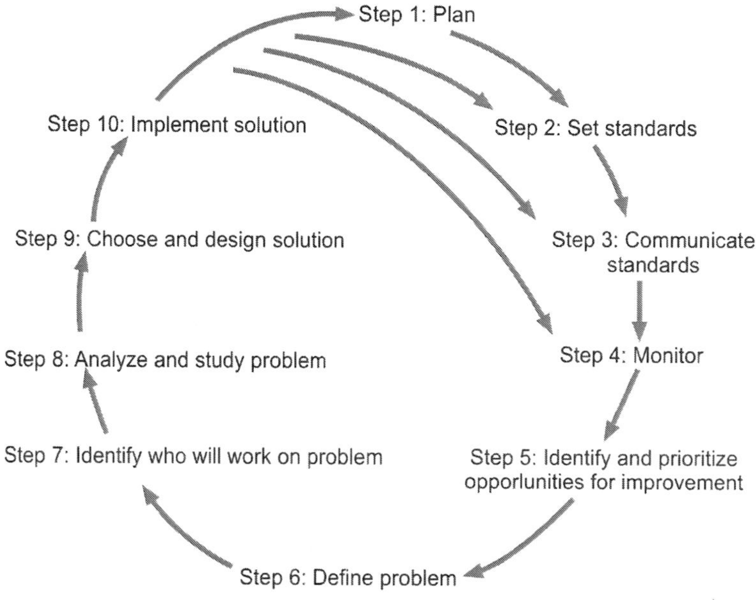

Fig. 53.2: Ten steps of quality assurance

5. **Identifying problems and selecting opportunities for improvement:** Program managers can identify quality improvement opportunities by monitoring and evaluating activities. Other means include soliciting suggestions from health workers, performing system process analyses, reviewing patient feedback or complaints, and generating ideas through brainstorming or other group techniques. Once a health facility team has identified several problems, it should set quality improvement priorities by choosing one or two problem areas on which to focus. Selection criteria will vary from program to program.
6. **Defining the problem:** Having selected a problem, the team must define it operationally-as a gap between actual performance and performance as prescribed by guidelines and standards. The problem statement should identify the problem and how it manifests itself. It should clearly state where the problem begins and ends, and how to recognize when the problem is solved. Developing a problem statement is a crucial step in the QA process, and its apparent simplicity is deceptive.
7. **Choosing a team:** Once a health facility staff has employed a participatory approach to selecting and defining a problem, it should assign a small team to address the specific problem. The team will analyze the problem, develop a quality improvement plan, and implement and evaluate the quality improvement effort. The team should comprise those who are involved with, contribute inputs or resources to, and/or benefit from the activity or activities in which the problem occurs. This ensures the involvement of those most knowledgeable about the process.
8. **Analyzing and studying the problem to identify the root cause:** Achieving a meaningful and sustainable quality improvement effort depends on understanding the problem and its root causes. Given the complexity of health service delivery, clearly identifying root causes requires systematic, in-depth analysis. Analytical tools, such as system modeling, flow charting, and cause-and-effect diagrams can be used to analyze a process or problem.
   Analytical tools alone will not always provide enough information. A problem-solving team may need to conduct an in-depth examination. Such studies can be based on clinical record reviews, health center register data, staff or patient interviews, service delivery observations.
9. **Developing solutions and actions for quality improvement:** The problem-solving team should now be ready to develop and evaluate potential solutions. Unless the procedure in question is the sole responsibility of an individual, developing solutions should be a team effort. It may be necessary to involve personnel responsible for processes related to the root cause.
10. **Implementing and evaluating quality improvement efforts:** Implementing quality improvement requires careful planning. The team must determine the necessary resources and time frame and decide who will be responsible for implementation. It must also decide whether implementation should begin with a pilot test in a limited area or should be launched on a larger scale. The team should select indicators to evaluate whether the solution was implemented correctly and whether it resolved the problem it was designed to address. In-depth monitoring should begin when the quality improvement plan is implemented. It should continue until either the solution is proven effective and sustainable, or the solution is proven ineffective and is abandoned or modified. When a solution is effective, the teams should continue limited monitoring.

53.9 ROLE OF NURSE IN QUALITY ASSURANCE

Nurses are responsible for managing the caseload of client with needs of varying degrees of urgency. Using the resources available, they must provide priority services that will promote the highest possible level of person and group functioning and health. Some quality improvement activities for nurses include daily prioritizing care needs, seeking supervision or skills development for a difficult case, systematizing charting so that needed documentation is effectively completed, proposing better ways to organize care of chronically ill client, or establishing new agency procedures. All these actions demonstrate that nurses are valuating their work and looking for ways to improve care. Staff meetings, quality circle meeting, peer review and case conferences are common settings for nurses to bring the lessons of their practices to the larger group for examination and potential adoption.

It is the role of nursing administrator to develop a formalizing tractor to develop a formalized quality program that includes a three-pronged focus based on a classic approach to quality management.

1. Review organizational structure, personnel and environment.
2. Focus on standards of nursing care and methods of delivering nursing care.
3. Focus on the outcomes of care.

Thus, any activities the nurse engages in to realize these goals contribute to the quality management program.

CONCLUSION

Quality assurance is a management system designed to give maximum guarantee and ensure confidence that the service provided is up to the given accepted level of quality, the standards prescribed for that service which is being achieved with a minimum of total expenditure. The QA program provides efficient method for gathering and maintaining information on the quality characteristics of products and on the source and nature of defects and their impact on the current operation. It permits decisions to be based on facts rather than on intuition or memory. It provides comparative data that will be useful long after the details of particular times or events have been forgotten. Quality assurance requires that certain individuals have both the authority and the responsibility for overseeing QA related actions.

54 Total Quality Management

54.1 INTRODUCTION

Total quality management (TQM) is the optimization and integration of all the functions and processes of a business in order to provide for excited customers through a process of continuous improvement. The 1990s are the decade of Globalization. In order for companies to be competitive in this environment they have seen the imperative need for Quality. However, through the decades leading to the 90s there have been many "gurus" who have explicitly underlined the need for total quality management systems in companies, but due to many factors these ideas have either gone unheeded, or been buzz word for a short time. It is possible that TQM, is once again a buzz word and a marketing tool, but nevertheless it is a tool that is being extensively used in the 90s to help companies gain and maintain a competitive edge over their rivals.

54.2 DEFINITION

1. Total quality management refers to management methods used to enhance quality and productivity in business organizations. TQM is a comprehensive management approach that works horizontally across an organization, involving all departments and employees and extending backward and forward to include both suppliers and clients/customers.
2. TQM is a management philosophy that seeks to integrate all organizational functions (marketing, finance, design, engineering, and production, customer service, etc.) to focus on meeting customer needs and organizational objectives.

54.3 OBJECTIVES OF TQM

1. Process improvement.
2. Defect prevention.
3. Priority of effort.
4. Developing cause-effect relationships.
5. Measuring system capacity.
6. Developing improvement checklist and check forms.
7. Helping teams make better decisions.
8. Developing operational definitions.
9. Separating trivial from significant needs.
10. Observing behavior changes over a period of time.

54.4 TOOLS OF TQM

1. **Quality improvement teams:** These are small groups of employees who work on solving specific problems related to quality and productivity, often with stated targets for improvement.

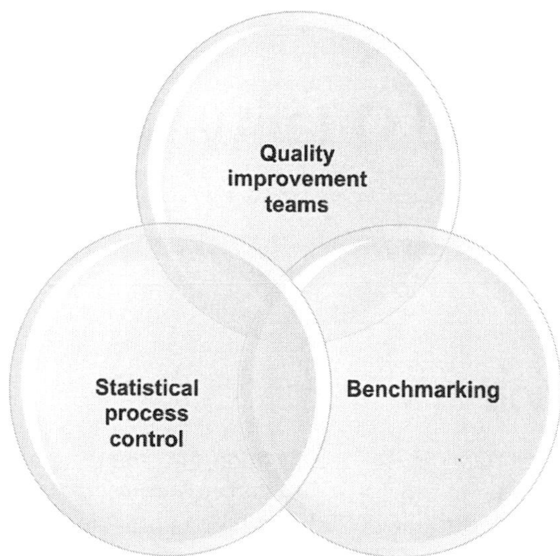

Fig. 54.1: Total quality management

Quality improvement teams are proving to be highly successful at tracking down the causes of poor quality as well as taking remedial action.

2. **Benchmarking:** This is the process of identifying the best practices and approaches by comparing productivity in specific areas within ones' own company to other organizations both within and outside the industry.
3. **Statistical process control:** This is a statistical technique that uses periodic random samples taken during actual production to determine whether acceptable quality levels are being met or whether production should be stopped in order to take remedial action. Because most processes produce some variation, statistical process control uses statistical tests to determine when variations fall outside a narrow range around the acceptable quality level. The emphasis when using SPC is on defect prevention rather than trying to inspect the quality into the product.

54.5 PRINCIPLES OF TQM

1. **Add values to the process:** Every action by every employee should add value to the process or product in every way all the time. Enhance your work by your actions.
2. **Deliver quality on time all the time:** Develop a pattern of delivering perfect products and services on time. Rate your sources by their ability to do this.
3. **Base business relationships on mutual trust and confidence:** Providers and suppliers build trust and confidence through quality and deliverability. Customers build it by quick payment and clear lines of communication. Reliability, forthrightness, and honesty are the basis of forming business relations.
4. **Train individuals and teams to solve problems:** Teach problem-solving tools/techniques and teaming as the means to solve quality, safety, productivity, and deliverability problems.
5. **Empower employees to be responsible:** For quality, safety, productivity and deliverability. Empowering means giving workers responsibility for their actions affecting their work. Share governance.
6. **Deed ownership of process to employees:** Who have proven their capability. Reward and reinforce empowerment with incentives, job security and equity sharing. Make employees owners of the process, not attendants.

7. **Implement the new technology**: Use modern information resources, internet, databases, telecommunications, applications software, and project scheduling as tools to improve productivity. Use Statistical Process Control (SPC) to eliminate errors and defects and continually improve the system.
8. **Collect, measure and evaluate data:** Before Making Decisions. "It never hurts to turn the light on." (J DeSimone). Make Decisions based on evidence. "If you can't measure it, you can't evaluate it."
9. **Apply the 80/20 principle:** Use this Problem-Solving Tool to put problems into 'Trivial Many' and 'Vital Few' Categories. Record the causes and frequencies of problems on a Tally Sheet. Develop this into a Pareto Chart which plots the frequencies (most- to least-important) of the problems. 20% of the causes create at least 80% of the problems. Importance of resolving vital problems first.
10. **Develop win-win scenarios:** Create solutions that will benefit all parties. Cooperation that develops synergism is the best solution.
11. **Develop a master plan:** Good Design Precedes Good Craftsmanship. A well-designed plan tracks and benchmarks an action through to its completion. "Quality begins at the Design Level." (Marty Madigan)
12. **Plan for all contingencies:** Prepare for all solutions by developing alternatives. If necessary, flowchart plans dealing with all possible alternatives. Apply 'If-Then-Else' type of logic to problems.
13. **Make zero defects and accidents:** Use the tools of TQM, SPC, and Problem-Solving to achieve these goals by detecting and eliminating the causes.
14. **Qualify your sources and supplies:** Use Quality and Deliverability as the basis for selecting the source of your materials and services.
15. **Deliverability:** The right product at the right place at the right time. In world-class Just-in-Time (JIT) delivery systems, source parts are used without delay and inspection in the process.
16. **Meet the needs of your customers:** Customers are anyone affected by your work: coworkers, team members, management, and especially the end-users. They are the rationale for your work. The justification for your work is to deliver products or services that meet or exceed their requirements.
17. **Improve continuously and always:** Institute continuous improvement & life-long education, principles based on the 14 Points by W Edwards Deming. Optimize your curve. They constitute an ever expanding continuum. Add to this list.

54.6 ELEMENTS OF TQM

Total Quality Management (TQM) is a management approach that originated in the 1950s and has steadily become more popular since the early 1980s. Total quality is a description of the culture, attitude and organization of a company that strives to provide customers with products and services that satisfy their needs. The culture requires quality in all aspects of the company's operations, with processes being done right the first time and defects and waste eradicated from operations.

To be successful implementing TQM, an organization must concentrate on the eight key elements:

1. Ethics
2. Integrity
3. Trust
4. Training
5. Teamwork
6. Leadership
7. Recognition
8. Communication

This paper is meant to describe the eight elements comprising TQM.

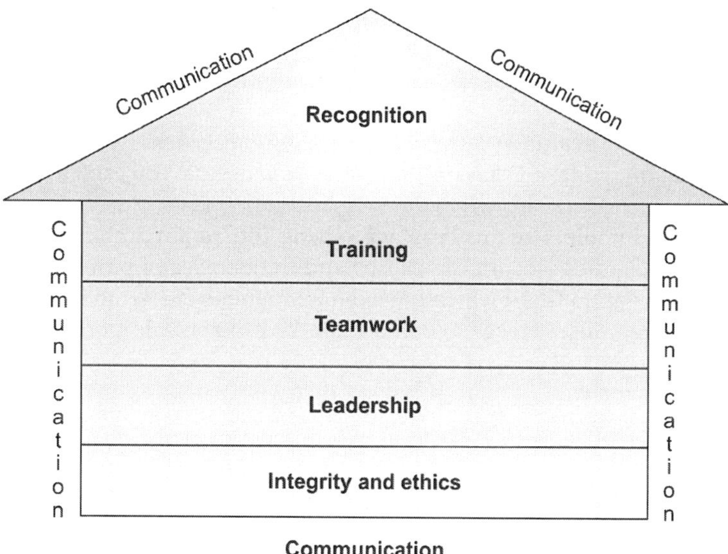

Fig. 54.2: Key elements of TQM

Key Elements

TQM has been coined to describe a philosophy that makes quality the driving force behind leadership, design, planning, and improvement initiatives. For this, TQM requires the help of those eight key elements. These elements can be divided into four groups according to their function. The groups are:
I. Foundation: it includes: Ethics, integrity and trust.
II. Building Bricks: it includes: Training, teamwork and leadership.
III. Binding Mortar: it includes: Communication.
IV. Roof: it includes: Recognition.

I. Foundation

TQM is built on a foundation of ethics, integrity and trust. It fosters openness, fairness and sincerity and allows involvement by everyone. This is the key to unlocking the ultimate potential of TQM. These three elements move together, however, each element offers something different to the TQM concept.

1. **Ethics:** Ethics is the discipline concerned with good and bad in any situation. It is a two-faceted subject represented by organizational and individual ethics. Organizational ethics establish a business code of ethics that outlines guidelines that all employees are to adhere to in the performance of their work. Individual ethics include personal rights or wrongs.
2. **Integrity:** Integrity implies honesty, morals, values, fairness, and adherence to the facts and sincerity. The characteristic is what customers (internal or external) expect and deserve to receive. People see the opposite of integrity as duplicity. TQM will not work in an atmosphere of duplicity.
3. **Trust:** Trust is a by-product of integrity and ethical conduct. Without trust, the framework of TQM cannot be built. Trust fosters full participation of all members. It allows empowerment that encourages pride ownership and it encourages commitment. It allows decision-making at appropriate levels in the organization, fosters individual risk-taking for continuous improvement and helps to ensure that measurements focus on improvement of process and are

not used to contend people. Trust is essential to ensure customer satisfaction. So, trust builds the cooperative environment essential for TQM.

II. Bricks

Basing on the strong foundation of trust, ethics and integrity, bricks are placed to reach the roof of recognition. It includes:

4. **Training:** Training is very important for employees to be highly productive. Supervisors are solely responsible for implementing TQM within their departments, and teaching their employees the philosophies of TQM. Training that employees require are interpersonal skills, the ability to function within teams, problem solving, decision-making, job management performance analysis and improvement, business economics and technical skills. During the creation and formation of TQM, employees are trained so that they can become effective employees for the company.
5. **Teamwork:** To become successful in business, teamwork is also a key element of TQM. With the use of teams, the business will receive quicker and better solutions to problems. Teams also provide more permanent improvements in processes and operations. In teams, people feel more comfortable bringing up problems that may occur, and can get help from other workers to find a solution and put into place. There are mainly three types of teams that TQM organizations adopt:
   A. **Quality improvement teams or excellence teams (QITs):** These are temporary teams with the purpose of dealing with specific problems that often recur. These teams are set up for period of three to twelve months.
   B. **Problem solving teams (PSTs):** These are temporary teams to solve certain problems and also to identify and overcome causes of problems. They generally last from one week to three months.
   C. **Natural work teams (NWTs):** These teams consist of small groups of skilled workers who share tasks and responsibilities. These teams use concepts such as employee involvement teams, self-managing teams and quality circles. These teams generally work for one to two hours a week.
6. **Leadership:** It is possibly the most important element in TQM. It appears everywhere in organization. Leadership in TQM requires the manager to provide an inspiring vision, make strategic directions that are understood by all and to instill values that guide subordinates. For TQM to be successful in the business, the supervisor must be committed in leading his employees. A supervisor must understand TQM, believe in it and then demonstrate their belief and commitment through their daily practices of TQM. The supervisor makes sure that strategies, philosophies, values and goals are transmitted down throughout the organization to provide focus, clarity and direction. A key point is that TQM has to be introduced and led by top management. Commitment and personal involvement is required from top management in creating and deploying clear quality values and goals consistent with the objectives of the company and in creating and deploying well-defined systems, methods and performance measures for achieving those goals.

III. Binding Mortar

7. **Communication:** It binds everything together. Starting from foundation to roof of the TQM house, everything is bound by strong mortar of communication. It acts as a vital link between all elements of TQM. Communication means a common understanding of ideas between the sender and the receiver. The success of TQM demands communication with and among all the organization members, suppliers and customers. Supervisors must keep open airways where employees can send and receive information about the TQM process. Communication coupled

with the sharing of correct information is vital. For communication to be credible the message must be clear and receiver must interpret in the way the sender intended.

There are different ways of communication such as:

A. **Downward communication:** This is the dominant form of communication in an organization. Presentations and discussions basically do it. By this the supervisors are able to make the employees clear about TQM.

B. **Upward communication:** By this the lower level of employees are able to provide suggestions to upper management of the affects of TQM. As employees provide insight and constructive criticism, supervisors must listen effectively to correct the situation that comes about through the use of TQM.

   This forms a level of trust between supervisors and employees. This is also similar to empowering communication, where supervisors keep open ears and listen to others.

C. **Sideways communication:** This type of communication is important because it breaks down barriers between departments. It also allows dealing with customers and suppliers in a more professional manner.

IV. Roof

8. **Recognition:** Recognition is the last and final element in the entire system. It should be provided for both suggestions and achievements for teams as well as individuals. Employees strive to receive recognition for themselves and their teams. Detecting and recognizing contributors is the most important job of a supervisor. As people are recognized, there can be huge changes in self-esteem, productivity, quality and the amount of effort exhorted to the task at hand. Recognition comes in its best form when it is immediately following an action that an employee has performed. Recognition comes in different ways, places and time such as,

Ways: It can be by way of personal letter from top management. Also by award banquets, plaques, trophies etc.

Places: Good performers can be recognized in front of departments, on performance boards and also in front of top management.

Time: Recognition can given at any time like in staff meeting, annual award banquets, etc.

54.7 TOTAL QUALITY MANAGEMENT PROCESS

TQM views an organization as a collection of processes. It maintains that organizations must strive to continuously improve these processes by incorporating the knowledge and experiences of workers. The simple objective of TQM is "Do the right things, right the first time, every time". TQM is infinitely variable and adaptable. Although, originally applied to manufacturing operations, and for a number of years only used in that area, TQM is now becoming recognized as a generic management tool, just as applicable in service and public sector organizations.

1. **Planning phase:** Planning is the most crucial phase of total quality management. In this phase, employees have to come up with their problems and queries which need to be addressed. They need to come up with the various challenges they face in their day to day operations and also analyze the problem's root cause. Employees are required to do necessary research and collect relevant data which would help them find solutions to all the problems.
2. **Doing phase:** In the doing phase, employees develop a solution for the problems defined in planning phase. Strategies are devised and implemented to overcome the challenges faced by employees. The effectiveness of solutions and strategies is also measured in this stage.
3. **Checking phase:** Checking phase is the stage where people actually do a comparison analysis of before and after data to confirm the effectiveness of the processes and measure the results.
4. **Acting phase:** In this phase, employees document their results and prepare themselves to address other problems. TQM is now becoming recognized as a generic management tool, just

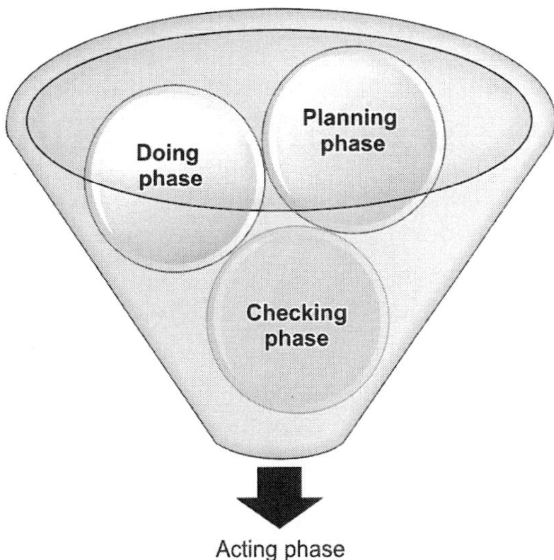

Fig. 54.3: TQM process

as applicable in service and public sector organizations. There are a number of evolutionary strands, with different sectors creating their own versions from the common ancestor. TQM is the foundation for activities, which include:

1. Commitment by senior management and all employees.
2. Meeting customer requirements.
3. Reducing development cycle times.
4. Just in time/demand flow manufacturing.
5. Improvement teams.
6. Reducing product and service costs.
7. Systems to facilitate improvement.
8. Line management ownership.
9. Employee involvement and empowerment.
10. Recognition and celebration.
11. Challenging quantified goals and benchmarking.
12. Focus on processes/improvement plans.
13. Specific incorporation in strategic planning.

CONCLUSION

Total quality management (TQM) is a comprehensive and structured approach to organizational management that seeks to improve the quality of products and services through ongoing refinements in response to continuous feedback. TQM processes are divided into four sequential categories: plan, do, check, and act (the PDCA cycle). In the planning phase, people define the problem to be addressed, collect relevant data, and ascertain the problem's root cause; in the doing phase, people develop and implement a solution, and decide upon a measurement to gauge its effectiveness; in the checking phase, people confirm the results through before-and-after data comparison; in the acting phase, people document their results, inform others about process changes, and make recommendations for the problem to be addressed in the next PDCA cycle.

55 Patient Assignment

55.1 INTRODUCTION

Planning of patient assignment is not a mere matter of dividing up the patients among the available members of the staff, but it is assigning an individual patient or group of patients to nurses according to the patient's nursing care needs and nurses ability to give care to those assigned patients.

55.2 OBJECTIVES OF PATIENT ASSIGNMENT

1. To promote the patient with the best possible nursing care.
2. To plan assignments which are interesting and stimulating to professional growth?
3. To provide a broad education and experience for each student nurse.
4. To achieve good ward management.

55.3 PRINCIPLES OF PATIENT ASSIGNMENT

1. Equal case load depending on staff ability and hours.
2. Patient assignment should be made according to the needs of each patient and of the nurse's ability to give him the care.
3. In hospital where student nurses are being educated, assignment must necessarily revolve round the requirements for the student's education.
4. For nurses to grow in professional competence, assignments must be varied and challenging to their ability.
5. Activities are better performed when each one is made responsible for a single person.
6. If there are not enough nurses on duty to carry the nursing load. It is preferable to overload the graduate staff nurses than the students or non professional works.
7. Assignments of patients and duties should not be changed frequently than is absolutely essential.
8. The care required by all patients in the group assignments to one nurse must be considered when making assignments.
9. Assignments planning are closely related to time planning. If patients are to receive good care in the late afternoon and early evening, usually as many nurses are required during these periods as during the morning hours.
10. The best use will be made of nurse's time, if the patients assigned to one nurse are geographically close together.

55.4 PATIENT ASSIGNMENT PROCESS

One important function of the professional nurse at the first-line management position of nursing service department is organizing the activities of the staff into a workable pattern to meet patient needs. She/he should establish effective relationships between the activities to be performed, the workers to perform them.

Definition of assignment: Assignment refers to "a written delegation of duties to care for a group of patients by trained personnel assigned to the unit".

Purposes of assignment:

1. To delegate the work to be done to the nursing personnel.
2. To gain the cooperation of the nursing personnel by knowing and accepting the acceptance of the work to be done.

Principles of personnel assignment:

1. Made by the head nurse or nurse in-charge for each individual nurse.
2. Based on:
   a. Nursing needs of each patient and approximate time required to care for him.
   b. The capabilities, skill level, previous experience and the interest of the staff members.
   c. Job description.
3. Planned weekly, and revised daily if necessary to assure continuity of care.
4. Take into account all the direct, indirect and unit activities.
5. Consider the geographical location of the unit and the assigned duties to save nurse's time and effort.
6. Must be balanced among nursing staff.
7. Never to assign the same task to more than one nurse.

Process of organizing patient care: The head nurse or the nurse in-charge should carry out their duties and responsibilities through applying the following steps:

1. **Planning:** It is a process of developing a course of action for meeting the needs of patient. In planning, the head nurse decides what should be done, when, how, where, by whom and to whom.
2. **Assigning:** Assignment of patient and nursing activities are written in the assignment sheet by the head nurse/nurse in-charge, based on the principles of assignment.
3. **Leading:** Includes issuing instructions, motivation, and coordination of activities, by making rounds, checking performance and conducting conferences.
4. **Evaluating:** By reviewing nursing performance and patient progress to be compared by the assignment and nursing care plan.
5. **Reporting:** The head nurse prepares a nursing unit report "e.g. shift report" which includes patient's needs, special observations, census, bed number, all critically ill and post operative patients.

Methods of patient care delivery: (methods of assignment)

I. **The traditional methods:**
   1. Case method.
   2. Functional method.
   3. Team method.
   4. Modular nursing.
   5. Primary nursing method.

II. **The advanced method:** Case management

55.5 CASE METHOD

It is the oldest mode of organizing patient care. In this method, nurses assume total responsibility for meeting all the needs of assigned patients during their time on duty. It involves the assignment of one or more clients to a nurse for a specific period of time, such as shift. Complete care, including treatments, medication administration and nursing care planning, is the assigned nurse's responsibility. Even though the case method is one of the earliest methods of nursing care delivery, it is still widely used in hospitals and in home health agencies. It is developed and communicated through written sources, its usage remains in contemporary practice. Students most frequently learn within this model, private duty nurses practice with this design, and specialty units, such as ICU, ICCU etc. most often use this model.

Case method nursing provides nurses with high autonomy and responsibility. Assigning patient is simple and direct and does not require the planning that other methods of patient care delivery do. The lines of authority and accountability are clear. The patient theoretically receives holistic and unfragmented care during the nurse's time on duty. Each nurse caring for the patient can, however modify the care regimen. The merits and demerits of this method are as follows.

Advantages

1. The nurse can see better and attend to the total needs of clients due to the time and proximity of interactors. Coordination of all aspects of care is the main responsibility of the nurse; which includes physical, emotional, medical regimen, teaching and all other aspects related to it.
2. Continuity of care can be facilitated with care.
3. Client/nurse interaction/rapport can be developed by virtue of intensity of time and proximity of those involved.
4. Client may feel more secure, knowing that one person is thoroughly familiar with the needs and the course of treatment of his/her disease.
5. Educational needs of the clients can be closely monitored.
6. Family and friends become better known by nurse and get more involved in the care of the client.
7. Work load for the unit can be equally divided among the available staff.
8. Nurse's accountability for their function is built-in.

Disadvantages

1. Many clients do not require the inherent care of intensity in this type of service.
2. This method must be modified if non-professional health workers are to be used effectively.
3. Nurses are not enough to comply the demand of this model; cost-effectiveness must be considered.
4. It is difficult for nurses to use this method to become involved in long-term planning and evaluation of care.
5. The greatest disadvantage to case nursing occurs, when the nurse is inadequately trained or prepared to provide total care to the patient.

55.6 FUNCTIONAL METHOD

Emerged during 1950s, due to shortage of nurses. This method focuses on getting the greatest amount of tasks in the least time. In this method, the nursing care is divided into tasks and each staff member is assigning to perform one or two tasks for all patients in the unit according to the level of skill required for performance as follows:

- **Registered professional nurses:** Responsible for administering medication to all unit patients, another for changing dressings and administering ordered treatments (such as postural drainage or warm compresses) for all patients.
- **Technical nurses:** Responsible for taking vital signs and recording intake and output for all patients in the unit, while another might be giving baths to all bedridden patients.
- **Nurse aides:** Responsible for making beds for all ambulatory patients and assisting mobility-impaired patients to move in bed or walk in the hall.
- **Unit clerk:** Responsible for answering telephone, delivering messages, recording admissions and discharges, etc.

Advantages

1. Care is provided economically and efficiently.
2. Minimum number of Registered Nurses (RNs) required, so it is efficient when there is a shortage in the staff or there is limited number of professional nurses.
3. Tasks are completed quickly.
4. Useful in emergency situations.

Disadvantages

1. Care may be fragmented.
2. Patient may be confused with many care providers.
3. Caregivers feel unchallenged.
4. Lack of communication among the different persons who care for the patient.
5. Neglecting the humanity of the patient and the individual needs of the patient will be lost in an effort to get the work done.

55.7 TEAM NURSING

Team nursing was developed because of social and technological changes in world war-II drew many nurses away from hospitals, learning haps, services, procedures and equipment became more expensive and complicated, requiring specialization at every turn. It is an attempt to meet increased demands of nursing services and better use of knowledge and skills of professional nurses.

Definitions

1. Team nursing is based on philosophy in which groups of professional and non-professional personnel work together to identify, plan, implement and evaluate comprehensive client-centered care. The key concept is a group that works together toward a common goal, providing qualitative comprehensive nursing care. *-Kron 1978*
2. Team nursing was designed to accommodate several categories of personnel in meeting the comprehensive nursing needs of a group of clients. *-Donavan 1975*

Concept of team nursing: The concept of team nursing was introduced in the early 1950s. It is a method of nursing assignment that binds professional, technical and nurse aides into small teams. This method allows for efficient utilization of technical and/or nurse's aide through the direct supervision, guidance, and teaching of professional nurses.

Objectives: The objective of team nursing is to give the best possible quality of patient care by utilizing the abilities of every member of the staff to the fullest extent and by providing close supervision both of patient care and of the individual who give it.

Process of implementing the team method: One registered nurse in the team is appointed by the head nurse to serve as a team leader. The team members commonly consist of at least one professional nurse, one technical nurse, nursing students and nursing aides. All team members may receive reports about their patients' care needs from the team leader or team member on previous shift.

The team leader usually assigns:

1. **Professional nurse** to care for the most seriously ill patients, to ensure informed observation and skilled interventions. Often, the team leader assigns the technical nurse to bath, feed, and move and change dressings for patients.
2. **Nurse aides** are assigned to make beds, assist ambulatory patients with bathing and grooming, testing urine and performing simple nursing care procedures.
3. **Team leader** usually administers medications and monitors parenteral fluid therapy for all patients assigned to the team. Without team planning and communication through the team conferences, team nursing may become in reality just a variation of the functional method.

Functions of team nursing: The two important functioning are:

1. The head nurse must know at all times the condition of the patients and the plan for their care and must be assured that assignments and workmanship contribute to quality nursing.
2. The team leader must have freedom to use their initiative and the opportunity to nurse, supervise, and teach unencumbered by the responsibility for administrative detail.

Functions of registered nurse:

1. In the team nursing, RN functions as a team leader and coordinates the small group (no more than four or five) of ancillary personnel to provide care to a small group of patients.
2. As coordinator of the team, the RN must know the condition and needs of all patients assigned to the team and plan for the individualized care for each patient. (Marquis and Huston, 2003)
3. The team leader is also responsible for encouraging a cooperative environment and maintaining clear communication among all team members.
4. The team leader's duties include planning care, assigning duties, directing and assisting team members, giving direct patient care, teaching and coordinating patient activities.
5. The team leader assigns each member specific responsibilities dependent on the role.
6. The members of the team report directly to the team leader, who then reports to the charge nurse or unit manager.
7. Communication is enhanced through the use of written patient assignments, the development of nursing care plans, and the use of regularly scheduled team conferences to discuss the patient status and formulate revisions to the plan of care.
8. However, for team nursing to succeed, the team leader must have strong clinical skills, good communication skills, delegation ability, decision-making ability, and the ability to create a cooperative working environment.

Advantages

1. High-quality, comprehensive care with a high proportion of ancillary staff.
2. Team members participate in decision-making and contribute their own expertise.

Disadvantages

1. Continuity suffers if daily team assignments vary.
2. Team leader must have good leadership skills.
3. Insufficient time for planning and communication.

55.8 MODULAR NURSING

Modular nursing assignment is used when the nursing staff includes technical and nurse aides, as well as professional nurses. Although, two or three persons are assigned to each module, the greatest responsibility for the care of assigned patients falls on the professional nurse. The professional nurse is also responsible for guiding and teaching nonprofessional nurse.

Definition

Modular nursing is a modification of team nursing and focuses on the patient's geographic location for staff assignments.

–Magargal 1980

1. The patient unit is divided into modules or districts, and the same team of caregivers is assigned consistently to the same geographic location.
2. Each location, or module, has an RN assigned as the team leader, and the other team members may include LVN/LPN or UAP.

   –Yoder Wise 2003
3. Just as in the team nursing, the team leader in the modular nursing is accountable for all patient care and is responsible for providing leadership for team members and creating a cooperative work environment.

4. The concept of modular nursing calls for a smaller group of staff providing care for a smaller group of patients.
5. The goal is to increase the involvement of the RN in planning and coordinating care.
6. Communication is more efficient among a smaller group of team members.

–Marquis and Huston, 2003

7. The success of the modular nursing depends greatly on the leadership abilities of the team leader.

Advantages: (Yoder Wise 2003)

1. Continuity of care is improved when staff members are consistently assigned to the same module.
2. The RN as team leader is able to be more involved in planning and coordinating care.
3. Geographic closeness and more efficient communication save staff time.

Disadvantages: (Yoder Wise 2003)

1. Costs may be increased to stock each module with the necessary patient care supplies (medication cart, linens and dressings).
2. Long corridors, common in many hospitals, are not conducive to modular nursing.

Special note

1. Modular nursing is similar to team nursing because professional and nonprofessional employees cooperate in caring for patients under the leadership of a professional nurse.
2. Module nursing is similar to primary nursing because each pair or trio of nursing personnel are responsible for the care of the patients in their caseload from admission to discharge, following discharge and during subsequent admissions to the agency.
3. As with primary nursing, the worker pair or trio arrange or another pair or trio to care for their assigned patients on alternate shifts and days off.

55.9 PROGRESSIVE PATIENT CARE

Progressive client care is a method in which client care areas or units provide various levels of care, e.g. (1) intensive care unit for the critically ill, (2) post intensive care unit, (3) regular care units, (4) convalescent unit, and (5) self care unit. Here, the clients are evaluated with respect to all level (intensity) of care needed. As they progress towards increased self care (as they become less ethically ill or in need of intensive care or monitoring) they are marked to units/wards staffed to best provide the type of care needed. The merits and demerits of progressive patient care are as follows:

Advantages

1. Efficient use is made of personnel and equipment.
2. Clients are in the best place to receive the care they require.
3. Use of nursing skills and expertise are maximized due to different staffing patterns of each unit.
4. Clients are moved towards self care, independence is fostered where indicated.
5. Efficient use and placement of equipment is possible.
6. Personnel have greater probability to function towards their fullest capacity.

Disadvantages

1. There may be discomfort to clients who are moved often.
2. Continuity care is difficult, even though possible.
3. Long-term nurse/client relationships are difficult to arrange.
4. Great emphasis is placed on comprehensive, written care plan.

5. There is often times difficulty in meeting administrative need of the organization, staffing evaluation and accreditation.

55.10 PRIMARY NURSING METHOD

This method is the best in an agency with an all-professional nurse staff. It is a comprehensive, continuous and coordinated nursing process for meeting the total needs of each patient.

Basic Concepts in Primary Nursing

1. **Patient assessment** by a primary nurse, who plans the care to be given by secondary or associate nurse when the primary nurse is off duty. The 24 hours responsibility for care is put into practice through the primary nurse's written directive on a preplanned communication assignment.
2. **Complete communication** of care given in the nursing staff daily reporting method.
3. **Discharge planning** including teaching, family involvement and appropriate references.

Process for Implementing Primary Nursing Method

1. **The head nurse:**
   a. Assigns primary nurse to patients by matching the skills of the nurse to the needs of the patients.
   b. Ensures proper scheduling for all shifts so that if primary nurse is off the unit an associate nurse is available for care.
   c. Guides, counsels and evaluates care given.
   d. May also assign herself to patients either as a primary nurse or associate nurse.
2. **Professional staff nurse:**
   1. **Primary nurse:** Functions of primary nurse include performing the following:
      1. Conducting an admission (initial) assessment.
      2. Developing, planning, implementing, and revising the nursing care plan.
      3. Directing care in her absence.
      4. Collaborating with physicians and families.
      5. Making referrals.
      6. Teaching health concepts.
      7. Making discharge plans.
   2. **Associate nurse:** Associate nurse may be professional or technical nurse. She carries out the nursing care planned by the primary nurse when she is not on duty.
   3. **Technical nurse:** Carry out the nursing tasks assigned by the primary or associate nurses in giving the care.
   4. **Nurse aides:** Their activities are focusing away from direct contact with the patient and can be utilized as messengers and transporters.
   5. **Ward clerk:** Responsible for the nonnursing functions of administrative duties.

Advantages

1. High-quality, holistic patient care.
2. Establish rapport with patient.
3. RN feels challenged and rewarded.

Disadvantages

1. Primary nurse must be able to practice with a high degree of responsibility and autonomy
2. RN must accept 24-hour responsibility.
3. More RNs needed; not cost-effective.

55.11 CASE MANAGEMENT

Case management is a process of monitoring an individual patient's healthcare by the case manger, for the purpose of maximizing positive outcomes and containing costs.

The case manger has graduate-level preparation or is at an advanced level of nursing practice. The case manager role requires not only advanced nursing skills but also advanced managerial and communication skills.

The case manager is an individual "professional nurse" assigned responsibility for this process.

1. The case manager may follow the patient from the diagnostic phase through hospitalization, rehabilitation and back to home care.
2. Case manager has responsibility and authority for planning, implementing, coordinating and evaluating care for the patient throughout the period of illness, regardless of the patient's movement among various units and services (such as emergency room, surgical unit, recovery unit, etc.).
3. The case manager ensures that plans are made in advance for the next needed step. Through this, the manager assists with decision-making and helps to ensure that the patient receives care that will achieve the most positive outcomes in the most efficient manner. This process helps to eliminate costly delays in progress.

Case Manager's Approaches

1. **Case managers employed by the hospitals** follow a patient from the time admission is planned through the time of discharge. This case manager might plan the admitting process to ensure that all preadmission work-ups are completed and that the patient is being admitted at the appropriate time to facilitate follow-up through on problems.
2. **Case managers in private practice** may focus on a particular group of client. For example, the geriatric case manager focuses on managing care for the older client. The private case manager is paid by the client or family usually based on the hours of service provided. The case manager may help the family to identify all the options for care and treatment, ask questions to obtain greater understanding of the overall problem, and work with the family in the decision-making process.

Case Management Tools

The case manager uses two tools, Case Manager Plan (CMP), and Critical Path Diagnosis (CPD) to, design, map, track, monitor, and adjust the patient's course through the care-treatment process.

1. **Case manager plan (CMP):** It is a multicolumn plan with accompanying time line that includes medical and nursing diagnosis, desired care outcomes, intermediate daily goals to supports each outcome, and the daily activities required of nurse, physicians, and other caregivers to achieve intermediate goal.
2. **Critical path diagnosis (CPD):** It is an abbreviated , one-page version of the required physician and nurse action listed in the CMP, together with the exact data on which all key events must occur to achieve the desired outcome by the target date. The case manager evaluates the patient's progress toward care and treatment goal daily by comparing signs, symptoms, and assessment data against information in the CMP and CDP then tracking variances from the expected course of progress.

Advantages

I. For the patient:

1. Establishing and achieving a set of "expected" or standardized patient care outcomes for each patient.

2. Facilitating early patient discharge or discharge within an appropriate length of stay.
3. Using the fewest possible appropriate healthcare resources to meet expected patient care outcomes.
4. Facilitating the continuity of patient care through collaborative practice of diverse health professionals.

II. For the nurse:

1. Enhancing nurse's professional development and job satisfaction.
2. Facilitating the transfer of knowledge of expert clinical staff of novice staff.

CONCLUSION

For the patients to receive good nursing care the nurse must have time to give him the physical and psychological care which his condition requires and to help him prepare to take his place in the life of his family and the community as quickly as possible.

56 Documentation in Nursing

56.1 INTRODUCTION

All professional persons need to be accountable for the performance of their duties to the public. Since, nursing has been considered as profession, nurses need to record their work on completion. A record is a permanent written communication that documents information's relevant to a client's healthcare management. A record is a clinical, scientific, administrative and legal document relating to the nursing care given to individual family or community. The records are a practical and indispensable aid to the doctor, nurse and paramedical personnel in giving the best possible service to their clients. Recorded facts have a value and scientific accuracy for more than mere impression of memory and there are guidelines for better administration of health services. Records are the means of communications between health workers and their clients.

56.2 PURPOSE OF RECORDS

1. Records provide data for programme planning and evaluation.
2. Records are the tools of communication between the health workers, the family and other development personnel.
3. Records indicate plans for the future.
4. Records provide baseline data to estimate the long-term changes related to the services.
5. Records provide an opportunity for evaluating the services.
6. Records help in the research for improvement of nursing care.

Every institution keeps some kinds of records. The hospital is no exception. The patients clinical record is a brief account of the personal and medical history of the patient, results of diagnostic tests, findings of medical examination, treatment and nursing care daily progress notes and advice on discharge.

56.3 IMPORTANCE OF RECORDS

1. Record provides an accurate and detailed account of treatments and care given to the patient. Therefore, it serves as a guide for follow up of the course of disease and future care.
2. The record provides accurate information of the results of medication and treatments given to the patient. So, through the records the physician gets accurate information about the patient's conditions from day to day.
3. Records are of great value in the diagnosis, treatments and nursing care.
4. A record of illness and treatment saves duplication of work in the future care especially when the patient is transferred from one department to another or from one institution to another or when an attending physician is transferred and other person takes charge. In such situations it helps the patient to get prompt treatment.

5. A well-written record has legal value. The records safeguard the patients, nurses, doctors and the hospital. It serves as evidence that the patient care is intelligently managed.
6. Records are tools of communication among the members of the health team. It is of great value for the doctors and nurses at the shifting of duty hours.
7. Records help the medical and nursing students in the clinical experience and provide data for care studies.
8. Records serve as a reference material for research work.
9. The patients record, registers and reports furnish the vital statistics and give information needed to evaluate the service rendered by hospital to the community.
10. Data taken from the patient's record points out the health problems of the country and it also provides a baseline in which local, state, national and international health services are planned.

56.4 PRINCIPLES OF RECORD WRITING

1. Since, the clinical record is a legal document, it is essential that they should be written clearly, accurately, appropriately and legibly.
2. The individual who writes them should sign all entries.
3. Care to be taken not to make any error on the records. If anything is crossed out, it should be dated and initialed.
4. All records should be written with black ink or typed for better legibility.
5. Records should be written in chronological order as to date and time. When recording medications and treatments, note exact time and date on which they are carried out.
6. Records are written continuously with no blank spaces. If any space is left out, it should be crossed out, dated and signed.
7. Lengthy corrections of records are written as amendments.
8. Each page of the record should be properly identified with the name, age, I.P. No. OP-No. Date, etc.
9. Use only standard abbreviations.
10. Records should be truthful, brief and complete. It should include all the services given to the patients, the observations made on the patient from day to day and the results of treatments etc.

56.5 TYPES OF RECORDS

1. Outpatient and inpatient records.
2. Nurse's recording.
3. Doctor's order sheet.
4. Graphic charts of Temperature, pulse and respiration (TPR).
5. Reports of laboratory examinations.
6. Diet sheets.
7. Consent form for operations and anesthesia.
8. Intake and output chart.
9. Reports of anesthesia, physiotherapy and other special treatment.
10. Registers.

56.6 GENERAL RULES OF RECORDING

1. Keep separate records or charts for each individual patient.
2. It is a legal document; write it, in English, clearly, accurately, appropriately and legibly.
3. Name, age, ward, date and in-patient number should be written on each page.
4. All entries should be signed by the individual who makes the entry.

5. All entries should be written in blue or black ink.
6. Chart nursing-care and medications and other treatments only after giving them.
7. It should be reliable and accurate.
8. Information about patients and their care must be factual.
9. Correct spelling is also important for accurate recording.
10. Nurses should not allow others to record for her.
11. Use only standard abbreviations.
12. Do not use ditto marks or chemical formula in charting.
13. Each patient should have a daily note, written by nurses on all shifts.
14. The information within a record should be complete.
15. Concise data are easy to understand.
16. Lengthy notes are difficult to read.
17. Record immediately after performing nursing activities. It should have currentness.
18. It should be organized in a logical format or order.
19. Nurses should maintain confidentiality of patents' record.
20. Do not use blank space in the record. Keep it crossed.

56.7 NURSES RESPONSIBILITY IN RECORDING

Generally, nurses' notes contain the following information:
1. Treatment and nursing care given by various members of the health team.
2. Doctor's orders carried out by nurses.
3. Nursing needs met by nurses as per doctor's order.
4. Observations, e.g. vital signs, physical signs and behavioral patterns of patient.
5. Response of patient to treatment and nursing care.
6. Health advice given by nurses and other staff
7. Independent nursing functions are also recorded.

56.8 PURPOSE OF REPORTS

Reports are oral or written exchanges of information shared between caregivers or workers in a number of ways. A report summarizes the services of the person or personnel and of the agency. Reports are usually written daily, weekly, monthly or yearly.
1. To show the kind and amount of services rendered over a specified period.
2. To illustrate progress in reaching goals.
3. As an aid in studying health conditions.
4. As an aid in planning.
5. To interpret the services to the public and to the other interested agencies.

Probably no other single factor is more vital for good administration than prompt and complete reports. They save duplication of efforts and eliminate the need for investigation to learn the facts in situation.

56.9 TYPES OF REPORTS

Reports may be classified as oral and written.
1. **Oral reports:** Oral reports are given when the information is for immediate use and not for permanency. For example, oral report is made by the nurse who is assigned to patient care, to another nurse who is planning to relieve her, and some of the oral reports may be made to charge nurses and nurse supervisors and also doctors. Reports are to be written when the information is to be used by several personnel, which is more or less of permanent value, for

example day and night reports, census, interdepartmental reports and other special reports, needed according to situation, events and conditions.

The reports used in hospital setting usually are change-of-shift reports, transfer reports, incident reports, day, evening and night reports, legal reports.

2. **Change-of-shift reports:** These may be given orally in person by audio taping, recording, or during rounds at the clients' bedside some of the points to be kept in mind while giving such reports are as follows:
   1. Provide only essential background information about client (name, sex, age, diagnosis and medical history) but do not review all routine care procedures or tasks.
   2. Identify clients' nursing diagnosis or healthcare problems and other related causes but do not review all biographical information on case sheets.
   3. Describe objective measurements or observations about clients 'condition and response to health problem. Stress recent change, but do not use critical comment about clients' behavior.
   4. Share significant information about family members, as it relates to clients' problems do not make any assumptions about relationship between family members.
   5. Continuously review ongoing discharge plan. Don't engage in idle gossip.
   6. Relay to staff significant changes in the way therapies are given. Do not describe basic steps of a procedure.
   7. Describe instruction given in teaching plan and clients' response. Do not explain detailed content unless staff members ask for clarification.
   8. Evaluate results of nursing or medical care measures. Do not simply describe results as good or poor. Be specific.
   9. Be clear on priorities to which oncoming staff must attend. Do not force oncoming staff to guess what to do first.
3. **Transfer-reports:** Patients will frequently be transferred from one unit to another to receive different levels of care. A transfer report involves communications of information about clients from the nurse on sending unit to the nurse on the receiving unit. When giving transfer request, nurse should include the following information.
   1. Client's name, age, primary doctor, and medical diagnosis.
   2. Summary of medical progress upto the time of transfer.
   3. Current health status—physical and psychosocial.
   4. Current nursing diagnosis or problems and care plan.
   5. Any critical assessment or interventions to be completed shortly.
   6. Needs for any special equipment etc.
4. **Incident reports:** Nurses usually become involved in client-related incidents as some point in their careers. They must understand the purpose of incident reports and the correct way to report information. While incident reporting, the following points are to be kept in mind:
   1. The nurse who witnessed the incident or who found the client at the time of incident should file the report.
   2. The nurse describes in concise what happened specifically objective terms, etc.
   3. The nurse does not interpret or attempt to explain the cause of the incident.
   4. The nurse describes objectively the clients, conditions when the incident was discovered.
   5. Any measures taken by the nurse, other nurses, or doctors at the time of the incident are reported.
   6. No nurse is blamed in an incident report.
   7. The report is submitted as soon as possible to the appropriate authority.
   8. The nurse should never make photocopy of the incident report.
5. **Legal reports:** Incident reports and reports on accidents, mistakes and complaints are legal in nature. There are times when a hospital is criticized for what is claimed to be negligence or

poor care because of a condition that resulted in discomfort and perhaps serious harm to a patient or client. In such reports, the content is stated briefly and objectively giving all pertinent information. Accuracy, timeliness, completeness and relevancy to the problems are maintained promptly while making such reports.

56.10 PRINCIPLES OF RECORD KEEPING

Records and reports must be functional, accurate, complete, current organized and confidential.

1. **Fact:** Information about clients and their care must be functional. A record should contain descriptive, objective information about what a nurse sees, hears, feels and smells. In the same way, anything happens during the managing the affairs in the institutions/hospital, manager should document inferences or construction with functional information to avoid misleading, misinterpretation and any error in administration.
2. **Accuracy:** A client record must be reliable. In other words, information must be accurate so that health team members have confidence in it. The use of correct measurements ensures that a record is accurate.
3. **Completeness:** The information within a recorded entry or a report should be complete, containing concise and thorough information's about a client care or any event or happening taking place in the jurisdiction of manager.
4. **Currentness:** Delays in recording or reporting can result in serious omissions and untimely delays for medical care or action legally, a late entry in a chart may be interpreted on negligence.
5. **Organization:** The nurse or nurse manager communicates information in a logical format or order. Health team members understand information better when it is given in the order in which it occurred.
6. **Confidentiality:** Nurses are legally and ethically obligated to keen information about client's illnesses and treatments confidential. In the same way certain information in management also should be kept confidential.

   Any information about clients care or event taking place in the healthcare agencies should be communication with careful thought. All members of health team depend on recorded and reported information. Accurate information ensures continuity and quality of care, and also smooth running of administration.

56.11 NURSES RESPONSIBILITY IN RECORD KEEPING

Nurses have legal responsibility for accurately reporting and recording patient's conditions, treatments and responses to care. The medical record is a written or computerized account of a patient's illness and treatment that includes information submitted by all members of the patient healthcare team. The medical record is an information source document that should be used to plan care, evaluate care, allocate costs, educate personnel, research care measure and substantiate legal claims.

Court decisions have stated that the patient's medical record is essential to proper care and the medical record is the property of the health agency. However, the patient has a property right to information contained in the report, the patient has a right to inspect and copy the record after being discharged. However, it is unadvisable to allow a patient to review his or her medical record without medical supervision and explanation because a patient is likely to misunderstand certain record notations.

Failure to record significant patient information on the medical record makes a nurse guilty of negligence when the patient is injured because of a doctor's ignorance of significant information about medical history, signs and symptoms.

The medical record must be accurate to provide a sound basis for care planning. Therefore, errors in nurses charting must be corrected promptly in a manner that leaves no doubt about the facts. Every health agency should have a policy and protocol that directs that an erroneous chart entry be crossed through labeled as erroneous signed by the employee who corrects the error, and retained in the patient's record. Correct information should then be documented to replace the erroneous and corrected entries should never be destroyed. Nurses who conspire with doctors and others to falsify a patient's record for purposes of concealing a criminal violation may be found criminally liable. Generally, the person who makes reports required by statute is immune from suit under the doctrine of the public's right to know. In many countries there are statutes that require health personnel to report instances of child abuse, ophthalmic neonatorum, communicable diseases, and births out of wedlock, gunshot wounds, suicide, rape, and use of unperceived narcotics. In reporting information about criminal acts obtained during patient care, the nurse must reveal such information only to the police, because it is considered a privileged communication. Several aspects of statutory, case, and administrative law control nursing practice and nursing management.

CONCLUSION

All professional persons need to be accountable for the performance of their duties to the public. Since nursing has been considered as profession, nurses need to record their work on completion. A record is a permanent written communication that documents information's relevant to a client's healthcare management. A record is a clinical, scientific, administrative and legal document relating to the nursing care given to individual family or community. The records are a practical and indispensable aid to the doctor, nurse and paramedical personnel in giving the best possible service to their clients. Recorded facts have a value and scientific accuracy for more than mere impression of memory and there are guidelines for better administration of health services. Records are the means of communications between health workers and their clients.

Section-10

Nursing Theories

57 Nursing Practice Theories

57.1 INTRODUCTION

As a science, nursing is in its infancy. Professional nurses are aware of this and conscious of the need for both nursing theory development and theory based practice. As nursing comes of age, not only as a practice discipline but also as a scholarly discipline, there will be increasing interest in delineating the theory base of nursing. Some believe that theory development is the most crucial task facing nursing (Chinn and Jacobs, 1978). This study of theory helps to develop analytical skills, challenge thinking, clarifies values and assumptions, and determines purposes for nursing practice, education, and research. The contributions of many theorists outside of nursing profession formed the knowledge based for nursing practice for many years. New disciplines are often slow to develop their own theories and nursing was no exteption. Even now, theories from the physical, biological, social, and behavioral sciences in addition to more recent nursing models and theories are used extensively in nursing practice.

57.2 MEANING

Theories are general explanations which scholars use to explain, control and understand commonly occurring events. Theories are best understood as preliminary explanations that reflect the current understanding of events. "Theory is defined as a set of propositions used to describe, explain, predict and control events". Here set refers to a group of circumstances, situations, and so on, joined and treated as a whole; propositions refers to statements about how two or more concepts are related; concepts refers to an abstract classification of data, temperature; describe means of tell about in details; explain means to offer reasons for; predict means to foretell/forecast; control means to exercise as regulating influence over; and phenomena refer to theory includes the joint functions of theory, i.e. description explanation, prediction and control.

57.3 IMPORTANCE OF NURSING THEORIES

Theory helps in providing knowledge to improve practice by describing, explaining, predicting, and controlling phenomena. Nurses power is increased through theoretical knowledge because systematically developed more likely to be successful. In addition, nurses will know why they are doing, what they are doing if challenged. Theory provides professional autonomy by guiding the nursing practice, education and research functions of profession. And also there has been interest in identifying a body of nursing knowledge that is essential to professional nursing practice. Theory development contributes to knowledge building and is seen a means of establishing 'nursing as a profession'.

The commitment to that nursing practice based on sound, reliable knowledge is intrinsically valuable to nursing. That is to say, knowledge is desirable by its very nature. The growth and enrichment of theory and of itself is an important goal for nursing as a scholarly discipline, to pursue. Now nursing practice settings are complex, and the amount of data available to nurses are virtually endless. Nurses must analyze a tremendous amount of information about each patient and decide what to do. If a theory helps practicing nurses categorize and understand what is going on in nursing practice, if it helps them predict patients responses to nursing care, and if it is helpful in clinical decision making, it is useful as a guide to nursing practice.

57.4 DEVELOPMENT OF NURSING THEORIES

The development of nursing science and theory is a scholarly activity. Developing this science involves generating knowledge; although this knowledge can be used with knowledge from other disciplines, it is designed to advance and support nursing practice and healthcare. As nursing continues to evolve, nurses theorize about the nature of nursing practice, the principles on which practice is based, and the proper goals and functions of nursing in society. Conceptional and theoretical nursing models are used to provide knowledge to improve practice, guide research and curricular and identify domain and goals of nursing practice. Nursing theories provide the nurse with goals of assessment, nursing diagnosis and intervention; common ground for communication; and professional autonomy and accountability. They also guide future directions for nursing research; practice, education, and administration.

Theories of nursing can help the nursing student to understand how the roles and actions of nurses fit together in nursing. The brief descriptions of selected nursing theories are as follows.

57.5 NIGHTINGALE'S THEORY (ENVIRONMENTAL MODEL)

Florence Nightingale, the matriarch of modern nursing, who is establishing the discipline of nursing, spoke with firm conviction about the 'nature of nursing as a profession that required knowledge distinct from medical knowledge'. The overall goal of this knowledge has been explained the practice of nursing as different and distinct from the practice of medicine, psychology, and social work. Nightingale conceptualized disease as a reparative process and described the nurses' role as manipulating the environment to facilitate this process. Her ideas regarding ventilation, warmth, light, diet, cleanliness, variety and noise are presented in her classic nursing textbook, i.e. Notes on nursing (1859).

Nightingale believed that every woman at one time or another would be a nurse, in the sense that nursing was to have the responsibility for someone's health. This she proved women with guidelines for nursing care and advice on 'how to think and how to nurse'.

The major concepts as defined by Nightingale are as follows:

1. **Patient,** viewed as individual or person, is responsible, creative in control of their lives and health, and desiring good health. However, the patient is regarded as being acted upon by the nurse or affected by the environment.
2. **Health** viewed as a state of being well; using ones power to the fullest.
3. **Illness** defined as the reaction of the nature against the condition in which we have placed ourselves. Disease is a reparative mechanism, an effort of nature of remedy, a process of delay.
4. **Environment** refers to that external to the persons, but affecting the health of both sick and well persons. Environment, one of the chief sources of infection, must include fresh air, fresh water, efficient drainage, cleanliness, and light.
5. **Nursing,** defined as a service to people, is intended to relieve pain and suffering. Goal of nursing is to promote the reparative process by manipulating the environment. Client's environment is manipulated to include appropriate noise, nutrition, hygiene, light, comfort, socialization, and hope. Nightingale's descriptive theory provides nurses with a way to think about nursing or a

frame of reference that focuses on patients and the environment. Her principles encompass the areas of practice, research, and education.

57.6 PEPLAU'S THEORY (1952)

Hildegard E Peplau was born on September 1, 1909, and graduated from Pottstown, Pennsylvania hospital, school of nursing in 1931. The nature of science and nursing refers to the body of verified knowledge found within the discipline of nursing, i.e. mainly knowledge from the biological and behavioral sciences. The synthesis, reorganization, or extension of concepts drawn from the basic and applied sciences, which is their reformation tend to become new concepts have led to the growth of nursing science. Then the evolution of Peplau's theory of interpersonal relations resulted. Peplau's theory focuses on the individual nurse and the interaction process; the result is the nurse-client relationship. The major concepts defined/viewed are as follows.

Psychodynamic Nursing

Psychodynamic nursing is being able to understand one's own behavior to help others identify felt difficulties, and to apply principles of human relations to the problems that arise at all levels of experience. She describes the structural concepts of interpersonal process and both the nurse-patient relationship to be based on psychodynamic nursing.

Nurse-Patient Relationship

Nurse-patient relationship described by the Peplau in four phases, i.e. orientation, identification, exploitation, and resolution:

1. **In orientation phase,** the individual has a felt need and seeks professional assistance. The nurse helps the patient recognize and understand his problem and determine his need for help.
2. **In identification phase,** the patient identifies with those who can help him (relatedness). The nurse permits exploration feelings to aid the patient in undergoing illness as an experience that reorients feelings and strengthens positive forces in the personality and provides needed satisfaction.
3. **In exploitation phase,** the patient attempts to derive full value from what is offered him through the relationship. Now goals to be achieved through personal efforts can be projected and power shifted from the nurse to the patient as the patient delays gratification to achieve the newly formed goals.
4. **In resolution phase,** old goals are gradually put aside and new goals are adopted. This is a process in which the patient frees himself from identification with the nurse.

Nursing Roles

Peplau describes six different nursing roles that emerge in the various phases of the nurse-patient relationship as given below:

Role of the stranger: In this role both nurse and patient are stranger to each other, the patient should be treated as he is and with ordinary courtesy. This coincides with the identification phase.

Role of resource person: In this role nurse provides specific answers to questions, especially health information, and interprets to the patient the treatment or medical plan of care. Here the nurse also determines what type of response is appropriate for constructive learning, either straight forward factual answers or providing counseling.

Teaching role: It is a combination of all roles. Peplau separates teaching into two categories, i.e. instructional which consists largely of giving information and is the form explained in educational literature and practical which is using the experience of the learner as a basis from which learning products are developed.

Leadership role: It involves the democratic process. The nurse helps the patient meet the tasks at hand through a relationship of cooperation and active participation.

Surrogate role: The patient casts the nurse in the surrogate role. The nurse's attitudes and behaviors create 'feeling tones' in the patient that reactivate feelings generate in a prior relationship. The nurse's function is to assist the patient in recognizing similarities between herself and the person recalled by the patient. She then helps the patient see the differences in her role and that of the recalled person. In this phase, nurse and patient defines areas of dependence, independence and finally interdependence.

Counseling role: Peplau believes the counseling role has the greatest emphasis on psychiatric nursing. Counseling functions in the nurse-patient relationship by the way nurses response to patient demands.

Nursing: Nursing is described by Peplau as a significant, therapeutic, interpersonal process. It functions comparatively with other human processes that make health possible for individuals in communities. When professional health teams offer health services, nurses participate in the organization of conditions that facilitate natural ongoing tendencies in human organism.

Nursing is an educative instrument, a maturing force that aims to promote forward movement of personality in the direction of creative constructive, productive, personal, and community living.'

Person: Person refers to man. Man is an organism that lives in an unstable equilibrium.

Health: Health is defined by Peplau as 'a word symbol that implies forward movement of personality and other ongoing human processes in the direction of creative, constructive, productive, personal and community living.'

Environment: Environment is defined in terms of 'existing forces outside the organism and in the context of cultures,' from which morals, customs, and beliefs are acquired. However, general conditions that are likely to lead to health always include the interpersonal process.

According to this theory, the client is an individual with a felt need, and nursing is an interpersonal and therapeutic process. Nursing goal is to educate the client and family and to help the client reach mature personality development. Therefore, nurse strives to develop a nurse-patient relationship in which the nurse serves as a research person, counselor and surrogate. This theory creates a 'making force' through which interpersonal effectiveness assists in meeting the client needs.

57.7 HENDERSON'S THEORY (1955)

Virginia Henderson was born in November 30, 1897, a native of Kansas city, Missouri, spent her developmental years in Virginia because her father practiced law in Washington DC. During World War I, she developed an interest in nursing. The major concepts defined by Henderson are as follows.

Nursing: Henderson defines nursing in functional terms, i.e. 'the unique function of the nurse is to assist the individual, sick or well, in the performance of those activities contributing to health or its recovery (or to peaceful death) that he would perform unaided if he had the necessary strength, will or knowledge. And to do this is such a way as to help him gain independence as rapidly as possible'.

Health: Henderson did not define health, but looking into several definitions of health. She views health in terms of patient's ability to perform unaided the 14 components of nursing care. She says it is 'the quality or health rather than life itself, that margin of mental physical vigor that allows a person to work most effectively and to reach his highest potential level of satisfaction of life'.

Environment: By using Webster's definition, Henderson's defines 'environment as the aggregate of all the external conditions and influence affecting the life and development of an organism'.

Person (Patient): Henderson views the patient as an individual who requires assistance to achieve health and independence or peaceful death. The mind and body are inseparable. The patient and his family are viewed as a unit.

Needs: Henderson did not define a need, but she identifies 14 basic needs of the patient, which comprises the components of nursing care. These include the need to:

1. Breathe normally.
2. Eat and drink adequately.
3. Eliminate body wastes by all avenues of elimination.
4. Move and maintain a desirable position.
5. Sleep and rest.
6. Select suitable clothing, i.e. dress and undress.
7. Maintain body temperature within the normal range by adjusting clothing and modifying the environment.
8. Keep the body clean and well groomed and protect the integument.
9. Avoid dangers in the environment and avoid injuring others.
10. Communicate with others in expressing emotions, needs, fears or opinions.
11. Worship according to one's faith.
12. Work in such a way that there is a sense of accomplishments.
13. Play or participate in various forms of recreation, and
14. Learn, discover or satisfy the curiosity that leads to normal development and health and use the available health facilities.

Henderson viewed nursing as an art and a discipline separate from medkine, and viewed the nurse's role as that of a substitute for the patient, a helper to the patient, and a partner with the patient. The fourteen basic needs compose Henderson's components of nursing care.

57.8 ABDELLAH'S THEORY (1960)

Faye Glenn Abdellah was born in New York City. Graduated from Fitkin Memorial Hospital, School of Nursing. She received BS, MA and EdD from Teachers College at Columbia University. She completed her doctoral work in 1955. The nursing theory developed by Faye Abdellah et al. emphasized delivering nursing care for the whole person to meet the physical, emotional, intellectual, social, and spiritual needs of the client and family. The major concepts defined by Abdellah are as follows:

Nursing: Abdellah defined nursing as 'service to individuals and families, therefore to society'. It is based upon an art and science which mould the attitudes, intellectual competencies and technical skills of the individual nurse into the desire and ability to help people sick or well to cope with their health needs, and may be carried out under general or specific medical direction.

Abdellah was clearly promoting the image of the nurse who was not only kind and caring, but also intelligent, competent and technically well prepared to provide service to the patient/mankind.

Nursing problem: Nursing problem is a problem that is presented by the patient in a condition faced by the patient of family which the nurse can assist him or them to meet through the performance of her professional function. The problem can be either an overt or covert nursing problem:

1. An overt nursing problem is an apparent condition faced by the patients or family which the nurse can assist him or them to meet through the performance of her professional functions.
2. A covert nursing problems is a concealed or hidden condition faced by the patient or family which then nurse can assist him or them to meet through the performance of her professional functions.

The functions of the nurses are to identify and solve the specific problems of clients. This identification and classification of problems was called the 'typology of 21 nursing problems, i.e. Abdellah 21 nursing problems were divided into the following three areas:

A. Physical, sociological, and emotional needs of the patient.
B. Type of interpersonal relationships between the nurse and patient.
C. Common elements of patient care.

The 21 nursing problems are as follows:

1. To maintain good hygiene and physical comfort.
2. To promote (achieve) optimal activity, exercise, rest, and sleep.
3. To promote safety through prevention of accidents, injury or other trauma and through the prevention of the spread of infection.
4. To maintain good body mechanics and prevent and correct deformity.
5. To facilitate the maintenance of supply of oxygen to all body cells.
6. To facilitate the maintenance of nutrition of all body cells.
7. To facilitate the maintenance to elimination.
8. To facilitate the maintenance of fluid and electrolyte balance.
9. To recognize the physiological responses of the body to disease conditions—pathological, physiological and compensatory.
10. To facilitate the maintenance or regulatory mechanisms and functions.
11. To facilitate the maintenance of sensory function.
12. To identify and accept positive and negative expressions, feelings, and reactions.
13. To identify and accept interrelatedness of emotions and organic illness.
14. To facilitate the maintenance of effective verbal and nonverbal communications.
15. To promote the development of productive interpersonal relationships.
16. To facilitate progress toward achievement of personal spiritual goals.
17. To create and/or maintain a therapeutic environment.
18. To facilitate awareness of self as an individual with varying physical, emotional and developmental needs.
19. To accept the optimal possible goals in the light of limitations, physical and emotional.
20. To use community resources as an aid in resolving problems arising from illness.
21. To understand the role of social problems as influencing factors in the cause of illness.

When using Abdellah's approach, the nurse needs knowledge and skills in interpersonal relations, psychology, growth and development, communication and sociology as well as knowledge of the basic sciences and specific nursing skills.

Problem-solving: Problem-solving refers to the process of identifying overt and covert nursing problems and interpreting, analyzing, and selecting appropriate causes of action to solve these problems. This process closely resembles the nursing problems.

The nurse is a problem solver and decision maker. The nurse formulates an individualized view of the client's needs, which may occur in the following areas:

1. Comfort, hygiene, and safety.
2. Physiological balance.
3. Psychological and social factors, and
4. Sociological and community factors.

The specific clients' needs, which are often referred to as Abdellah 21 nursing problems, that is useful in identifying the needs and plan and implement the nursing intervention, accordingly.

57.9 ORLANDO'S THEORY (1961)

Ida Jean Orlando was born in August 12, 1926. In 1947, she received a diploma in nursing later on received B S (PHD), and MA in mental health consultation. From Machen College, Columbia University, she worked as a staff nurse, nursing supervisor, teacher, research associate.

Orlando describes her model as revolving around five major interrelated concepts:

1. Function of professional nurses.
2. Present behavior of the client.
3. Immediate reaction or internal response to nurse.
4. Nursing process discipline, and
5. Improvement.

Major concepts of her model defined are as follows:

1. Nurses responsibility means whatever help the patient may require for his needs to be met.
2. Need situational, defined as requirement of the patient which is supplied, relieves or diminishes his immediate distress or improves his immediate sense of adequacy or well-being.
3. Personal behavior means any observable, verbal or nonverbal behavior.
4. Immediate reactions include both the nurse and patients' individual perceptional, thoughts and feelings.
5. Nursing process discipline includes the nurse communicating to the client, his or her own immediate reactions, clearly identifying that the item expressed belongs to the nurse, then asking for validation or correction.
6. Improvement means to grow better, to turn, to profit, to use, to advantage.
7. Purpose of nursing refers to supply the help a patient requires in order for his needs to be met.
8. Automatic action, i.e. those nursing actions decided upon for research other than the patient immediate need.
9. Deliberate action, i.e. those actions decided upon after ascertaining a need and then meeting this need.
10. Orlando views that nursing should be a distinct profession that functions autonomously. Although, nursing has been historically aligned with medicine and continuous to have close relationship with medicine, nursing and practice of medicine are clearly separate profession. She states that 'function of professional nurse is conceptualized as finding out and meeting the patients immediate need for help. Accordingly, the goal of nursing is to respond to client's behavior in terms of immediate needs. To interact with client to meet immediate needs by identifying client behavior, reaction to nurse and nursing action to be taken.

To Orlando, the client is an individual with a need that when met, diminishes distress, increase adequacy or enhances well-being. Her theory focuses on nurses' reactions to client behavior in terms or the client immediate need. This theory contains those main elements—client behavior, nurse reaction and nurse action which compose the nursing situation. After nurses thoroughly assess the client's needs, they recognize the impact that need on the clients level of health and then act automatically or deliberately to meet the need, ultimately reducing client distress.

57.10 HALL'S THEORY (1962)

Lydia E Hall began her career in nursing as a graduate of the York Hospital, School of Nursing in York, Pennsylvania. She then earned her BS and MA degrees from Columbia University in New York. Nursing circles of care (body), core (person) and cure (disease) are the central concepts of Hall's theory:

1. Care alludes to the 'hands on' intimate bodily care of the patient and implies a comforting; nurturing relationship (the body-natural and biological sciences intimate bodily care- aspects of nursing 'the cure).
2. Core involves the therapeutic use of self in communicating with the patient. The nurse reflects questions appropriately and helps the patient clarify motives and goals facilitating the process of increasing the patients self awareness (the person-social science therapeutic use of self aspects of nursing—the core).
3. Cure is the aspects of nursing involved with the administration of medications and treatments. The nurse functions in this role as an investigator and potential painer.' (The disease—pathological and therapeutically sciences-seeing the patient and family through medical care aspects of nursing 'the cure). According to this theory, the goal of nursing is to provide care and comfort to client during disease process. The client is composed of the following overlapping parts, i.e. person (core) pathological state and treatment (cure), and body (care). Nurse is a caregiver. The professional nurses function most therapeutically when patients have entered the second stage of their hospital stay. This stage is the recuperating or nonacute phase of

illness. The first stage of illness is the time of biological crisis, with nursing being an ancillary to medicine. After the crisis period the patient is more able to benefit and learn from the teaching that nurses can offer.

57.11 WIEDENBACH THEORY (1964)

Ernestine Wiedenbach's interest in nursing began with her childhood experiences with nurses. She earned master's degree from Columbia University. The major concepts defined by Wiedenbach are as follows:

1. **Patient:** She defines patient as an individual who is receiving help of some kind, be it care, instruction or advice, from member of the health profession or from worker in the field of health.
2. **Need for help:** A need is anything that individual may require maintaining or sustaining himself comfortably or capably in his situation. A need for help is a any measure or action required or desired by the individual, which has potential for restoring or extending his ability to cope with the demands implicit in his situation.
3. **Nurse** is a functioning human being. For the nurse whose actions are directed toward achievement of a specific purpose, thoughts and feelings, a discipline role to play.
4. **Purpose** that nurse wants to accomplish through what she does—in the overall goal.
5. **Philosophy:** An attitude toward life and reality evolves from each nurse beliefs and code of conduct, motivates the nurse to act, guides her thinking about when she is to do and influences her decisions. It stems from both her culture and subculture and is integral part of her. It is personal in character, unique to each nurse, and expressed in her way of nursing.
6. **Practice:** Overt action, directed by disciplined thoughts and feelings toward meeting the patients need for help. It constitutes the practice of clinical nursing; it is goal direction deliberately carried out and patient curaterd. Knowledge, judgment skills are necessary for effective practice. Identification, administration, validation are three competence of practice directly related to the patient care.

According to Wiedenbach's theory 'nursing is a practice which is related to the individuals who need help because of behavioral stimulus. The goal of nursing is to assist individuals in overcoming obstacles that interfered with the ability to meet demands or needs brought about by condition, environment, situation or time. Clinical nursing has following component, i.e. philosophy, purpose, practice and art.

Wiedenbach identifies five essential attributes to professional person (nurse). These characteristics are as follows:

1. Clarity of purpose.
2. Mastery of skill and knowledge essential for fulfilling purpose.
3. Ability to establish and sustain purposeful working relationship with others, both professional and nonprofessional.
4. Interest in advancing knowledge in the area of interest and creating new knowledge.
5. Dedication of furthering the goal of mankind rather than to self aggrandizement. She also stated the following four assumptions related to person:
   a. Each human being is endorsed with unique potential to develop within himself—resources which enable him to maintain and sustain himself.
   b. The human being basically strives toward self direction and relative independence and desires not only to make best use of his capabilities and potentialities but to fulfill his responsibilities.
   c. Self awareness and self acceptance are essential to the individual sense of integrity and self worth.
   d. Whatever the individual does represents his best judgment at the amount of his doing it.

57.12 LEVINE'S THEORY (1966)

Myra Estrin Levine obtain diploma from Cook Country, School of Nursing in 1944, and Master Science of Nursing (MSN) from Wayne State University in 1962. She views the person is who we know ours if to be or a sense of identity and views the client as an integrated being who instructs with and adapts to the environment.

In her view 'nursing is a human interactions'. The essence of Levine's theory is that 'when nursing intervention influence adaption favorably or toward renewed social being, then the nurse is acting in a therapeutic sense, when response is unfavorable, the nurse adds supportive care. The goal of nursing is to promote wholeness. Whole, health, hale is all derived from Anglo-Saxon word 'hal'. Wholeness (Holistic) emphasizes a sound, organic, progressive, mutually between diversified functions and parts with an entirety, the boundaries which are open and fluent. 'Holism' means that human beings are more than the different from the sum of their parts. Perceiving the 'wholes' depends upon recognizing the organization and interdependence of observable phenomena.

Levine believes that nursing intervention is a conservation activity, with conservation of energy as a primary concern. Health is viewed in terms of the conservation of energy in the following areas, i.e. which Levine calls the 'four conservation principles of nursing':

1. Conservation of client energy.
2. Conservation of structural integrity.
3. Conservation of personal integrity.
4. Conservation of social integrity.

Integrity is from Latin integer, meaning 'being control of one's life'. Conservation is also from the Latin word 'conservation' meaning to keep together. Conservation describes the way by which complex system are able to continue to function even when severally challenged.

The brief description of conservation principle of nursing is as follows:

Conservation of energy: The individual requires a balance of energy and constant renewal of energy to maintain life activities. That energy is challenged by process such as healing and aging. Conservation of energy has long been used and nursing practice even with the most basic procedures.

Conservation of structural integrity: Healing is the process of restoring structural integrity. Nurses should limit the amount of tissue involved in disease by early recognition of functional changes and by nursing interventions.

Conservation of personal integrity: Self worth and a sense of identity are important. Nurses can show patients respect by calling them by name, respecting their wishes, valuing personal possessions, providing privacy during procedures, supporting their defenses, and teaching them. The nurse goal is always to impart knowledge and strength so that the individual can resume a private life—no longer patient, no longer dependent.

Conservation of social integrity: Life gains meaning through social communities and health is socially determined. Nurses fulfill professional roles, provide family members, asses with religious needs, use interpersonal relation to conserve social integrity.

Adaptation is a process of change whereby the individual retains his integrity within the relation of his environment. In Levine's approach, nursing care involves conservation activities aimed at the optimal use of the client's resources.

57.13 JOHNSON'S THEORY (1968)

Dorothy E Johnson was born on August 21, 1919, in Savannah and received BA from Armstrong Junior College and got MPh degree from Harward University in Boston, 1948. Johnson's perceives nursing is an external force aiming to preserve the organization of the patient behavior. While the patient is under stress by means of imposing regulatory mechanism or by providing resources. As an art and science, it supplies external assistance both before and during system or balance disturbance and therefore requires knowledge of order, disorder, and control.

She views man as a behavioral system with patterned, repetitive and purposeful ways of behaving that link him to the environment. Person is a system of interdependent parts that requires some regularity and adjustment to maintain balance. She perceives health as an inclusive dynamic state influenced by biological, psychological, and social factors. Health is the desired value by health professionals and focuses on the person rather than illness.

Johnson theory of nursing focuses on how the client adapts to illness and how actual or potential stress can affect the ability to adapt. The goal of nursing is to reduce stress, so that the client can move more easily through recovery. This theory focuses on basic needs in terms of the following categories of behavior:

1. Security-seeking behavior.
2. Nurturance-seeking behaviors.
3. Master of oneself and ones environment according to internalize standards of excellence it.
4. Taking nourishment by socially and culturally acceptable ways.
5. Ridding the body of nurse and socially and cultured acceptable way.
6. Sexual roles identify behavior.
7. Self protected behavior.

According to Johnson, nurses assess the client's needs in these categories of behavior, called behavioral subsystem and plan, and provides nursing care to resolve problems in meeting the clients' needs.

57.14 ROGER'S THEORY (1970)

Martha E Rogers was born on May 12, 1914 in Dalls, Texas. She began her collegiate education at the University of Jannesse and Knoxville and acquired Doctorate degree (Ed.D) from John Hoplun University, Balmier.

Roger felt that historically the term 'nursing' most often has been used as a verb simplifying 'to do' when nursing is perceived as a science. The term 'nursing' being a noun, signifies body of knowledge. She describes nursing as a learned profession that is both a science and an art. 'Nursing is a humanistic science dedicated to compassionate concern for maintaining and promoting health, preventing illness and caring for and rehabilitating the sick and disabled.' Nursing seeks to promote symphonic interactions between the environment and man, to strengthen the coherence and integrity of the human beings and do direct and redirect patterns of interaction between man and his environment for the realization of maximum health potential.

Roger considers man (unitary human being) as an energy field coexistence within the universe. An energy field constitutes the fundamental unit of both the living and nonhiving. Field is unifying concept and energy signifies the dynamic nature of the field. Energy fields are infinite, so she identified only two, i.e. the human field and the environment field:

- The unitary human being (human field) is defined as an irreducible, indivisible, pandimensional energy field identified by pattern and manifested characteristics that are specific to the whole and which cannot be predicted from knowledge of the parts.
- The environment field is defined as an irreducible pandimensional energy field identified by pattern and integral with human field. Each environmental field is specific to its given human field. Both change continuously and creatively. Unitary man evolves along life process. Client continuously changes and coexists with environment.

Roger viewed the terms health and illness as value leader, arbitrarily defined but as part of the same continuum, i.e. health occurs when patterns of living are in harmony with environmental change and illness occurs when patterns of living conflicts with environmental change and are deemed unacceptable.

The four dimension used in Roger's theory of energy fields, openness (universe of open system) pattern and organization and to derive principles about how human beings develops. Her views on nursing primarily as a science and is committed to nursing research. Nursing, therefore, corporate knowledge of the basic sciences and physiology, as well as nursing knowledge. The science of nursing aims to provide a body of abstract knowledge growing out, of scientific research and logical analysis and capable of being translated into nursing practice. Nursing body of knowledge is a new product specific to nursing.

According to this theory, the goal of nursing is to maintain and promote health, prevent illness and care for and rehabilitate ill and disabled client through humanistic science of nursing.

57.15 OREM'S THEORY

Dorothea Elizabeth Orem, one of the American foremost nursing theorists was born in Baltimore, Maryland. She began her nursing career at Providence Hospital, School of Nursing, Washington DC, where she received diploma in nursing and she also recipient of BSN and MS of Catholic University of America. Orem's self-care deficit' theory of nursing as a general theory consists of three related theories:

1. Theory of self-care (describes and explains self-care).
2. Theory of self-care deficit (describes and explains why people can be helped through nursing).
3. Theory of nursing system (describes and explains relationship that must be brought about and maintained for nursing to be produced).

The major concepts defined by Orem's are as follows:

Self-care: Self-care is a learned good oriented activity of individuals. It is behavior that exists in concrete life situations directed by persons to self or to the environment to regulate factors that affects their own development and functioning in the interests of life, health, or well-being.

Self-care requisites are expression of purposes to be attained, results desired from-deliberate engagement in self-care. They are the reasons for doing actions that constitute self-care. There were three categories of self-care requisite as given below:

Universal self-care requisites: These are common to all human beings and include the maintenance of air, water, food elimination, activity and rest, and solitude and social interaction, prevention of hazards and promotion of human functioning.

Development self-care requisites: These are self-care requisites that they promote processes for life and maturation and prevent conditions deleterious to maturation or mitigate those effects.

Health deviation self-care requisites: These are defined by Orem that disease or injury affects not only specific structures and physiologic or psychological mechanisms, but also integrated human functioning. When integrated functioning is seriously affected the individuals' developing or developed powers of agency are seriously inspired either permanently or temporarily— discomfort, frustration resulting from medical care also create a requisites for self-care to bring relief.

Self-care deficit: Self-care deficit refers to a relationship between the human properties therapeutic self-care demand and self-care agency in which constituent developed self-care capabilities within self-care agency are nonoperable or not adequate for knowing and meeting some or all components of the existent or projected therapeutic self care demand.

Nursing agency: Nursing agency refers to the complex property or attribute of persons educated and trained as nurses that is enabling when exercised for knowing and helping others, know their therapeutic self-care demands, for helping others meet or in meeting their therapeutic self-care demands, and in helping other regulate the exercise or development of their self-care agency or their dependent care agency. Therapeutic demand is a humanly constructed entity, with an objective basis in information that describes in individual structurally, functionally, and developmentally.

Nursing system: Nursing system refers to a continuing series of actions produced when nurses link one way or a number of ways in helping to their own actions or the actions of the persons under care that are directed to meet these persons' therapeutic self-care demands or to regulate their self-care agency. Self-care agency is the complex acquired ability to meet one's continuing requirement for care them regulated life processes, maintains or promotes integrity of human structures and functioning, and human development and promotes well-being.

Three types of nursing system (described by Orem) are as follows:

Wholly compensatory nursing systems: These are needed when the nurse should be compensating for a patients total inability for (or prescription against) engaging and self-care activities that require ambulation and manipulation of movements.

Partially compensatory nursing system: It exists when both nurse and patient perform care measures or other actions involving manipulative tasks or ambulation.

Supportive educative nursing system: These are for situations when the patient is able to perform or can and should learn to perform required measures for externally or internally oriented self-care but cannot do so without assistance. The methods of assistance will include acting or doing for guidance, i.e. teaching, supporting, and providing a developmental environment.

In Orem's self-care deficit theory, nursing care becomes necessary when client is unable to fulfill biological, psychological, developmental and/or social needs. The goal of nursing is to care for and help client within total self-care. She viewed person/patient in an individual unable to continuously maintain self-care in sustaining life and health, in recovering from disease or injury or in coping with their effects.

According to Orem, health is an ability to meet self-care demands that contribute to the maintenance and promotion of structural integrity, functioning, and development. Illness occurs when a individual is incapable of maintaining self-care as a result of health related limitations. She perceived environment that any setting in which a patient has unmet self-care needs. And nursing is service of deliberately selected and performed actions to assist individuals to maintain selfcare, including structural integrity, functioning, and development. Accordingly, nursing care is necessary when the client is unable to fulfill biological, psychological, developmental and/or social needs. The nurse determines why a client is unable to meet these needs, what must be done to enable the client to meet them and how much self-care the client is able to perform.

Orem describes her philosophy of nursing as follows:

Action and the provision and management of it on continuous basis in order to sustain life and health, recover from disease or injury, and cope with their effects. Self-care is a requirement of every person — man, women, and child. When self-care is not maintained, illness, disease or death will occur. Nurses sometimes manage and maintain required self-care continuously for persons who are totally incapable. In other instance, nurses help persons to maintain required self-care by performing some but not all care measures, by supervising others who assist patients and by instructing and guiding individuals as they gradually move toward self-care.

Orem suggests that a person needs nursing when the person has a health related self-care deficit. The areas of nursing practice are:

1. Entering into and maintaining nurse-client relationships with individuals families or groups.
2. Determining if and how clients can be helped through nursing.
3. Responding to clients' requirements and needs.
4. Giving direct help to clients and families.
5. Coordinating and integrating nursing with the clients' daily living, other healthcare activities, and social or educational services required.

57.16 KING'S THEORY (1971)

Imogene M King earned her diploma in nursing from St John's hospital of Nursing in St Louis in 1945, and earned Master in Science of Nursing (MSN) at St Louis University and Doctor of Education degree from Columbia University, New York.

The major concepts in her theory of goal attainment are interaction, perception, communication, transaction, role stress, growth and development and time and space. The definition, of these concepts by King is as follows.

Interaction is defined as a process of perception and communication between person and interaction environment and between person to person, represented by verbal and nonverbal behaviors that are goal directed. Each individual in an interaction (Nurse and client) brings different knowledge, needs, goals, post experiences and perceptions which influence the interactions.

Perception: Perception is defined as 'each persons' representation of reality. This includes import and transformation of energy, and processing, storing, and exporting information's. Perceptions are related to post experiences, concept of self socioeconomic group, biological inheritance, and educational background.

Communication: Communication is a process whereby information is given from one person to another either directly or indirectly. It is the information component of the interactions. The exchange or verbal and nonverbal signs and symbols between nurse and client, or between client and environment are communications.

Transaction: Transaction is defined as purposeful interaction that leads to goal attainment. It includes observable behavior of human beings interacting with their environment, the valuation components of human interaction.

Role: Role is defined as a 'set of behavior's expected to persons occupying a position in a social system; rules that define rights and obligations in a position. If expectations of role differ, then role conflict and role confusion exists.

Stress: Stress is a 'dynamic state' whereby a human being interacts with the environment. It involves an exchange of energy and information between the person and the environment for regulation and control of stressors and energy response of an individual to person, objects, and events. An increase in the stress of the individual leads to narrow perception and decrease rationality, and also affects nursing care.

Growth and development: Growth and development are defined as continuous changes in the individuals at the cellular, molecular, and behavioral levels of activities-conducive in helping individuals to move toward maturity.

Time: Time is defined as a sequence of events moving onward to the future — time is duration between one event and another as uniquely experienced by each human being.

Space: Space is defined as existing in all directions and is the same everywhere. It is immediate environment in which nurse and client interact.

King's personal philosophy about human beings and life influenced her assumptions. Her theory of goal attainment based on those assumptions that focus on nursing is human beings interacting with their environment leading to a state of health for individuals, which is an ability to function in social roles.

Her assumptions are nursing, person's health and environment as given below:

1. Nursing is an observable behavior found in healthcare system in society. The goal of nursing is to help individuals maintain their health so that they can function in their roles. Nursing is viewed as an interpersonal process of action, reaction, interaction, and transaction. Perception of nurse and client also influences the interaction process.
2. Persons refer to individuals that they are social beings, sentient beings, rational beings, perceiving beings, controlling being, purposeful beings, action oriented beings, and time oriented beings.

Health: Health is viewed as a dynamic state in the life-cycle; illness is interference in the lifecycle. Health implied continuous adaptation to stress in the internal and external environment through optimum use of one's resources to achieve maximum potential for daily living. Health is the function of nurse, patient, physician, family and other interaction.

Environment: King states that an understanding of the ways that human beings interact with their environment to maintain health is essential for nurses. Adjustment to life and healthcare influenced by an individual's interaction with environment.

King's theory focuses on the interpersonal relationship between client and the nurse. The nurse-client relationship is vehicle for the nursing process, which is a dynamic interpersonal process in which the nurse and client are affected by each other's behavior, as well as by the health-care system. The nurses goal is to use communication to assist the client in re-establishing maintaining positive adaptation to environment.

57.17 TRAVELBEE'S THEORY (1972)

Joyce Travelbee was a psychiatric nurse practitioner, educator and writer, born on 1926. She had basic nurse preparation at Charity Hospital School of Nursing and earned BSN from Louisiana State University New York University and MSN from Yale in 1959.

Major concepts defined by Travelbee in her theory are as follows:

1. Nursing is defined as an 'interpersonal process whereby the professional nurse practioner assists an individual, family or community to prevent or cope with the experience of illness and suffering and if necessary, to find meaning in these experiences.' Nursing is an interpersonal process because it is an experience that occurs between the nurse and an individual or group of individuals.
2. Person defined as human being, both the nurse and patient are human beings.
3. Health refers to the criteria of subjective and objective health. A person's 'subjective' health states in an individually defined state of well-being in accordance with self-appraisal of physical, emotional, spiritual status. Objective health is an absence of discernible disease, disability, or defect as measured by physical examination, laboratory test, assessment by spiritual director, or psychological counselor.

Travelbee viewed interpersonal process as human-to-human relationship formed during illness and 'experience of suffering.' The goal of nursing is to assist individual or family to prevent or cope with illness, regain health, find meaning in illness, or maintain maximum degree of health.

57.18 NEUMAN'S THEORY (1972)

Betty Neuman was born on 1924, completed her initial nursing education at Akron, Ohio in 1947, then earned master degree in mental health in 1966 and received doctorate degree in clinical psychology in 1985. She was a pioneer of nursing involvement in mental health.

The major concepts identified in her model are; holistic client approach, open system, basic structure, environment, created environment, stresses, lines of defense and resistance, degree of reaction, prevention as intervention, and reconstruction. Further included the concepts of scholastic approach, content, process input and output, negontrophy, entropy, stability, wellness and illness.

To Neuman, the persons are dynamic composite of physiological, socio-cultural, and developmental variables that function as an open system. As an open system, the person interacts with adjusts to and it adjusted by the environment, which is viewed as stressor. Stressors disrupt the system. She includes intrapersonal, interpersonal and extrapersonal stressor.

Neuman believes that nursing is concerned with the whole person. She views nursing as a 'unique profession in that it is concerned with all of the variables affecting an individual response to stress.' Because the nurses perception influences the care program. Neuman equates health to wellness and defines health and/or wellness as 'the condition in which all parts and subparts (variables) are in harmony with the whole of the client. So, health is a dynamic equilibrium on the normal line of defense. Illness occurs due to reaction to stressor with lines of resistance, internal and external stressors and restrictive factors are the environment. The reduction of the stressors through prevention acts at three levels of nursing.

The goal of nursing is to assist individual, families, and groups in attaining and maintaining maximal level of total wellness. The nurse assesses managers and evaluates client systems. Nursing focuses on the variables affecting the client response to the stressor. Nursing action are earned out on three levels. When the stressor is identified but no reaction has occurred; interventions can decrease the degree of reaction or increase the line of defense. This is called primary prevention. When the reaction has already happened, secondary prevention is carried out, with intervention aimed at treating symptoms and reducing reactions. After active treatment, tertiary prevention strengthens the lines of defense through education and uses the systems total resources to prevent further occurrence.

Neuman model is applicable to all phases of the nursing process. It can be applied across all clinical areas and is especially useful for individuals and families. It is a holistic approach because each system or subsystem cannot be isolated; rather, the influence of each system on the whole must be considered. The three levels of prevention are useful guidelines for planning nursing interventions.

57.19 ROY'S THEORY (1979)

Sister Callista Roy, a member of the Sisters of St Joseph of Carondelet, was born on October 14, 1939 in Los Angeles, California. She was the receiver of BA in Nursing, MSc Nursing, MA and PhD in Sociology.

The major concepts defined by Roy are as follows:

1. **Person:** According to Roy, a person is a biopsychosocial being in constant interaction with a changing environment. She defined the person, the recipient of nursing care, as a living complex, adaptive system with internal processes (the cognator and regulator) acting to maintain adaptation in the four adaptive modes, i.e. physiological needs, self-concept, role functions, and interdependence. The person as a living system is 'a whole' made up of parts or subsystems that function as a unity for some purpose, patient is a person or family with unusual stressor or ineffective coping mechanism.
2. **Health:** It is a state and a process of being and becoming an integrated and whole person. Lack of integration represents lack of health.
3. **Environment:** According to Roy, environment is all the conditions, circumstances, and influences surrounding and affecting the development and behavior of persons or groups. Factors in the environment that affect the person are categorized as focal, contextual, and residual stimuli.
4. **Nursing:** It is defined broadly as 'a theoretical system of knowledge which prescribes a process of analysis and action related to the care of the ill or potentially ill person.'

Roy differentiates nursing as a science from nursing as a practice discipline. Nursing science is a developing system of knowledge about person that observes, classifies, and relates the processes by which persons positively affect their health status. Nursing as a practice discipline is nursing scientific body of knowledge used for the purpose of providing an essential service to people, that is, promoting ability to affect health positively.

Roy's goal of nursing is to help man adapt to change in his physiological needs, his self concept, his role function, and his interdependent relations during health and illness. Nursing fills a unique role as a facilitator of adaptation by assessing behavior in each of these four adaptive modes and intervening by managing the influencing stimulants.

As defined by Roy, response to a decrease in body integrity creates a need state, and the individual responds with an act or behavior. The physiologic mode involves oxygenation, and circulation, fluid and electrolyte balance, nutrition, rest and activity and regulations of temperature, hormones and sensory function. The self concept mode concerned with perceptions of one's physical self and personal self including personality, moral ethical beliefs and values. The interdependent mode involves social relationships, including both the need to be interdependent and the need for support by others. The role function involves the behaviors of a person in each role taken on life.

In this model, all nursing activities are aimed at promoting the individuals adaption to health and illness in all four adaptive modes. The nurse determines what demands are causing problems for a client and assess how well the client is adapting to them. Nursing care is then directed at helping the client adapt.

57.20 ZEININGERS THEORY (1978)

Madeleine M Zeininger is the founder of transcultural nursing and a leader in transcultural nursing and human cure theory.

The major concepts defined in her theory are as follows:

1. **Care:** It refers to phenomenon related to assistive, supportive or enabling behavior toward or for another individual (or group) with evident or anticipated needs to ameliorate or improve a human condition or life way.
2. **Caring:** It refers to action directed towards assisting, supporting or enabling another individual (or group) with evident or anticipated needs to ameliorate or improve a human condition or life way.
3. **Culture:** It refers to the learned, shared and transmitted values, beliefs, norms and life-ways practices of a particular group that guides thinking, decisions, actions and patterned ways.
4. **Cultural care:** It refers to the cogruitively known values, beliefs, and patterned expressions that assist, support, or enable another individual or group to maintain well-being, improve a human condition or life way, face death and disabilities.
5. **Nursing:** It is a learned humanistic art and science that focuses upon personalized (individual group) care behaviors, functions, and processes directed toward promoting and maintaining health behaviors or recovery from illness which have physical, psycho cultural and social significance or meaning or those being assisted generally by a professional nurse or one with similar role competencies. The goal of nursing is to provide care consistent with nursing emerging science and knowledge with caring as a central focus. According to his theory, caring is central and unifying domain for nursing knowledge and practice.

57.21 WATSON'S THEORY (1979)

Jean Watson was born on June 10, 1940 in Williamson in Southern West Virginia. She earned a BSc in 1964, an MS in psychiatric and mental health nursing in 1966 and a PhD in educational psychology and counseling in 1973. Watson's philosophy of caring attempts to define outcome of nursing activity in regard to the humanistic aspects of life. Her theory and philosophy of caring is based on the values of kindness, concern, love of self and others and respect for the spiritual dimensions of the person.

Watson defined human caring in nursing as "an art and a science in which caring is a human-to-human process demonstrated through a therapeutic interpersonal interactions". The action of nursing is directed at understanding the interrelationships, with health, illness, and human behavior. Nursing is concerned with promoting and restoring health and preventing illness.

Formation of a humanistic-altruistic system of values: Humanistic and altruistic values are learned early in life but can be greatly influenced by nurse education. This factor can be defined as satisfaction through giving and extension of the sense of self.

Instillation of faith and hope: This factor incorporating humanistic and altruistic values facilitates the promotion of holistic, nursing care and positive health within the client population. It also describes the nurses' role in developing effective nurse-client interrelation and in promoting wellness by helping the client adopt health seeking behavior.

Cultivation of sensitivity to one's self and to others: The recognition of feelings leads to self actualization through self acceptance for both the nurse and the client. As nurses acknowledge their sensitivity and feelings, they become more genuine, authentic and sensitive to others.

Development of helping trust and relationship: The development of helping trust relationships between the nurse and client is crucial for transpersonal caring. A trusting relationship promotes and accepts the expression of both positive and negative feelings. It involves congruence, empathy, nonpossessive warmth, and effective communication.

Promotion and acceptance of the expression of positive and negative feelings: The sharing of feeling is a risk taking experience for both nurse and client. The nurse must be prepared for either positive or negative feelings. The nurse must recognize that intellectual and emotional understandings of a situation differ.

Systematic use of scientific problem solving method of decision-making: Use of the nursing process brings a scientific problem solving approach to nursing care.

Promotion of interpersonal teaching learning: It is an important factor in which nurse facilitates the process of teaching-learning techniques that are designed to enable the client to provide self-care, determining personal needs, and to provide opportunities for their personal growth.

Provision for supportive, protective and/or corrective mental, physical, sociocultural and spiritual environment: The nurses must recognize the influences that internal and external environment have on the health and illness of individual. Accordingly, they should make arrangement to create such conducive environment for the patient in positive direction.

Assistance with gratification of human needs: The nurse recognizes the biophysical, psycho-physical, psychosocial, and interpersonal needs of self and client. Client must satisfy lower order needs before attempting to attain higher order ones, i.e. food elimination, ventilation (biophysical lower needs), activity/inactivity; sexuality (lower psychological needs) and achievement, affiliation, self actualization (higher ones).

Allowance for existential phenomenological force: Phenomenology describes data of the immediate situation that help people understand the phenomena in question. This analysis of human existence in a situation provides a thought provoking, experience leading to better understanding of ourselves and others. As stated above each factor describes the earning prices of how client attain or maintains health or dies peacefully. Caring represents all of the factors the nurse uses to deliver healthcare to the client.

CONCLUSION

To be in a simple term it can be said or compared to a frame of a house just as the foundation supports a house, a conceptual frame work provides a rationale for prediction about relationship among variable in the research study. It's also a frame of reference that is a base for observation, definitions of concepts, research designs, interpretations and generalization much as the frame that rests on a foundation defines the overall design of a house.

58 Metaparadigms of Nursing

58.1 INTRODUCTION

A metaparadigm is a concept that is extremely general, one that serves to define an entire world of thought. "Meta" means "that which is behind," in Greek, and refers to that which under girds something else, serving as a conceptual basis. In her seminal (1984, cited in Slevin) work, "Analysis and Evaluation of Conceptual Models of Nursing," Jacqueline Fawcett developed the basic four metaparadigms of nursing. More recently, these have been revised by Basford and Slevin (2003) and serve to underpin the entire conceptual universe of the nursing profession.

58.2 DEFINITION

1. The nursing metaparadigm embodies the knowledge base, theory, philosophy, research, practice, and educational experience and literature identified with the profession. These given concepts vary in accordance to the experiences and views of different nursing theorists.
2. A nursing paradigm is a model that describes the relationship between a person, their health and the environment. The model has developed over a long period of time from the beliefs and practices of healthcare professionals.
3. Nursing metaparadigm is a nursing statement or group of statements that identifies phenomena which encompass a series of philosophical assumptions and also guides the approach to those assumptions. It has four interrelated central concepts which are person, environment, health, and nursing. Nursing metaparadigm serves to strengthen the entire conceptual field of the nursing profession.

58.3 CONCEPT OF METAPARADIGM

A nursing program is identified as a single entity (program) when it can be demonstrated that all of the following criteria are met:

1. The program is within one governing organization that holds an appropriate institutional accreditation from an agency recognized by the Accreditation Commission for Education in Nursing (ACEN).
2. The program is within the jurisdiction of one State Board of Nursing and/or other identified regulatory body exclusive of clinical learning experiences.
3. There is one set of student learning outcomes for the program offered.
4. There is one nurse administrator who has responsibility and authority for the program which may include: the hiring and evaluation of faculty; the development or revision of the curriculum; the assignment/approval of faculty responsibilities; the establishment of program specific admission/progression criteria; and development and administration of the program budget.

5. The faculty can demonstrate that they function as a faculty of the whole within a set of established faculty policies through their organization and decision-making processes, and methods of input into the curriculum development, delivery, and evaluation.
6. There is a systematic evaluation plan that addresses the student learning outcomes, program outcomes, and the ACEN Standards.
7. A single degree, certificate, or diploma is offered to students successfully completing the program.
8. All students are governed by a single set of policies.

58.4 MEANING OF METAPARADIGMS

Metaparadigm is the combination of two words, meta and paradigm. According to Mosby's (1994) definition, Meta, can mean either "after or next" or "change or exchange." Mosby's (1994) defines Paradigm as "a pattern that may serve as a model or example. Chinn and Jacobs (1987) identify paradigm as, a generally accepted world view or philosophy, a framework or structure within which theories of the discipline are organized. According to Fawcett (1984), "a metaparadigm of a discipline is a group of statements identifying its phenomena in a global rather than specific way." Metaparadigm is "the most global perspective of a discipline and acts as an encapsulating unit or framework, within which the more restrictive structures work".

A metaparadigm is the most global perspective of a discipline and "acts as an encapsulating unit, or framework, within which the more restricted ...structures develop" (Eckberg and Hill, 1979, p. 927). Each discipline singles out phenomena of interest that it will deal with in a unique manner. The concepts and propositions that identify and interrelate these phenomena are even more abstract than those in the conceptual models. These are the concepts that comprise the metaparadigm of the discipline (Fawcett, 1994).

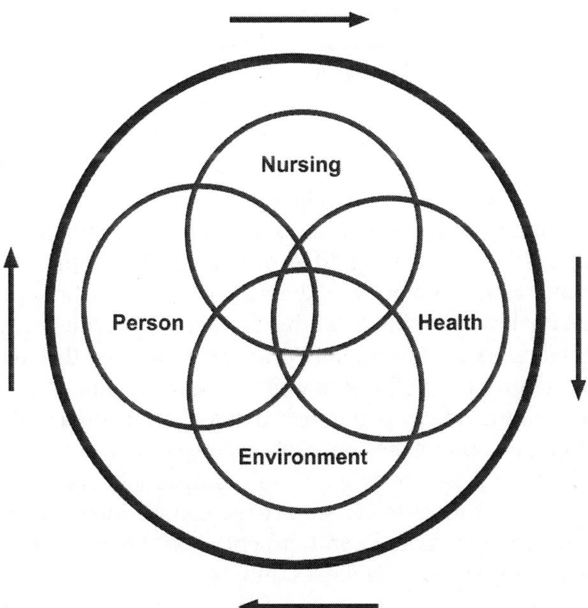

Fig. 58.1: Metaparadigm of nursing

58.5 COMPONENTS OF METAPARADIGMS

I. **Human beings:** Human beings are viewed as open energy fields with unique life experiences. As energy fields, they are greater than and different from the sum of their parts and cannot be predicted from knowledge of their parts. Humans, as holistic beings, are unique, dynamic, sentient, and multidimensional, capable of abstract reasoning, creativity, aesthetic appreciation and self-responsibility. Language, empathy, caring, and other abstract patterns of communication are aspects of an individually high level of complexity and diversity and enable one to increase knowledge of self and environment. Humans are viewed as valued persons, to be respected, nurtured and understood with the right to make informed choices regarding their health.

For the purpose of study in nursing, biological, psychological, spiritual, intellectual and sociocultural dimensions of human beings and stages of human development are delineated as they affect behavior and health. These dimensions operate within and upon the human being in an open, interrelated, interdependent, and interactive way. The nursing client is an open system, continually changing in mutual process with the changing environment. Recipients of nursing actions may be well or ill and include individuals, families and communities.

II. **Environment:** Environment is the landscape and geography of human social experience, the setting or context of experience as everyday life and includes variations in space, time and quality. This geography includes personal, social, national, global, and beyond. Environment also includes societal beliefs, values, mores, customs, and expectations. The environment is an energy field in mutual process with the human energy field and is conceptualized as the arena in which the nursing client encounters aesthetic beauty, caring relationships, threats to wellness and the lived experiences of health. Dimensions that may affect health include physical, psychosocial, cultural, historical and developmental processes, as well as the political and economic aspects of the social world.

III. **Health:** Health, a dynamic process, is the synthesis of wellness and illness and is defined by the perception of the client across the life span. This view focuses on the entire nature of the client in physical, social, aesthetic, and moral realms. Health is contextual and relational. Wellness, in this view, is the lived experience of congruence between one's possibilities and one's realities and is based on caring and feeling cared for. Illness is defined as they lived experience of loss or dysfunction that can be mediated by caring relationships. Inherent in this conceptualization is each client's approach to stress and coping. The degree or level of health is an expression of the mutual interactive process between human beings and their environment.

IV. **Nursing practice:** Nursing is an academic discipline and a practice profession. It is the art and science of holistic healthcare guided by the values of human freedom, choice, and responsibility. Nursing science is a body of knowledge arrived at through theory development, research, and logical analysis. Nursing and other supporting theories are essential to guide and advance nursing practice. The art of nursing practice, actualized through therapeutic nursing interventions, is the creative use of this knowledge in human care. Nurses use critical thinking and clinical judgment to provide evidence-based care to individuals, families, aggregates, and communities to achieve an optimal level of client wellness in diverse nursing settings/contexts. Clinical judgment skills are therefore essential for professional nursing practice.

Human caring as the moral ideal of nursing is the central focus of professional practice. It involves concern and empathy, and a commitment to the client's lived experience of human health and the relationships among wellness, illness, and disease. The nurse, as a person, is engaged as an active partner in the human care transactions with clients across the life span.

Human care and human care transactions seek to protect, enhance, and preserve human worth and dignity. Human caring involves values, a will and a commitment to care, communication, knowledge, caring actions and consequences. Human care is an epistemic endeavor that defines both nurse and client and requires study, reflection, and action. Caring is contextual, specific and individual and involves organized, specific practice that is related to caring for and about others. Caring is nursing's source of power.

58.6 NURSING AND METAPARADIGM

Nurses function autonomously and use power to shape the profession and empower clients through caring partnerships and other transactions. Within this framework, power is defined as the capacity to participate knowingly in the nature of change and is characterized by awareness, advocacy, choice, freedom to act intentionally, healing and involvement in creating changes.

Nurses use critical thinking to facilitate translation of knowledge and skill into professional nursing practice. The nursing process, a form of critical thinking, is a methodology for nursing practice, deliberate, systematic, and goal-oriented. Deliberative behaviors for the process are observation, intuition, reflection, caring, empowering, communication, assessment, and choice of alternative actions. Nursing practice incorporates intellectual, interpersonal, communication and psychomotor skills in the care of individuals, families, aggregates and communities, regardless of setting, and emphasizes a collaborative relationship with other healthcare providers.

Multiple aspects of the complex role of the humanitarian nurse, such as learner, clinician and leader derive from the responsibility to provide diagnostic, technologic, supportive and therapeutic care; to protect the rights, safety and welfare of clients; to improve healthcare delivery, to influence health and social policy, and to contribute to the development of the profession. The goal of nursing is humanistic enhancement of health potential in human beings as well as caring for the well, ill and the dying. Excellence in nursing requires commitment, caring and critical thinking in terms of mastery, status and control over practice.

CONCLUSION

Nursing metaparadigm is a nursing statement or group of statements that identifies phenomena which encompass a series of philosophical assumptions and also guides the approach to those assumptions. It has four interrelated central concepts which are person, environment, health, and Nursing. Nursing metaparadigm serves to strengthen the entire conceptual field of the nursing profession. The concepts and propositions that identify and interrelate these phenomena are even more abstract than those in the conceptual models. These are the concepts that comprise the metaparadigm of the discipline.

Section-11

Advancement in Nursing

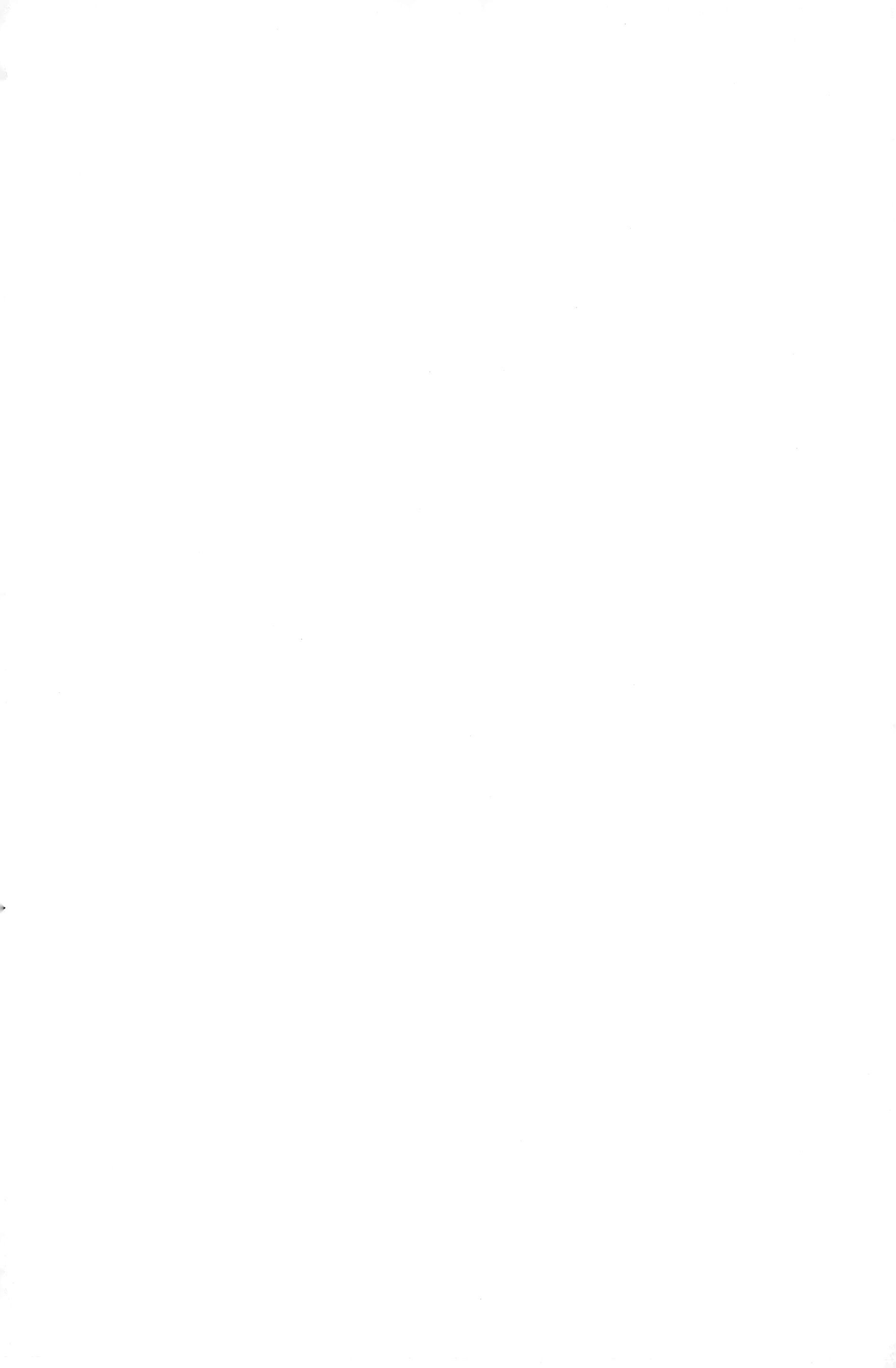

59 Computer in Nursing

59.1 INTRODUCTION

The word computer comes from the word Compute which means 'to calculate'. So, a computer generally considered to be calculating device that can perform operations at very faster rates. Computer is programmable, that means we can instruct the computer to perform a variety of tasks through programs (a program is a set of instructions). Computer on its own cannot think or perform any task. As a user we have to specify the task. Computer is a machine that simply follows the instructions given to it. So, a computer can be defined as an electronic device which processes input based on the instructions provided and generals the desired output.

59.2 DEFINITION

A computer is an electronic machine that processes data according to a set of instructions that are stored internally either temporarily or permanently. The computer and all equipment attached to it are called hardware. The instructions that tell it what to do are called "software". A set of instructions that perform a particular task is called a "program" or "software program".

59.3 BASIC OPERATION SYSTEM

All computer systems perform the following five basic operations:

1. **Inputting:** The process of entering data and instructions into the computer system is called inputting.
2. **Storing:** Saving data and instructions so that they are available later is called storing.
3. **Processing:** Processing means performing operations on data to get the result.
4. **Outputting:** Output is the result of processing.
5. **Controlling:** Controlling means directing the manner and sequence in which all of the above operations are performed.

59.4 USES OF COMPUTER

Computers influence every sphere of human activity and bring in many changes in industry, education, healthcare, scientific research, social science, law and even in arts, music and painting. In India, the impact of computer technology can be felt only in certain fields whereas in developed countries computers have become part of every man's life. Although, computers have been used in healthcare since 1960's, the use of computer by nurses has increased rapidly in developed countries. Computers can perform a wide range of activities that save time and help nurses to provide quality nursing care.

59.5 COMPUTER IN CLINICAL PRACTICE

Computer is used in nursing for admission, discharge and transfer (ADT). ADT system allows nurses to obtain basic biographical information on clients before they arrive to the unit. When a discharge or transfer is entered in the computer, all the appropriate departments (e.g. dietary, housekeeping, pharmacy) are automatically notified, thus, saving the nurses from many phone calls. Information about beds and a client's location on the unit is also readily available.

Uses of computer in nursing documentation: Nursing assessments, clients' care plans, medication, administration records, nursing notes and discharge plans are some of the forms of nursing documentation that are computerized. Computerized documentation has many advantages. It is typed and therefore legible. The computer can be programmed to identify the data and time of all entries as well as the initials or the name of the person making the entry. The computer can store standard nursing care plans in a format determined by the institution, to be used by nurses as the basis for developing individualized client care plan. The computer is often programmed to automatically print a list of medication to be administered at pre determined times, during the day. A nurse using a printout for a particular client, administers the medication and then charts it on the computer (If the medication is not charted and given within a specified time after the scheduled time, the computer prints a reminder that the medication is overdue). Computer can perform drug dosage calculation faster and more accurately. Nurses' notes can be entered quickly by choosing statements, appropriate for a particular client from multiple preprogrammed choices.

Uses of computer in nursing education: Computer is a useful tool in Education because it allows for an individual a self paced learning. Computed assisted instruction (CAI) is a method of teaching that involves interaction between the learner and the computer. The computer takes on the role of a teacher.

59.6 CAI PROGRAMS

There are three different types of CAI programs:

1. **Drill and practice:** It is the most common and least complex type of CAI. A learner is presented with a series of questions or problems about materials that have already been learnt. Drug dosage calculation, intravenous drip rate calculation and medical terminology and abbreviations are some of the topics that drill and practice CAT is well suited for.
2. **Tutorial programs:** Display new materials that are similar to programmed instructions. Tutorials present information and provide the learner the feedback.
3. **Simulations:** Present before learners the 'real-life situations that are designed to assist learners in developing problem solving and decision-making skills in a safe environment. Interactive video instruction (IAV) can provide learners, with "true-to-life" simulation. IAV combines CAI with a videotape or videodisc player so that video pictures as well as graphics can be incorporated in the design of the software.

59.7 COMPUTER IN NURSING RESEARCH

Computers facilitate the research process in a number of ways. Computerized literature searches are a particular advantage to the researchers because they save time and can increase the scope of the search and the number of data base that can be searched. The computer can also help researchers collect and analyze data, prepare research reports, and disseminate research findings.

59.8 COMPUTER IN NURSING ADMINISTRATION

Computers are useful tools for nurse administrators. A number of computers programmes are designed to assist nurse administrators. Computerized patients' classification system can be used to assign nursing staff based on how severely ill clients are. Clients are assessed on a number of criteria and their abilities or need for nursing care is rated. A client's total rating score indicates how much nursing care the client requires computerized inventory system keeps track of supplies received and disbursed. They can also be integrated with the client billing system. General computer application software such as word processing, electronic spread sheets and database management system help nurse administrator to prepare reports and letters, create budgets and maintain personnel records and mailing lists. Computers can calculate daily the number of nurses needed on each unit, computer can be used to schedule nurses' days off so that an optional number of nurses are working at one time.

CONCLUSION

Computers influence every sphere of human activity and bring in many changes in industry, education, healthcare, scientific research, social science, law and even in arts, music and painting. In India, the impact of computer technology can be felt only in certain fields whereas in developed countries computers have become part of every man's life. Although, computers have been used in healthcare since 1960's. The use of computer by nurses has increased rapidly in developed countries. Computers can perform a wide range of activities that save time and help nurses to provide quality nursing care.

60 Health Information System

60.1 INTRODUCTION

Information is what is used in the act of informing or the state of being informed. Information includes knowledge acquired by some means. In the 1960s and 70s, it became necessary to formalize an educational approach to systems for business so that individuals and work groups and businesses who crossed boundaries in the various operations of business could have appropriate information. Technical developments in computers and data processing and new theories of systems analysis made it possible to computerize systems. Much of this computerization of systems was an outgrowth of basic research by the federal government.

60.2 DEFINITION

Health information is defined as a mechanism for the collection, processing, analysis and transmission of information required for organizing and operating health services and also for research and training.

60.3 MEANING OF HEALTH INFORMATION SYSTEM (HIS)

Management is usually defined as planning, organizing, directing, and controlling the business operation. This definition, which evolved from the work of Henri Fayol in the early 1900s, defines what a manager does, but it is probably more appropriate to define what management is rather than what management does. Management is the process of allocating an organization's inputs, including human and economic resources, by planning, organizing, directing, and controlling for the purpose of producing goods or services desired by customers so that organizational objectives are accomplished. If management has knowledge of the planning, organizing, directing, and controlling of the business, its decisions can be made on the basis of facts, and decisions are more accurate and timely as a result. Management information systems are those systems that allow managers to make decisions for the successful operation of businesses. Management information systems consist of computer resources, people, and procedures used in the modern business enterprise. The term MIS stands for management information systems. MIS also refers to the organization that develops and maintains most or all of the computer systems in the enterprise so that managers can make decisions.

60.4 OBJECTIVES OF HIS

1. To provide reliable, latest and useful health information to all levels of health officers and administrators.

2. To contribute towards achievement of objectives of health policies and programs.
3. To increase efficiency and quality in health management.
4. To provide information about periodically and time bound programs.
5. To amend health policies and working system on the basis of feedback.

WHO Expert committee criteria:

1. Health information system should be population based.
2. Health information system should be problem oriented.
3. Health information system should employ functional and operational terms (e.g. episodes of illness, treatment regimens, laboratory tests).
4. The health information system should avoid the unnecessary agglomeration of data.
5. The health information system should express information briefly and imaginatively (e.g. tables, charts, percentages).
6. The information system should make provision for the feedback of data.

60.5 COMPONENTS OF HIS

1. Demography and vital events.
2. Environmental health statistics.
3. Health status—morality, morbidity, disability and quality of life.
4. Health resources—facilities, beds, manpower.
5. Utilization and nonutilization of health services attendance, admission, and waiting lists.
6. Financial statistics (cost, expenditure) related to the particular objective.
7. Indices of outcome of medical care.

60.6 USES OF HEALTH INFORMATION

1. To measure the health status of the people.
2. To quantify health problems, medical and healthcare needs.
3. To compare local, national and international health status of the people.
4. To plan effective management of health services and programs.
5. To assess the effectiveness and efficiency of accomplishing their objectives of health services.
6. To assess the attitudes and degree of satisfaction of the beneficiaries with the health system.
7. To conduct research on particular problems of health and disease.

60.7 SOURCES OF HEALTH INFORMATION

1. **Census:** The total process of collecting, compiling and publishing demographic, economic and social data pertaining at a specific time or times, to all persons in a country or delimited territory.
2. **Registration of vital events:** It is a legal registration, statistical recording and reporting of the occurrence of statistics and the collection, compilation, presentation, analysis and distribution of statistics pertaining to vital events, i.e. live births, deaths, fetal deaths, marriages, divorces, adoptions, legitimations, recognitions, annulments and legal separations.
3. **Sample registration systems:** It is used to provide reliable estimates of birth and death rates at the national and state level. It is also a dual records system, consisting of continuous enumeration of births and deaths by an enumerator and an independent survey every 6 months by an investigator—supervisor.
4. **Notification of disease:** Notification provides valuable information about fluctuations in disease frequency. It also provides early warning about new occurrence or outbreaks or disease.

5. **Hospital records:** The hospital records provides information about age, sex, diagnosis, time interval between occurrence and hospital admission and distribution of patients according to different social and biological characteristics.
6. **Disease register:** Morbidity register exist only certain disease and conditions. It also provides information about duration of illness, case fatality and survival. These register allow follow-up of patients and provide a continuous account of the frequency of disease in the community.
7. **Record linkage:** Medical record linkage implies the assembly and maintaince for each individual in a population, of a file of the more important records relating to his health. The events commonly recorded are birth, marriage, death, hospital admission and discharge.
8. **Epidemiological surveillance:** It is a system used to report on the occurrence of new cases and on efforts to control diseases.
9. **Other health service records:** It includes outpatient departments, primary health centers, subcenters, polyclinics, private practitioners, Medical Center Hospital (MCH), school health records, diabetic and hypertensive clinics etc.
10. **Environmental health data:** It is helpful in the identification and quantification of causative factors of disease. Collection of environmental data plays a essential role to remain a major problems for the future.
11. **Manpower statistics:** It is a information about physicians, dentists, pharmacists, veterinarians, hospital nurses, medical technicians etc. Their records are maintained by the state medical/dental/nursing councils and the directorates of medical education.

CONCLUSION

Health information is any quantifiable and non-quantifiable information that can be used by health decision-makers and clinicians to better understand disease processes and healthcare issues, and to prevent, diagnose or treat health problems. A health information system refers to inter-related component parts for acquiring and analyzing data and providing information (management information, health statistics, and health literature) for the management of a health program or system and for monitoring health activities. (WHO).

61 Nursing Informatics

61.1 INTRODUCTION

Nursing informatics (NI) is a specialty that integrates nursing science, computer science, and information science to manage and communicate data, information, knowledge, and wisdom in nursing practice. NI supports consumers, patients, nurses, and other providers in their decision-making in all roles and settings. This support is accomplished through the use of information structures, information processes, and information technology.

61.2 DEFINITION

"Nursing informatics is defined as combining nursing science, information management science, and computer science to manage and process nursing data, information, and knowledge to deliver quality care to the public". [Health Resource and Services Administration (HRSA), 2008]. "Nursing informatics facilitates the integration of data, information, and knowledge to support patients, nurses, and other providers in their decision-making in all roles and settings. This support is accomplished through the use of information structures, information processes, and information technology. The goal of NI is to improve the health of populations, communities, families, and individuals by optimizing information management and communication." [American Nurses Association (ANA), 2008].

61.3 MEANING OF NURSING INFORMATICS

Nursing informatics is the "science and practice (that) integrates nursing, its information and knowledge, with management of information and communication technologies to promote the health of people, families, and communities worldwide." (IMIA Special Interest Group on Nursing Informatics, 2009). The application of nursing informatics knowledge is empowering for all healthcare practitioners in achieving patient centered care.

Nurse informaticians work as developers of communication and information technologies, educators, researchers, chief nursing officers, chief information officers, software engineers, implementation consultants, policy developers, and business owners, to advance healthcare. Core areas of work include:

1. Concept representation and standards to support evidence-based practice, research, and education.
2. Data and communication standards to build an interoperable national data infrastructure.
3. Research methodologies to disseminate new knowledge into practice.
4. Information presentation and retrieval approaches to support safe patient centered care.
5. Information and communication technologies to address inter-professional work flow needs across all care venues.

6. Vision and management for the development, design, and implementation of communication and information technology.
7. Definition of healthcare policy to advance the public's health.

61.4 NURSING INFORMATIC PROCESS

The informatics perspective can provide insights and opportunities to improve each of the seven ongoing elements of any public health surveillance system. Examples include the following:

1. **Planning and system design:** Identifying information and sources that best address a surveillance goal; identifying who will access information, by what methods and under what conditions; and improving analysis or action by improving the surveillance system interaction with other information systems.
2. **Data collection:** Identifying potential bias associated with different collection methods (e.g. telephone use or cultural attitudes toward technology); identifying appropriate use of structured data compared with free text, most useful vocabulary, and data standards; and recommending technologies (e.g. global positioning systems and radio-frequency identification) to support easier, faster, and higher-quality data entry in the field.
3. **Data management and collation:** Identifying ways to share data across different computing/technology platforms; linking new data with data from legacy systems; and identifying and remedying data-quality problems while ensuring data privacy and security.
4. **Analysis:** Identifying appropriate statistical and visualization applications; generating algorithms to alert users to aberrations in health events; and leveraging high-performance computational resources for large data sets or complex analyses.
5. **Interpretation:** Determining usefulness of comparing information from one surveillance program with other data sets (related by time, place, person, or condition) for new perspectives and combining data of other sources and quality to provide a context for interpretation.
6. **Dissemination:** Recommending appropriate displays of information for users and the best methods to reach the intended audience; facilitating information finding; and identifying benefits for data providers.
7. **Application to public health programs:** Assessing the utility of having surveillance data directly flow into information systems that support public health interventions and information elements or standards that facilitate this linkage of surveillance to action and improving access to and use of information produced by a surveillance system for workers in the field and healthcare providers.

The evolving field of surveillance informatics presents both challenges and opportunities. The challenges include finding efficient and effective ways of combining multiple sources of complex data and information into meaningful and actionable knowledge (e.g. for situational awareness). As these challenges are met, opportunities will arise for faster, better, and lower cost surveillance and interpretation of health events and trends. The domain of public health informatics designs and evaluates methods appropriate for this complex environment.

61.5 ROLE OF NURSE IN NURSING INFORMATICS

Much like nursing, nursing informatics has applications in the areas of clinical information, education, and administration. The most successful information technology implementations take advantage of the user-perspective. Users play a critical role in every phase from the needs assessment through the post-implementation review. Frequently, one challenge for information technology projects is gaining the involvement and support of the end-users. In the case of clinical systems, those end-users are clinicians—nurses and physicians. With the time of caregivers at a precious premium, it is not easy to balance the time requirements of the project with the demands of their "day job". But without clinician input to the requirements, the design, and the deployment, the technology implementation project stands a good chance of failing.

Nursing informatics can help vendors design better technology solutions and healthcare organizations select and implement solutions that will help nurses as well as have the potential to improve patient care. If you were to survey the vendors of electronic health record systems, you would find that each has hired nurses to provide input, assist in the sales and help with the project implementation of their solutions. You will find nurses in the technology departments of healthcare organizations. And, where there is a technology implementation project, there are consultants. Consulting firms are no exception; they too are hiring nurses with nursing informatics interest and/ or training.

61.6 ROLE OF NURSE-SPECIALIST IN INFORMATICS

Just like any other nursing specialty, a nurse who decides to take the role of an Informatics Nurse Specialist, will undergo formal academic preparation (masters degree), testing and certification, and practical experience in using computers in patient care settings. From ANA (1994), the following are expected functions of the Informatics Nurse Specialist (INS):

1. **Theory development:** The INS contributes to the scientific knowledge base of nursing informatics.
2. **Analysis of information needs:** The identification of information that nurses' need to in order to accomplish their work; client care, education, administration, and research
3. **Selection of computer systems:** The INS, guides the user in making informed decisions related to the purchase of computer systems.
4. **Design of computer systems and customizations:** The INS collaborates with users and computer programmers to make decisions about how data will be displayed and accessed.
5. **Testing of computer systems:** Systems must be checked for proper functioning before they are made available for use in patient care.
6. **Training users of computer systems:** Users need to be trained in how the system works, the importance of accurate data entry, and how the system will benefit them, and more importantly how it will improve patient outcomes.
7. **Evaluation of the effectiveness of computer systems:** The unique role of the INS makes them the ideal person to evaluate the effectiveness of computer systems.
8. **Ongoing maintenance and enhancements:** The INS makes sure the computerized system functions properly and explores possible enhancements to the system that will better serve the users and the patients.
9. **Identification of computer technologies that can benefit nursing:** The INS must keep abreast of the changes in the fields of computers and information technology, including new hardware and software that will benefit the nurse and patient.

CONCLUSION

Technical developments in computers and data processing and new theories of systems analysis made it possible to computerize systems. Much of this computerization of systems was an outgrowth of basic research by the federal government. Management information systems are those systems that allow managers to make decisions for the successful operation of businesses. Management information systems consist of computer resources, people, and procedures used in the modern business enterprise. The term MIS stands for management information systems. MIS also refers to the organization that develops and maintains most or all of the computer systems in the enterprise so that managers can make decisions.

Section-12

Staff Welfare

62 Staff Development Program

62.1 INTRODUCTION

Staff development activities consist of the training and education provided by an employer to improve employee's occupational knowledge, skills and attitudes and to provide the employee with the opportunity to grow professionally. Professional nurses one education in a variety of ways staff development program have greater responsibility to develop characteristics, abolition work assignments and uptake knowledge among staff. Nursing managers are challenged to provide creative and consistent high guilty education to learner she frequently perform the staff development role, sometimes a director of nursing in a healthcare organizations as nurse manger or from other management positions.

62.2 DEFINITION

1. Staff development program (SDP) are designed to motivate learner in the way of the train and education to improve their knowledge, skills and attitudes.
2. A process that assists individuals in an agency or organization in attaining newskills and knowledge, gaining increasing levels of competence, and growing professionally. Various resources outside the agency employing the individuals may are used. The process may include such programs as orientation, in-service education, and continuing education.

62.3 MEANING OF STAFF DEVELOPMENT

Staff development refers to the continuing improvement of the nursing personnel. It also includes setting standards for jobs, providing on the job growth experiences, considering potential growth opportunities in all assignment planning, supervising and appraising performance proficiencies and assuming responsibility for reparative or corrective training measures. Staff development program arc designed to motivate learner in the way of the train and education to improve their knowledge, skills and attitudes.

62.4 OBJECTIVES OF STAFF DEVELOPMENT

1. To assist each employee to improve performance in present position.
2. To keep in pace with medical sciences.
3. New development in medical science and technology.
4. New diagnostic and treatment techniques.
5. To motivate each staff member and create a sense of security and loyalty.
6. To improve work productivity and for promotion.
7. To reduce staff turnover, absenteeism and tardiness.
8. To acquire personal and professional abilities that maximizes the possibility of career advancement.

62.5 STAFF DEVELOPMENT PROCESS

The major processes involved in the staff development programs are presented graphically in the following chart prepared by Silver (1981): The goals and objectives of the training program must first of all be defined. This will give focus and guidance to the entire program. Then, the strengths and weaknesses of staff must be identified. This will be useful in developing long-term plans and specific training programs which will involve specific outlines of major annual training goals, the number of individuals who will benefit from such training and the cost implication of the plan.

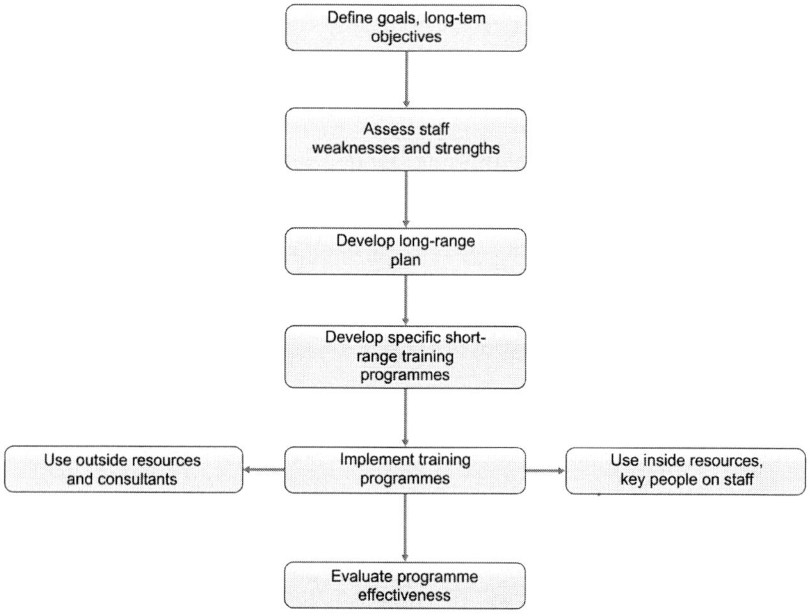

Fig. 62.1: Staff-development process

The next stage involves detailed training programs which will be undertaken. The acquisition of text and training materials, the preparation of teaching or instructional aides, the selection and appointment of instructors and their remunerations are determined. This stage is followed by the implementation of the program which will involve the use of consultants and resource persons. Meeting places are provided. The trainees are released from their regular duties for the training programs. The last stage is the evaluation of the efforts and performance of the training programs with a view to detecting the need for improvement in certain areas of the program.

62.6 FUNCTIONS OF STAFF DEVELOPMENT

Personnel assigned to staff development should provide the following consultative functions for healthcare agency:

1. Determination of the administrative structure of the staff development program.
2. Determination and establishment of organizational methods, policies and procedures for a staff development program.
3. Determination and establishment of lines of communication for the utilization of facilities and resources personnel for a staff development program.
4. Determination of organizational and individual staff development needs and priority.
5. Development of measurable short- and long-term objectives for staff development programs.

6. Promotion, development, implementation and evaluation of programs to meet these objectives.
7. Planning, coordination, and utilization of community resources to assist in meeting these objectives.
8. Provision of a consultative service and a resource for information relative to staff development.

62.7 STAFF DEVELOPMENT ACTIVITIES

Staff development includes formal and informal, group or individual training and education. Staff development activities include:
1. Induction training.
2. Orientation.
3. In-service education.
4. Continuing education, and
5. Training for special functions such as management, team building, and budgeting method.
1. **Induction training (3 days):** Is a brief introduction to agency philosophy, purpose, administrators, programs, policies and regulations that is given to new employee during the first three days of employment.
2. **Orientation (2–24 weeks):** Is individualized training given each employee during the first period of his job to familiarize him with his job's duties, work place, clients and coworker.
3. **In-service education (2–8 hours):** Includes all on-the-job instruction and training that is given to enhance employee's present job performance.
4. **Continuing education (1–5 days):** Includes all planned learning that is intended to increase employee's knowledge or skills beyond that needed for satisfactory performance in the present job.

62.8 IMPORTANCE OF STAFF DEVELOPMENT

1. It is focus on developing nursing skills and knowledge.
2. Introduce the employees to new situations and orientated to philosophy, soils, politics, and physical sanities.
3. It provider job-relate counseling, which involves promoting the professional growth of employees.
4. It provides learning experiences in the work setting for the purpose of refining and developing new skills and knowledge related to job performance.
5. It is planned and organized around learning experiences in variety of setting.
6. To reduce staff turnover and absenteeism.

62.9 STAFF DEVELOPMENT ORGANIZATION

The staff development program philosophy based on nursing organization. It includes:
1. How learning takes place.
2. Various teaching methods.
3. Responsibility for their learning.
4. Rights of the clients.
1. **Organization:** There are two methods of organization.
   a. Centralized model: Here, all department collaborating determining and planning the job needs of their staff.
   b. Decentralized model: Each department has its own organized staff development programs.
2. **Committees:** Committees identifying needs and resources for program committees member maintain relationship and communicable between each one to accomplish the goal.

3. **Budgets:** Budgets based on staff size, no of new employees and resource person, programme manager is responsible for budget preparation.
4. **Personnel:** Staff development manager to work on planning, implementing and evaluating staff development programs. The size of staff depends on the size of the agency.

62.10 STAFF DEVELOPMENT ASSESSMENT METHODS

Staff development planning, organizers to assessment needs of participants. Following faction should be considered to assess needs of the program:

1. Population.
2. Time.
3. Cost/financial.
4. Analysis time.
5. Objectivity.

Various Methods of Needs Assessment

1. Questionnaire method.
2. Survey.
3. Interview.
4. Observation.
5. Group meeting.
6. Performance appraisal.
7. Individual need assessment method.

62.11 GOALS OF STAFF DEVELOPMENT

Staff development includes formal and informal group and individual training and education. The goals of staff development programs are to assist each employee to improve performance in her or

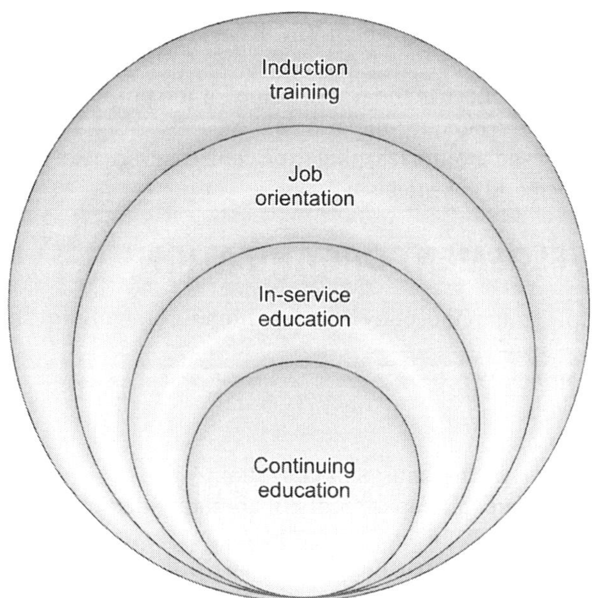

Fig. 62.2: Goal of staff development

his present position and to acquire personal and professional abilities that maximize the possibility of career advancement. Staff development activities include the following: 1. Induction training, 2. Job orientation, 3. In-service education, 4. Continuing education.

1. **Induction training** is a brief, standardized indoctrination to an agency's philosophy, purpose, policies and regulations given to each worker during her or his first two or three days of employment in order to ensure his or her identification with agency's philosophy, goals and norms.
2. **Job orientation** is an individualized training program intended to acquaint a newly hired employee with job responsibilities work place, clients and coworkers.
3. **In-service education** refers to an ongoing-on-the-job instruction that is given to enhance, the workers' performance in their present job. In-service education is a planned educational experience provided in the job setting and closely identified with service in order to help the person to perform more effectively as a person and as a worker. In-service education is defined as a continued program of education provided by the employing authority, with the purpose of developing the competence of personnel in their functions appropriate to the position they hold, or to which they will be appointed in the service.
4. **Continuing education** is "any extension of opportunities for reading, study and training to any person and adult following their completion of or withdrawal from full time school and/or college programs". It is there education for adults provided by specific schools, centers, colleges or institutions that emphasize flexible rather than traditional or academic programs. Adult education is a formal and informal instruction and aids to study for mature persons; all activities with educational purposes carried on by mature persons on a part time basis; any voluntary, purposeful effort towards the self development of adults conducted by public or private agencies, for informational, cultural, remedial, vocational, recreational, and professional and other purposes (Dictionary of Education).

62.12 ADMINISTRATIVE STRUCTURE OF SDP

The major factors that determine the administrative structure of an agency-wide staff development program are:

1. Administrative philosophy, policies and practices of healthcare agency.
2. Policies, practices and standards of nursing and other health professions.
3. Human and material resources within a healthcare agency and the community.
4. Physical facilities within a healthcare agency and the community.
5. Financial resources within a healthcare agency and the community.

Centralization v/s Decentralization: In some cases, a centralized structure will be more effective than a decentralized structure. There are advantages and disadvantages to both types of structure. Usually, the coordination of staff development is more readily facilitated in a centralized structure. However, in a decentralized structure, it is possible to involve a larger number of personnel in planning and implementing programs. One alternative is a centralized structure for an agency-wide staff development program and decentralized structure for programs related to learning a specific job skill. Whatever be the administrative structure, it is vital to circumvent redundancy, repetition and ineffective utilization of personnel and facilities.

62.13 ROLE OF HEAD NURSE IN SD

1. Involves staff members in developing high standards of patient care and in establishing objectives and criteria for their attainment.
2. Discover leadership's skills and creative abilities among staff and arrange for their development.

3. Encourage staff to participate in planning for the improvement of nursing care and to apply findings of nursing practice research.
4. Provide learning opportunities for professional advancement of staff in order to develop to their highest potential.
5. Share in planning and participate in staff educational programs of professional and non-professional personnel.
6. Allot time for discussions, observations and questions.
7. Set a good example in everyday practice.

CONCLUSION

Staff development includes formal and informal group and individual training and education. The goals of staff development programmes are to assist each employee to improve performance in her or his present position and to acquire personal and professional abilities that maximize the possibility of career advancement. Staff development is the process directed towards the personal and professional growth of nurses and other personnel while they are employed by a healthcare agency. Staff development refers to all training and education provided by an employee to improve the occupational and personal knowledge, skills and attitudes of vested employees.

63 Staff Welfare

63.1 INTRODUCTION

The institution should serve various facilities for the staff members to enable them to function effectively at their work. The institution expects from its staff a commitment to serve, in the spirit of god, the patients and others who come in search of the services. Some of the provisions provided are unique to the institution and we believe will faster a fellowship and friendship amongst the staff to develop a team spirit which is critical for successful medical services.

63.2 PURPOSES OF STAFF WELFARE

1. It motivates the staff to work effectively.
2. It improves interest to serve to the particular institution.
3. It facilitates the staff member to participate with full involvement.
4. It improves the team work in the institution.
5. It helps to meet the psychological, social and educational need of the employee.

63.3 FACULTY IMPROVEMENT TECHNIQUES

1. Encourage and stimulate faculty.
2. Take positive attitude towards problems of teachers.
3. Provide resources and facilities for the implementation of instructions.
4. Give recognition to abilities.
5. Create a climate which stimulates creative participation by faculty members.
6. While making changes in the curriculum, invite suggestions from the faculty.
7. Given opportunity to plan, experiment and explore.
8. Assist in developing teaching techniques.
9. Maintain good relation with faculty members.

63.4 STAFF WELFARE ACTIVITIES

The conditions under which the teaching staff have an effect on the implementation of the program besides contributing towards the stability of the staff. Frustrations, conflicts, resignations and frequent requesting for transfer can often be reduced when there are clearly defined policies related to hours of work, teaching load, welfare of the staff and other matters. The policies should be written down known to everyone. Employee welfare activities are social security measures provided by the institution for the welfare of the employees. Some of them are:

1. Employees provident fund.
2. Gratuity benefit.

3. Maternity benefit.
4. Risk allowances.
5. Compensations for work injuries.
6. Family pension schemes.
7. Employee state insurance.

Types of faculty welfare include:

1. Opportunity for leave on the basis of leave rules by the institution policies
   These leave rules incorporate existing Annual Leave, maternity leave, sabbatical leave, study leave, leave on loss of pay, official leave.
2. Gratuity - cum - retirement benefit scheme
3. Hospital concessions.
4. Staff special superannuation benefit scheme for long-term service.
5. Provident fund.
6. Death benefit schemes.
7. Providing opportunity to develop cognitive skills by staff development programs, in-service program and continuing education programs.

63.5 FORMULATION OF POLICIES

Condition under which the teaching staff work, has an effect n the implementation on the program besides contributing towards the stability of the staff trust rations, conflicts, resignations and frequent requests for transfer, can often be reduced when there are clearly defined policies relating to hour of work, teaching load, welfare of staff and other matters. Such policies are particularly effective when the staff have been involved in formulating them, when they are known to everyone. The following are some of the matters in which it would be helpful to have stated policies and some of the factors to be considered in formulating them are.

i. **Hours of work:** The policy should given direction on
   1. The maximum number of working hours per week.
   2. The number of days off per month, to which the staff is entitled.
   3. The procedure to be followed regarding public holidays.

ii. **Teaching load:** The policy regarding the maximum teaching load to be carried by each tutor should allow time for preparation for classes and laboratory sessions, student guidance and counseling, evaluation of student assignments, committee work, record keeping and all other functions expected of a tutor. A teaching load of 14–16 hours per week will permit attention to these functions. In cases where this in not possible, 20 hours of formal teaching per week should not be exceeded.

iii. **Residence:** There should be policy regarding the residence of staff quarters facilities. Residence for some staff is essential if student's curricular and extracurricular activities are implemented satisfactorily. The accommodation for married and unmarried staff including family quarters depends on institution's policy.

iv. **Leave:** The College should have clear policy about leaves.
   1. Time of year during which annual leave may normally be taken.
   2. How many leaves may be taken at one time?
   3. The purpose for which casual or special leave may be granted.
   4. The provision for maternity leave.

v. **Sickness:** In regard to the care which will be given to staff members who are sick the college policy should state clearly about sick leave, medical expenses, reimbursement facility etc.

vi. **Attendance at conference and study care:** The College should state policies regarding the selection and deputation of the staff for further education, including attendance at formal courses, refresher courses, work shop and conferences.

vii. **Promotion and transfer:** Promotion is the transfer of an employee to a job that pays more money or one that enjoys some preferred status. A promotion is the advancement of an employee to a better job better in terms of greater responsibilities, more prestige or status, greater skill, and especially increased pay or salary.
There should be a promotion policy in a college of nursing to motivate the teacher for higher productivity. The cadre of promotion must be clearly established and communicated to the employees. The promotion policy must consider the merit, potential for advancement and seniority of the employees. It should not be merely on the basis of year of experience.
Transfer involves the shifting of an employee from one job to another without special reference to changing responsibilities or compensation, placing employees to position more appropriate to their interest or abilities or filling vacancies in a department.

viii. **In-service education:** Service education is an organized educational program which is offered to trained staff during their period of employment and related to improvement of their performance. It should contain the element of orientation, training of special skills and continuing education.

ix. **Continuing education:** One of the basic aspects of continuing education for teachers is that it covers all those organized and informal means where by teachers of all ages are encouraged to learn from one another and from society around them. Continuing education is very essential for the faculty because there as been an explosion of knowledge in medical science and other allied areas. Also the growth of science and technology has mostly contributed to the development of new knowledge in the field of teaching. The scope of continuing education for nursing teachers is very broad and comprehensive. It refers to the education a teacher receives after she has entered into the teaching profession.

63.6 LEAVE FACILITIES

Leave facilities incorporate existing annual leave, casual leave, compensatory holidays, sick leave, maternity leave, sabbatical leave, study leave, leave on loss of pay, official level.

General rules of taking leave:

1. Leave shall be granted in accordance with the leave rules of institution.
2. Leave cannot be claimed by any employee as right.
3. The administrative officer concerned shall be the competent authority to sanction by the administrative officer concerned depending up on the necessities.
4. Ordinarily no employee shall absent himself or herself from work unless leave is sanctioned. Employees remaining absent unauthorisedly shall be subjected to disciplinary action.
5. Normally, leave application shall be made in prescribed forms.
6. All leave applications forwarded to the administrative officer concerted for sanctioning shall contain the recommendation of the head of the department.
7. The administrative officer concerned shall arrange to intimate the unveiled leave to the credit of the employees of each department.

I. Annual Leave

The quantum of annual leave shall be on the following scale.

Council appointees-35 days, Non-council appointees-25 days. Annual leave for unconfirmed employees shall be calculated on prorate basis on the number of days spent on duty by on employee in the leave year. For arriving at the number of days spent on duty the days availed on annual leave, casual leave, and sick leave, maternity leave will be taken into account.

Annual leave cannot follow casual leave. However, casual leave up to a maximum of five days can be added on to the annual leave by prior permission of administrative officer concerned. Annual leave shall not be granted in more than three installments in a leave year.

II. Casual Leave

Casual leave may be granted to a employees for a total of 10 days in each year subject to the necessities and exigencies of work. Casual leave may be either prefixed or suffixed to Sundays or holidays. Casual leave may be availed for half a day.

Unexpected casual leave up to 2 day may be carried over to the following year to be used within the first six months.

III. Compensatory and Institutional Holidays

If any member of staff is on any leave other than official leave on a declared holiday of the institution, no compensatory leave shall be given to him/her. However, if the day off given to a staff member falls on a declared. If Christmas, New Year's Day, Rupublic Day, Good Friday and Independence day, which are National and Institutional holidays falls on a Sunday, compensatory leave will be given which may be taken with in 6 months.

IV. Sick Leave

Sick leave with full pay for a total of 15 days may be granted in a leave year. In addition to 15 days sick leave full pay as above, sick leave with half pay for a further period up to 18 days may be granted in a leave year. However, this cannot be converted to 9 days sick leave with full pay.

Sick leave normally be granted only on production of a sick leave recommendation slip issued by the medical officer, staff student health service. Sick leave shall be sanctioned according to the number of days indicated in the sick leave slip issued by the staff student health service.

V. Maternity Leave

Women employees in the institution shall be granted maternity leave for 8 weeks with full pay. Part of the maternity leave may be availed just prior to delivery.

63.7 INCENTIVES

Incentives are provided by some organization in order to attract and retain good employees. Incentives may be monetary and non-monetary. The monetary incentives may be the form of payment of bonuses, merit increments, housing facilities, medical care, loans, provision of transportation, education of children etc. The non-monetary incentives are also used to motivate the employees for higher education. They are in the form of status and recognition, job security, responsibility; participation is decision-making, training facilities, promotion, discipline, team spirit etc., negative incentives are in the form of fine, demotion, suspension etc.

CONCLUSION

The conditions under which the teaching staff have an effect on the implementation of the program besides contributing towards the stability of the staff. Frustrations, conflicts, resignations and frequent requesting for transfer can often be reduced when there are clearly defined policies related to hours of work, teaching load, welfare of the staff and other matters. The policies should be written down known to everyone. The following are some of these matters.

64 Nursing Conference

64.1 INTRODUCTION

The individual and group conferences are methods of supervision. In fact, they are among the most valuable of supervisory technique. In group conferences the workers have an opportunity to inform the authorities about the activities of the hospital and ward. If meeting are held every two to four weeks with the workers collectively or in interest group, it helps to know about the problem of individuals.

64.2 DEFINITION

1. The act of consulting together involving a two way flow of conversation is called a group conferences.
2. Any coming together of two or more individuals in an informal meeting for the purpose of giving or exchanging ideas.

64.3 TYPES OF NURSING CONFERENCES

1. **Individual nursing conference:** It is a conversation between two persons, which may include the head nurse, physician, nurses, clinical instructor and the nursing students in order to solve a nursing problem.
2. **Group nursing conference:** It includes the conversation between large groups by discussing about his/her care. The patient may both be directly involved in the conference.

64.4 NURSING CONFERENCE AREAS

1. Specific points in the nursing care of individual patients.
2. Gaps in nursing care.
3. Reports on one or more patients who were admitted during the past 24 hours.
4. The importance of accurate or detailed charting on a patient whose diagnosis is not established.
5. An unusual or new drug or treatment which is being used on the ward for one or more patients.
6. Routine diagnostic tests/measures in relation to specific patients having such tests that day.
7. New hospital or ward routines.
8. Changes in nursing procedures.
9. Review of procedures which are unfamiliar or which are not being performed well.
10. Equipment which has been damaged by improper care, misuse or carelessness with discussion of cases, methods of prevention, costs etc.

64.5 TIME FOR CONFERENCE

1. When staff is free to attend.
2. Three times a week or daily according to the situation.
3. Some hour of the day once a week.
4. Preferably in the early morning.

64.6 SKILLS REQUIRED IN CONFERENCE

1. Skill in observation.
2. Skill in use of setting.
3. Skill in establishing resistance.
4. Skill in meeting resistance.
5. Skill in recognizing ambivalent feelings.
6. Skill in establishment of authority.
7. Skill in use of questions.
8. Silence as a skill.

64.7 USES OF NURSING CONFERENCES

1. It assists the nursing student to correlate between the class content and its practical application in the clinical area.
2. It is used to clarity class material for individual students.
3. It is a method of solving the patient's problems by discussion.
4. It acts as a means of communication among the health team members.
5. It helps in all round development of the personnel by keeping them up date on knowledge.
6. It helps to build up the group moral and interpersonal relationship.
7. It helps to pass on skill and knowledge to nursing students.
8. It encourages the team member to add their own to contribute in the profession.
9. It helps to refresh the mind of the participants.

64.8 PREPARATION FOR NURSING CONFERENCE

1. The nurse/student should gather all information regarding the patient, his history, nursing care etc.
2. The nurse/student should prepare the patient if he/she is to be presented to the group.
3. The nurse/student should be able to arrange for seating arrangements and a proper physical set up.
4. The nurse/student should be able to give up. To data information in relation to the patients conditions.

64.9 CONFERENCE TOPICS

1. A subject which probably needs to be discussed periodically with the ward housekeeping staff is the responsibility of the hospital towards the public.
2. Suggestion for improvement in their work in relation with coworkers may be proposed by the workers and by the head nurse.

3. Some groups will be benefited by a discussion on personnel hygiene and appropriateness of dress.
4. The ward and hospital policies which affect the coworkers should be carefully explained to them.
5. Some other activities like plans for building a hospital wing or a new arrangement in the obstetric departments can be discussed with the housekeeping personnel. Conferences should be held on a working day and should be scheduled for an hour which will not affect the work.

CONCLUSION

The individual and group conferences are methods of supervision. In fact they are among the most valuable of supervisory technique. In group conferences the workers have an opportunity to inform the authorities about the activities of the hospital and word. If meeting are held every two to four weeks with the workers collectively or in interest group, it helps to know about the problem of individuals.

65 In-Service Education

65.1 INTRODUCTION

In-service education is defined as learning experiences provided in the working setting for the purpose of assisting staff in performing their assigned functions in that particular agency.

65.2 DEFINITION

The American Nurses Association defined as "Planned education activities intended to build upon the educational and experiential bases of the professional nurse for the enhancement of practice, education, administration, and research or theory development to the end of improving the health of the public".

65.3 AIMS AND OBJECTIVES

1. The primary objective of in-service education is the improvement of professional practice, development of person as an individual and a responsible citizen.
2. It keeps enthusiastic in their learning and makes them to seek latest knowledge.
3. It enables to implement the knowledge with skill and ability.
4. It improves the healthcare delivery to the public enhancing the quality of effective nursing practice.
5. It develops interest and job satisfaction.
6. By acquiring current and up to date knowledge, confidence is developed among them.

65.4 NEED FOR IN-SERVICE PROGRAM

Need for in-service education for professional nurses is influenced by research and advances in healthcare. Nursing science and technology. In the current health environment, the quality appropriateness and effectiveness of interventions assume increasing importance.

1. **General in-service education:** This program is short-term learning experiences related to topics required to all staff. For example, Cardiopulmonary resuscitation (CPR), Fire safety.
2. **Specific in-service education:** This type of education programs are also short-term but are designed to meet the needs of a particular group of staff in a clinical area.

65.5 COMPONENTS OF IN-SERVICE

1. **Orientation:** The orientation influences the structure and content of individualized orientation of various groups of nursing service people. The goal of the orientation program is to enhance the competencies of nursing service personnel so that employees may continuously improve the quality of care provided to patients.

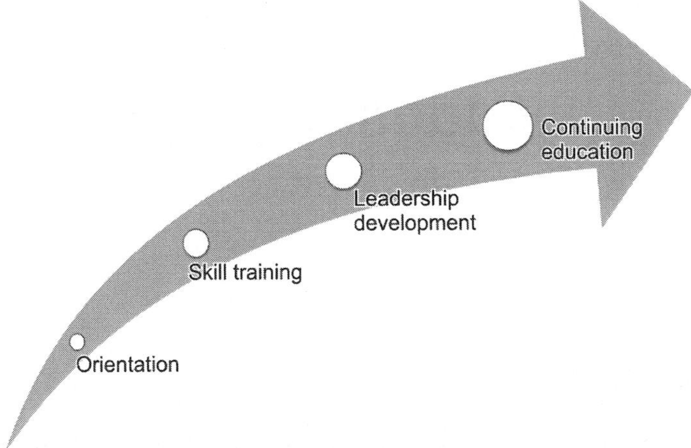

Fig. 65.1: Components of in-service

2. **Skill training:** For the new employee skill training provides an idea about how to carry out the assigned function complex ones. It enables to meet the standards established for quantity and quality of the performance and job satisfaction. It improves the new employees skill in the routine and special procedures.
3. **Leadership development:** The staff should have skills in leadership and management in order to guide a new employee in caring outpatient care activities. At present the hospitals are recognizing the development of leadership and management qualities among the staff members.
4. **Continuing education:** The International Council of Nurses emphasized the importance of continuing education for nurses in order to ensure safe and effective nursing care. It consists of a large number of educational programs and activities. It is the necessary for all the level of nursing personnel to deal with the needs of nursing oneself aware of all the development in the field of the specialization.

CONCLUSION

In service education program for the nursing staff are frequently planned by the nursing service administration. The most effective programmes give emphasis on outcome rather than on staff development. If result is considered valuable the individual's participation will be active. Some hospitals have found that staff development, personal and professional reaches its highest level when members work together to achieve a common purpose. Even when the hospital has not in-service program it would be better for the staff to have such program it would be better for the staff to have such programmes within their wards. Well-qualified staff nurses can make a worthy contribution to the students education both by assisting in the planned program and by their e.g. as nurses. The head nurse can help medical students in their adjustment to the hospital wards by holding orientation conferences and teaching them some of the fundamentals of nursing care. The increased knowledge owing to this program assists in maintaining an efficient ward. Housekeeping workers will also be taught on the ward.

66 Continuing Education

66.1 INTRODUCTION

Continuing education (CE) means the phenomenon of ever learning which does not stop at any particular stage. It includes all learning opportunities which would be taken up after full time education has stopped. It is the resumption of the process of studying or learning which might have interrupted because of some economic, professional and personnel compulsion of the individual. Continuing education program provide teaching and learning strategies that are based upon the learning theory which states that adult learners should participate in the development of their learning objectives.

66.2 DEFINITION

1. The American Nurses Association (ANA) has defined continuing education as "learning activities", intended to build upon the education and experience bases of the professional nurse for the enhancement of practice education, administration, and research or theory development.
2. Continuing education is a formal, organized educational programs designed to promote the knowledge, skills and professional attitudes of nurses.

66.3 OBJECTIVES OF CONTINUING EDUCATION

Continuing education helps the employee to:

1. Keep up-to-date with new concepts and development in the health field.
2. To increase their basic knowledge and skills and develop positive attitudes.
3. Develop an ability to analyze problems and to work with others.
4. Meet the challenge of changes in technology.
5. Maintain standards of healthcare at acceptable level.
6. Help in setting standards within the healthcare team.
7. Help in career development.
8. Motivate staff for better patient care.
9. Meet new needs of the community.

66.4 PURPOSES OF CONTINUING EDUCATION

1. Documenting attendance at the designed seminars or course of institution. Licensing bodies in a number of fields impose continuing education requirements on members who hold licenses to practice within particular profession.
2. These requirements are intended to encourage professionals to expand their knowledge base and up-to-date them on new departments.

3. Depending on the field, these requirements may be satisfied through college or university course work, extension courses or conferences and seminars attendance.

66.5 NEED FOR CONTINUING EDUCATION

1. Kothari Education Commission also suggested that education institutions should arrange adhoc courses which will make people to understand and solve their problems in life and to train wider knowledge and experience.
2. Learning through continuing education is also essential for the rural people, who must acquire full knowledge about rapid advancement of agricultural and economic techniques just as urban people have to acquire commercial techniques.
3. Indian Education Commission has rightly stated about it, "Education does not end with school, but it is a lifelong process.
4. Continuing education programmed provide teaching and learning strategies that are based upon learning theory which states that adult learners should participate in the development of their learning objectives.
5. Continuing education is the most essential requirement of the adult today. He can enjoy a better, healthier and more successful life only if he continues his education up to end of his life.

66.6 NATIONAL POLICY ON CONTINUING EDUCATION

According to National Policy on Education (NPE), Adult education can be successfully implemented by involving continuing education. Hence, these kinds of implemented by involving continuing education. Hence, these kinds of education are to be combined. It is possible to implement adult and continuing education programs through various ways, such as
1. To setup continuing education centers in rural areas.
2. To educate workers through their employers trade unions and concerned agencies of government.
3. To provide post secondary education institutions.
4. To provide books, libraries and reading rooms.
5. To use radio, television and film as mass and group learning media.
6. To create learners groups and organizations.
7. To design programs of distance learning.
8. To organize assistance in self-study.
9. To organize vocational training programs based on needs and interests of learners.

66.7 PROGRAMS OF ACTION ON NPE

Continuing education is any training or classes that one takes after completing formal education. Continuing education can be college classes taken after completing a formal degree program or seminars and training taken to improve one's job skills.
1. **Program of action** given by the ministry of Human Resource Development, Government of India has been fully formulated. First of all it is considered that continuing education is regarded as an indispensable aspect of the strategy of human resource development and the goal of creation of learning society.
2. **Continuing education** aims at post literacy for neo literates and school drop outs for retention of literacy skills continuation of learning beyond elementary literacy and application of this learning to improve their living conditions. However, the continuing education goes beyond post literacy and its instruments.

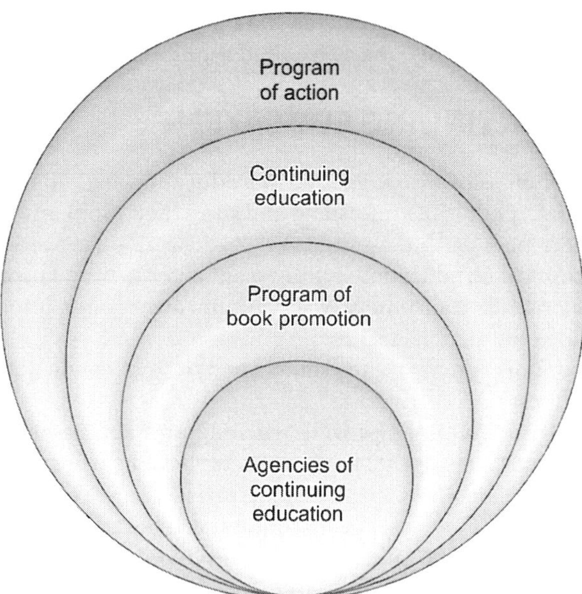

Fig. 66.1: Program of action on NPE

3. **Program of book promotion** will be undertaken on the lines indicated in the policy. Libraries and reading rooms in educational institutions should be opened to the public in the evening and necessary additional grants should be provided to them for this purpose. The voluntary efforts for establishment of reading room and libraries should be encouraged. Radio, TV films should be encouraged for sub serving the objectives of education and recreation.
4. **Agencies of continuing education** are parallel system of education, adhoc or short-term courses, open universities, distance education scheme, libraries, special part-time courses, special institutions and mass medias.

CONCLUSION

Many professions require that members of their profession continue learning new and changing skills to retain their credentials or even licenses. For example, Certified Public Accountants in most states are required to take continuing education hours every year to keep their licenses current. Continuing education is any course of study offered by an educational institution, association, professional society or organization for the purpose of providing continuing education for nursing home administrators. Continuing education program are usually short-term and specific, a certificate may be offered for completion of a course. It is not to be confused with academic degree-granting programs such as advanced education or post graduate education.

Section-13

Professional Organizations

67 Professional Organizations

67.1 INTRODUCTION

Organizations provide a means through which united efforts are made to elevate standards of nursing education and practice. It also offers a means of voicing and opinions, developing our abilities and keeping informed of new trends. Nursing regulatory bodies are also known as 'Professional Associations which are responsible for the licensing of nurses within their respective province or territory. These regulatory bodies set the enforced standards of nursing practice, monitor and enforce standards for nursing education, monitor and enforce standards for nursing practice and set the requirements for registration of nursing professionals. The professional nurse must be aware of these associations so as to participate in various nursing professional activities of these organizations. To be a part of these associations, the nurse must have life membership with these organizations through proper registration which is must.

67.2 FUNCTIONS OF PROFESSIONAL BODIES

1. These associations provide a means through which the professional development of a nurse can be channeled with the authority because of its representative character.
2. These associations also provide the nurses with the opportunities for expression of their viewpoints, development of their leadership qualities and abilities.
3. These associations keep the nurses informed of professional news and trends throughout the country and worldwide.

67.3 INDIAN NURSING COUNCIL

The Indian Nursing Council (INC) is an autonomous body under the Government of India, Ministry of Health and Family Welfare was constituted by the Central Government under Section 3(1) of the Indian Nursing Council Act, 1947 of Parliament in order to establish a uniform standard of training for nurses, midwives and health visitors.

Aims of INC: The aim of legislation in nursing is best achieved through introduction of a 'Nurse Practice Act' having statutory regulation which makes provision for establishment of nursing council. Since, health is a state subject, there is Nursing council at the state level which formulates their policy as per the guidelines provided by the Indian Nursing Council.

The members of the State Nursing Council is majority from the nursing profession. Nursing Council functions with enactment of an act by the state legislature. The act prescribes the licensures and the state council has to register the members of the profession.

The Central Government has established Indian Nursing Council which is a central council of the country established by an Act of Parliament in 1947.

The purpose of Indian Nursing Council (INC) is to formulate a national policy for training and practice of nursing depending mainly on the culture and philosophy of the country. Thus, INC is required to prescribe the syllabus for the training of nurses of all levels, e.g. MSc. BSc (N), General Nursing and Midwifery (GNM). Auxilliary Nurse Midwife Government (ANM), LHV, etc. and the minimum requirements for the recognition of any institution offering such a course. Nursing personnel has to be identified with an appropriate educational program for each level in the system of the country. The council has the authority to prescribe training institutions periodically to ensure its functioning abiding the standard prescribed. If any amendment of act of INC to be made following process is needed:

1. A proposal is to be sent to Government of India Ministry of Health and Family Welfare.
2. Ministry of Health will consult Ministry of Law.
3. It will go to cabinet (Legal Cell).
4. When it is approved by cabinet (Legal cell), it will be placed before Lok Sabha.
5. When the Lok Sabha approves it, then it will be placed before Rajya Sabha.
6. When the amendments are approved by the Rajya Sabha then it will be Gazeted and notified.

The Indian Nursing Council was authorized by the Indian Nursing Council Act of 1947. It was established in 1949 to provide uniform standards in nursing education and reciprocity in nursing registration throughout the country.

Objectives and Functions of Indian Nursing Council

1. To establish and monitor a uniform standard of nursing education for nurses midwife, auxiliary nurse midwives (ANM) and health visitors by doing inspection of the institutions.
2. To recognize the qualifications under section 10(2)(4) of the Indian Nursing Council Act, 1947 for the purpose of registration and employment in India and abroad.
3. To give approval for registration of Indian and Foreign Nurses possessing foreign qualification under section 11(2)(a) of the Indian Nursing Council Act, 1947.
4. To prescribe the syllabus and regulations for nursing programs.
5. Power to withdraw the recognition of qualification under section 14 of the Act in case the institution fails to maintain its standards under Section 14 (1)(b) that an institution recognized by a State Council for the training of nurses, midwives, ANMs or health visitors does not satisfy the requirements of the council.
6. To advise the State Nursing Councils, Examining Boards, State Governments and Central Government in various important items regarding Nursing Education in the Country.

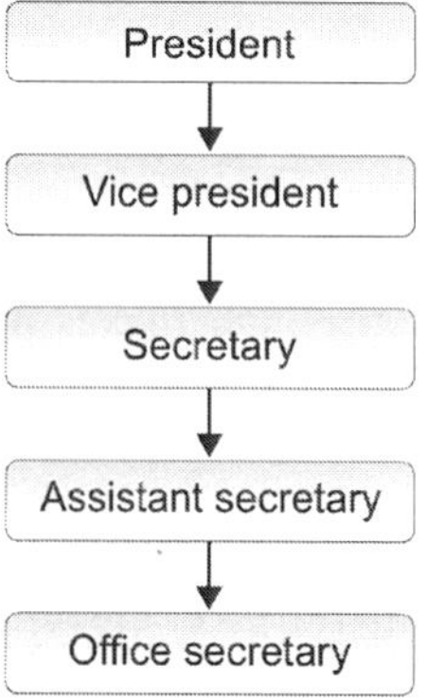

Fig. 67.1: Organizational structure of Indian Nursing Council

Organizational Structure of Indian Nursing Council Committee

1. **Executive Committee** of the Council is constituted to deliberate on the issues related to maintenance of standards of nursing programs.
2. **The Nursing Education** Committee is constituted to deliberate on the issues concerned mainly with nursing education and policy matters concerning the nursing education.
3. **Equivalence Committee** is constituted to deliberate on the issues of recognition of foreign qualifications, which is essential for the purpose of registration under section 11(2)(a) or (b) of the INC Act, 1947, as amended.

Functions of INC

1. It provides uniform standards in nursing education and reciprocity in nursing registration.
2. It has authority to prescribe curriculum for nursing education in all states.
3. It has authority to recognize program of nursing education or to refuse recognition of a program if it did not meet the standards required by the council.
4. It is registering the foreign nurses.
5. It also maintains the Indian Nurses Register.
6. The INC authorizes State Nurses Registration Council and examining boards to issue qualifying certificates.
7. Recognizes nurses as a separate branch in health service.
8. Regulates nursing training sets uniform standard types of training for nurses throughout the country.
   (a) Construct syllabus, e.g. ANM, GNM, BSc (N), MSc (N) etc.
   (b) Laid down requirements for admission of students.
   (c) Set up minimum standard of a schools and colleges of Nursing.
   (d) Certificates on completion of training.
9. Recognition of qualifications (basic and higher).
10. Effect of recognition any recognized qualification shall be sufficient qualification for enrolment in any state register.
11. Power to enquire information as to course of study and training and examination from any state from time to times as required.
12. Inspection of the schools and colleges of nursing.
13. Withdrawal of recognition of nursing institutions.
14. Maintenance of Indian Nurse Registers.
15. Power to make regulations.
16. To regulate nursing practice.
17. Permits title, badges, uniforms for registered nurses.
18. Uphold the standard of nursing.
19. Publications.

67.4 INTERNATIONAL COUNCIL OF NURSES (ICN)

The International Council of Nurses was founded in 1899 by Mrs Bedford Fenwick. It is a federation of nonpolitical and self-governing national nurses association. The ICN is the global voice of nursing. The main purpose of the ICN is to provide the means through which the national associations can share their interests in the promotion of health and care of the sick.

In 1900, the Council's Constitution was adopted and the first meeting was held at the World Exposition in Buffalo, New York. Their headquarter is established at Geneva in Switzerland.

Objectives of ICN

1. To promote the development of the strong National Nurses Association.
2. To assist National Nurses Association to improve the standards of nursing education and practice.
3. To assist National Nurses Association to improve the status of nurses within their countries.
4. To serve as the authoritative voice for nurses and nursing internationally.

Activities

1. The ICN has published the Code for Nurses.
2. It makes the policy statement on health and social issues.
3. It also maintains and improves the status of nurses and standard of nursing around the world.
4. The council works to improve the nursing education and practice by publishing the guidelines for National Nurses Association.

The governing body of the ICN is the Council of National Representatives, which is made up of the ICN honorary officers and the presidents of the National Member Associations.

The ICN publishes the International Nursing Review and the News Letter, which give the news of the ICN and the National Member Association.

The governing body: The council of national representatives which consists of INC honorary officers and president of the National Member Association. International exchange privileges for nurses have been provided through the INC. This gives the individual nurse the opportunity to observe and obtain employment in other countries and also contributes to improvement of standards.

The Activities of ICN

1. Making the code of nurses.
2. The worldwide accepted definition of a nurse.
3. A book of ethics "The nurses Dilemma".
4. Policy statement on health and social issues.
5. Arrange exchange program for study and employment.
6. Maintain a register on professional qualification of people.
7. Conducting seminars around the world to maintain relationship.

The International relationships: The International council of nursing has close relationship with many of the world's major international organizations such as WHO, ILO, UNESCO, UNICEF, Red cross and its allied leagues. This relationship helps ICN to have related concerns in the healthcare field and allows keeping abreast of trends affecting the future of nursing.

Functions of ICN

1. The division of nursing education.
2. The division of nursing service.
3. The division of social and economic welfare.

67.5 TRAINED NURSES ASSOCIATION OF INDIA

The Trained Nurses Association of India (TNAI), is a national professional association of nurses. The present name and organization were established in 1922, but its history of development goes back to 1905. The TNAI had its beginning in the Association of Nursing Superintendent which was founded for all nurses to participate at same level.

The level of organization moves to the district state and national levels. Members of the TNAI are usually most active on the level of the local unit. Activities and conferences however are planned regularly by the estate branches and provide opportunities for valuable professional participation and development of the individual member.

Governing body of TNAI: The governing body of the TNAI is the council which is assisted by standing committees for economic welfare, nursing research and finance. A fulltime salaried secretary was first appointed in 1935. A salaried assistant secretary who also serves as the advisor to the student nurses Association was appointed in 1983.

The aims of TNAI: The aims of TNAI center upon needs of the individual member and problems in the nursing profession as a whole, such aims include up grading, development and standardization of nursing education, improvement of living and working conditions for nurses in India and registration for qualified nurses.

Various activities of the TNAI implement its aims. It was active in helping to formulate basic nursing curricula when it first organized. More recently, it has promoted the development of courses in higher education for nurse. It gives scholarship for nurses who wish to go on for advanced study either in India or abroad.

The Trained Nurses Association of India also stimulates action to organize the state nurses and midwives registration councils. It also helps to remove discrimination against male nurses and initiates study and improvement of economic condition for nurses.

Membership of TNAI: The trained nurses Association of India membership is obtained by application and submission of a copy of your state registration certificate. Transfer of membership from the Student Nurses Association (SNA) by having a certificate sent from the institution in which the student studied within six months after completing the course. A reduced fee is offered to those who transfer membership directly from SNA.

Publications of TNAI: The Trained Nurses Association of India publishes. "The Nursing Journal of India", monthly. Another impressive publication is the "Indian Nursing Year book". This contains important reports, trends and statistics about the nursing profession in India.

67.6 STATE NURSING COUNCIL

State Nurses Registration Council is independent and recognized as a body that can make statues and prescribe by laws for trained nurses and prospective nurses who are undergoing various nursing programs. Although, it is an independent body but it has to obtain approval from state government for all the laws passed by it and decision taking. This council helps to maintain a register of names of professional nurses. Registration is must for the diploma and degree courses in nursing. Registration system helps to maintain the high standard amongst the professional nurses. Registration serves a legal protection to the nurse and also to the public as it prevents disqualified and incompetent persons to practice nursing.

The training of nurses, midwives, health visitors and ANMs is to a large extent controlled by the Nurses Registration Councils in the states. Registration in state nursing council is very necessary to be registered in order to practice officially as a professional nurse. Registration councils are functional in all the states of India and they are affiliated to INC.

Each state nurse registration council maintains a register of names of professional nurses. The names of these nurses are also put into Indian Nurses Registration Council. All the diploma and degree holder nurses have to register with State Nurses Registration Council.

Functions of State Nurses Registration Council

1. To accredit and inspect schools of nursing in their state.
2. To conduct examinations for General Nursing and Auxiliary Nursing courses.
3. To prescribe rules of conduct and take disciplinary actions.
4. Registration of nurses and midwives in their state.
5. Maintenance of register of nurses, midwives and others.
6. To renew registration and upgrade registration.

The state nursing council is an autonomous statutory registration body for registering qualified nurses, midwives, ANMs Multi purpose health workers (MPHWs) and health visitors. A council has president/vice president, registrar and staff of the council. The functions of the council includes the registration of qualified nursing professionals, regulation of training programs by conducting inspection, checking malpractice and maintaining professional ethics, foreign verification, coordinating with the INC and with various other government departments and universities. The council conducts inspection for the institution, who are conducting the programs such as ANM, MPHW, Diploma in General Nursing and Midwifery (DGNM), BSc (N), Post basic BSc (N), MSc (N) and Diploma in nursing education and administration. The council ensures that all facilities are available for conducting any of the nursing program before granting permission. It also conducts the surprise and periodical inspection to identify the deficiencies in that institution. If necessary, it also conducts reinspection to ensure that the deficiencies are rectified. It periodically sends communication to all the educational institutions to inform the issues of importance to nursing and health.

Activities

1. To look after the various nursing educational programs run under its territory.
2. To conduct exams of GNM and ANM in its areas.
3. To issue certificates of registered nurse and registered midwife to the qualified nurses.
4. Maintenance of various records such as the names and addresses of all-registered nurses, registered health visitors, registered midwives, registered nurse dais, registered trained dais in Punjab.

Renewal of Registration

The registration once done has to be renewed after a specific period of time or after attainment of higher education in nursing. It is done in respect to keep a control on registered persons practicing the profession in the state. The renewal process includes sending a dually filled form certified by the training institution with the copies of all the academic certificates and the required process fees. It is important to renew the registration in order to upgrade the status of the nurse within the state register.

67.7 STUDENT NURSE ASSOCIATION

The Student Nurses Association (SNH) organized in 1929 is associated under the jurisdiction of the TNAI, in addition to providing a means of personnel and professional development for the nursing students. It serves as a source of membership for the parent organization. In addition, the TNAI serves as the advisor for the SNA.

Objectives of SNA

1. To help the students to uphold the dignity and ideals of the profession for which they are qualifying.
2. To promote a corporate spirit among students for the common good for all.
3. To furnish nurses in training with advance in their courses of study leading to professional qualifications.
4. To encourage leadership ability and help students to gain a wide knowledge of nursing profession in all of its different branches and aspects.
5. To increase the students social conducts and general knowledge in order to help them to take their place in the world when they have finished their training.
6. To encourage both professional and recreational meeting, games, and sports.
7. To provide a special section in the nursing journal of India for the benefits of students.
8. To encourage students to participate in the student nurses exhibition and to attend national and regional conferences.

Functions of SNA

1. Project undertaking.
2. Socio cultural activities.
3. Exhibitions, public speaking and writing.
4. Organization of conferences.
5. Maintenance of SNA diary.
6. Propagation of profession.
7. Improvement of nursing education to improve healthcare.
8. Aid in the development of the nursing student.
9. Encourage optimal achievement in the professional role of the nurse.
10. Fund raising.

Organization activity: Organization activities in the SNA are similar to that of the TNAI. The beginning level of organization is the local unit established in a teaching institution. It then moves on to the state and national level as in the TNAI. Members of the local unit are guided and assisted by the president of their unit who is a professional nurse, member of the TNAI and serves only as an advisor. The vice-president, who presides at all meeting and secretary of the unit must be students. State level advisors are active members of the TNAI elected by the state branches. There is a salaried full time secretary on the national level who also a member of the TNAI and who is appointed by the TNAI council.

Membership: Membership fees in the SNA is minimal and easily met by the nursing student. The arrangement for transfer of membership to the TNAI has made in convenient for the new professional nurse to establish membership in the parent organization immediately.

67.8 CHRISTIAN MEDICAL ASSOCIATION OF INDIA

The Nurse's League of the Christian Medical Association (CMAI) was founded in 1930. CMAI is a registered, nonprofit, charitable organization. CMAI is the health arm of National Council of Churches in India (NCCI). They undertake programs in training, researcher community service, institutional consultancy, policy advocacy, interface of theology and medicine, information dissemination and others.

Objectives of CMAI

1. Prevention and relief of human suffering irrespective of caste, creed, community, religion and economic status.
2. Promotion of knowledge of the factors governing health.
3. Coordination of activities for training doctors, nurses, allied health professionals and others involved in the ministry of healing.
4. Implementation of schemes for comprehensive healthcare, family planning and community welfare.
5. Rendering health in calamities and disasters of all kinds.

Functions of the Nursing Examination Board

1. To coordinate and bring a uniform standard of nursing education, in accordance with the requirements of the Indian Nursing Council and State Nursing Council.
2. To verify the eligibility requirements of the students before each examination.
3. To arrange to conduct examination and issue diploma certificates to successful candidates.
4. To maintain and enhance the educational standards of Schools of Nursing by arranging continuing education programs/workshops/exhibitions.
5. To prepare the calendar of events at the beginning of each academic year.

6. To decide the disciplinary action against students/concerned staff in case of malpractice in examinations.
7. To nominate members for the panel of examiner's for 1st, IInd and IIIrd year of GNM nursing examinations.
8. To appoint the examiners before annual and supplementary examination.
9. To appoint an auditor to audit the board accounts.

The current objectives

1. To promote cooperation and encouragement among Christian nurses.
2. To promote efficiency in nursing education and services.
3. To secure the highest standard possible in Christian Nursing Education through the Christian Schools of Nursing.
4. To consider the special work and problems of Christian nurses working. Nursing considered to be an occupation now attains the status of profession.

CONCLUSION

Professional organizations and associations in nursing are critical for generating the energy, flow of ideas, and proactive work needed to maintain a healthy profession that advocates for the needs of its clients and nurses, and the trust of society. The goal of advocacy efforts by professional associations is to educate association members, all professional nurses, and the public about the importance of broad-base membership, creative ideas, esprit de corps, and energetic participation in helping the profession improve and move to higher levels. In prior eras, visionary nurses realized the need for associations in order to meet the changes occurring in the social, cultural, and economic sectors of their world. Elected association leaders today remain responsive to their members and incorporate members' input by devising new mechanisms to advance healthcare through the nursing profession, thus allowing members to contribute to the accountability and voice of the profession to society.

Section-14

Alternative Therapies

Complimentary/Alternative System of Medicine

68.1 INTRODUCTION

Therapies are used in addition to conventional treatment to provide healing resources and focus on the mind-body connection. Included are high-risk therapies (some that are invasive) and low-risk therapies (those that are non-invasive). The national center for complementary and alternative medicine proposed a classification system that includes five categories of complementary and alternative therapies.

68.2 CATEGORIES OF COMPLIMENTARY AND ALTERNATIVE THERAPIES

Table 68.1: Categories of alternative therapies

S.N	Categories	Description
1	Alternative medicinal medical system	**1. Environmental medicine:** Focuses on preventing the harmful effects of environment toxins and interventions include teaching, therapeutic diets, detoxification, immunotherapy, counseling and use of environmentally safe products. **2. Traditional Chinese medicine:** Focuses on restoring and maintain a balanced flow of vital energy and interventions include acupressure, acupuncture, herbal therapies, diet, meditation, tai-chi and qigong (exercise that focus on breathing visualization and movement). **3. Ayurveda:** Focuses on the balance of mind-body and spirit and intervention includes diet, medicinal herbs, detoxification, breathing exercises, meditation and yoga. **4. Homeopathy:** Focuses on healing and interventions consists of small doses of specially prepared plant and mineral extracts that assist in the innate healing process of the body. **5. Naturopathy:** Focuses on enhancing the natural healing responses of the body and interventions include nutrition, herbology, hydrotherapy, homoeopathy, acupunctures, physical therapies and counseling and psychotherapy.
2	Mind-body interventions	Mind-body interventions focus on controlling physical functions through positive mental process. Interventions include biofeedback, hypnosis, relaxation therapy, mediation, music or art therapy, qigong, prayer and mental healing.
3	Biological based therapies	Therapies include natural and biological-derived products, interventions and practices. Interventions include aromatherapy, herbal therapies, macrobiotic diet and orthomolecular therapy. **1. Aromatherapy:** The use of topical or inhaled oils (plant extract) that will promote and maintain health. **2. Herbal therapies:** The use of herbs from mostly plants sources that will maintain and restore balance and health. **3. Microbiotic diet:** Diet high in whole grain cereals, vegetables, beans and sea-vegetables and vegetarian soups. Elimination of meat, animal fat, eggs, poultry, dairy products sugars and artificially produced food from the diet. **4. Orthomolecular therapy:** Focus on nutritional balance, including the use of vitamins, essential amino acids, essential fats and minerals.

Contd...

Contd...

4	Manipulative and body-based interventions	Interventions involved manipulation and movement of the body by a therapist. Interventions include acupressure, movement reduction techniques, chiroparactic therapy and therapeutic massage.
5	Energy therapies	Energy therapies focus on energy originating within the body or on energy from other sources. Interventions include therapeutic touch and magnetic therapy.

68.3 INDIAN SYSTEM OF MEDICINE

In large part of our population have faith in ayurveda, yoga, siddha, unani, naturopathy, and homeopathy systems of treatment and takes medical help from these. Both in villages and cities, dispensaries of Indian system of medicine and homeopathy are found. In Indian context, this is significant that better healthcare can be provided by a suitable or safe combination of Indian Systems of Medicine and Allopathy.

Ayush: India, an ancient civilization, has varied community supported living traditions including medical traditions. Indian medical traditions include folk medicine and classical medical system. The folk medicine implies local health traditions which are practiced in rural and tribal communities. The folk medicine is based on locally available herbs, flora, fauna and minerals. The folk medicine is widespread. It is practiced by indigenous dais who are about 7 lakh in number and who conduct majority of the deliveries in rural and tribal areas; the bone setters (60000 in number) who deal with the problems of joint dislocation and bone fracture etc; herbal healers (80000 in number) who deal with all sorts of common ailments. In addition, millions of housewives who practice folk medicine for minor ailments. But, this system did not receive any support from the Government though it has a scope of attaining self-sufficiency to achieve the goal of Health for All (HFA).

Name of pathy/facilities	Hospitals	Dispensaries	Beds	Practitioners (Registered)
Ayurveda	2957	14755	43555	430263
Yoga	8	65	150	-
Naturopathy	23	56	832	482
Unani	312	961	5023	43330
Siddha	238	354	1991	17392
Homeopathy	306	7405	13593	200003

68.4 CLASSIFICATION OF INDIAN SYSTEM OF MEDICINE

The classical medical stream of Indian medical traditions is theory based having body of knowledge on all branches of medicine and surgery and documented in several regional manuscripts. By and large its practice is noninstitutionalized but a few Government and private hospitals and nursing homes do exist to provide institutionalized service when required. Ayurveda is the main indigenous classical medical system in India. Apart from main stream. Ayurveda, there are its regional streams, e.g. Sidha (in Tamil Nadu) and the Tibetan medical systems; other important traditional medical systems include yoga, naturopathy, unani and homeopathy. These systems are known as Indian Systems of Medicine (ISM). These are practiced in Government as well as in private sector. However, the Government sector gave very marginal support to these because of its bias towards Western System of Medicine which got Government support and flourished during British rule in India. The Indian Government after Independence continued with the same system of medicine which it inherited from the British Government. Only 4 percent of the National health budget is allocated to traditional medicine, while State Government budget for the same ranges from less than 1 percent (in West Bengal) to 13 percent (in Kerala). On an average most of the states provide less than 2 percent of their health budget for Indigenous Systems of Medicine. Therefore, the growth of ISM in Independent India has not been very satisfactory. There has been resurgence of interest in traditional systems of medicine as a result of search in the west for alternatives to allopathic system of medicine. This has regenerated the interest in ISM in India. It has been realized to involve a large number of traditionally trained human resources to contribute to achieve the goal of HFA by 2000 which was set forth in 1977. The important role of Indian Systems of Medicine and Homeopathy (ISM and H) in the delivery of primary health.

68.5 AYURVEDA

Life in Ayurveda is conceived as the union of body, senses, mind and soul. The living man is a conglomeration of three humours (Vata, Pitta and Kapha), seven basic tissues (Rasa, Rakta, Mansa, Meda, Asthi, Majja and Shukra) and the waste products of the body such as faeces, urine and sweat. Thus, the total body matrix comprises of the humours, the tissues and the waste products of the body. The growth and decay of this body matrix and its constituents revolve around food which gets processed into humours, tissues and wastes. Ingestion, digestion, absorption, assimilation and metabolism of food have an interplay in health and disease which are significantly affected by psychological mechanisms as well as by bio-fire (Agni).

Heath and Illness: Health or sickness depends on the presence or absence of a balanced state of the total body matrix including the balance between its different constituents. Both the intrinsic and extrinsic factors can cause disturbance in the natural equilibrium giving rise to disease. This loss of equilibrium can happen by dietary indiscrimination, undesirable habits and nonobservance of rules of healthy living. Seasonal abnormalities, improper exercise or erratic application of sense organs and incompatible actions of the body and mind can also result in creating disturbance of the existing normal balance. The treatment consists of restoring the balance of disturbed body-mind matrix through regulating diet, correcting life-routine and behavior, administration of drugs and resorting to preventive Panchkarma and Rasayana therapy.

Diagnosis: In Ayuveda, diagnosis is always done of the patient as a whole. The physician takes a careful note of the patient's internal physiological characteristics and mental disposition. He also studies such other factors as the affected bodily tissues, humors, the site at which the disease is located, patients resistance and vitality, his daily routine, dietary habits, the gravity of clinical conditions, condition of digestion and details of personal, social, economic and environmental situation of the patient. The diagnosis also involves the following examinations:

1. General physical examination.
2. Pulse examination.
3. Urine examination.
4. Examination of the feces.
5. Examination of tongue and eyes.
6. Examination of skin and ear including tactile and auditory functions.

Treatment: The basic therapeutic approach is, that alone is the right treatment which makes for health and he alone is the best doctor who frees one from disease. This sums up the principal objectives of Ayurveda, i.e. maintenance and promotion of health, prevention of disease and cure of sickness. Treatment of the disease consists in avoiding causative factors responsible for disequilibrium of the body matrix or of any of its constituent parts through the use of Panchkarma procedures, medicines, suitable diet, activity and regimen for restoring the balance and strengthening the body mechanisms to prevent or minimize future occurrence of the disease.

Normally, treatment measures involve use of medicines, specific diet and prescribed activity routine. Use of these three measures is done in two ways. In one approach of treatment the three measures antagonize the disease by counteracting the etiological factors and various manifestations of the disease. In the second approach the same three measures of medicine, diet and activity are targeted to exert effects similar to the etiological factors and manifestations of the disease process. These two types of therapeutic approaches are respectively known as Vipreeta and Vipreetarthkari treatments. For successful administration of a treatment four things are essential. These are the physician, the medicaments, the nursing personnel, and the patient, the physician comes first in order of importance. He must possess technical skill, scientific knowledge, purity and human understanding. The physician should use his knowledge with humility, wisdom and in the service of humanity. Next in importance comes food and drugs. These are supposed to be of high quality; wide application, grown and prepared following approved procedures and should be available adequately. The third component of every successful treatment is the role of nursing personnel who should have good knowledge of nursing, must know the skills of their art and be affectionate, sympathetic, intelligent, neat and clean and resourceful. The fourth component is the patient himself who should be cooperative and obedient to follow instructions of the physician, able to describe ailments and ready to provide all that may be needed for treatment.

68.6 YOGA

Yoga is a discipline to improve or develop one's inherent power in a balanced manner. It offers the means to attain complete self-realization. The literal meaning of the Sanskrit Word Yoga is 'Yoke'. Yoga can therefore be defined as a means of uniting the individual spirit with the universal spirit of God. According to Maharishi Patanjali, Yoga is the suppression of modifications of the mind.

Types of Yoga

1. **Japa Yoga:** To concentrate one's mind on divine name or holy syllable, mantra etc. like 'OM', 'Rama', 'Allah', 'God', 'Vahe Guru', etc. through repeated recitation or remembrance.
2. **Karma Yoga:** Teaches us to perform all actions without having any desire for their fruit. In this sadhana, a Yogi considers his duty as divine action, perform it with whole-hearted dedication but shuns away all desires.
3. **Gyana Yoga:** Teaches us to discriminate between self and nonself and to acquire the knowledge of one's spiritual entity through the study of scriptures, company of Saints and practices of meditation.
4. **Bhakti Yoga:** Bhakti Yoga, a system of intense devotion with emphasis on complete surrender to divine will. The true follower of Bhakti Yoga is free from egoism remains humble and unaffected by the dualities of the world.
5. **Raja Yoga:** Raja Yoga popularly known as "Ashtanga Yoga" is for all-round development of human beings. These are Yama, Niyama, Asana, Pranayama, Pratyahara, Dharana, Dhyana and Samadhi.
6. **Swara Yoga:** Swara Yoga is the science which is about the realization of cosmic consciousness, through the awareness/observation then control/manipulation of the flow of breath in the nostrils. Swara Yoga involves the systematic study of the breath flowing through the nostril (or Swara) in relation to the prevailing phases of the Sun, Moon, time of day and direction. It is the association of the breath in relation to the activities or phases or positions of the Sun, Moon, Planets, Seasons, Time of day, with the physical and mental conditions of the individual and then taking the appropriate action according to these subtle relations.
7. **Kundalini:** Kundalini Yoga is a part of Tantric Tradition. Since, the dawn of creation, the Tantrics and yogis have realized that in this physical body, there is a potential force residing in Muladhara Chakra, the first of seven Chakras. The seat of Kundalini is a small gland at the base of the spinal

cord. In the masculine body, it is in the perineum between the urinary and excretory organs. In the female body its location is at the root of the uterus in the cervix. Those people who have awakened this supernatural force have been called Rishis, Prophets, Yogis, Siddhas and other names according to the time, tradition and culture. To awaken the Kundalini, you must prepare yourself through yogic techniques such as Shatkriya, Asana, Pranayama, Bandha, Mudra and Meditation. Awakening of Kundalini results in an explosion in the brain as the dormant or sleeping areas start blossoming like flowers.

8. **Nadi:** As described by Yogic texts, Nadis are flow of energy which we can visualize at the psychic level as having distinct channels, light, color, sound and other characteristics. The entire network of nadis is so vast that even yogic texts differ in their calculations of the exact number. Reference in the Goraksha Sataka or Goraksh Samhita and Hatha Yoga Pradipika place their number at 72,000; emerged from the navel center—the Manipura Chakra. Of all the thousands of nadis, Sushumna is said to be the most important. The Shiva Swarodaya enumerates ten major nadis which connect to the 'doorways' leading in and out of the body. Of these ten, Ida, Pingala and Sushumna are the most important, they are the high voltage wires which conduct the energy to the substations or Chakras situated along the spinal column.

68.7 NATUROPATHY

Naturopathy is a system of man building in harmony with the constructive principles of nature on physical, mental, moral and spiritual planes of living. It has great health promotive, disease preventive and curative as well as restorative potential. According to the manifesto of British Naturopathic Association, "Naturopathy is a system of treatment which recognizes the existence of the vital curative force within the body." It therefore, advocates aiding human system to remove the cause of disease, i.e. toxins by expelling the unwanted and unused matters from human body for curing diseases.

Salient features of naturopathy: The main features of Naturopathy are as under:

1. All diseases, their causes and treatment are one. Except for traumatic and environmental conditions, the cause of all diseases is one, i.e. accumulation of morbid matter in the body. The treatment of all diseases is elimination of morbid matter from the body.
2. The primary cause of disease is accumulation of morbid matter. Bacteria and virus enter and survive in the body only after the accumulation of morbid matter when a favorable atmosphere for their growth is established in body. Hence, the basic cause of disease is morbid matter and bacteria secondary causes.
3. Acute diseases are self-healing efforts of the body. Hence, they are our friends, not the enemy. Chronic diseases are outcome of wrong treatment and suppression of the acute diseases.
4. Nature is the greatest healer. The human body itself has the healing power to prevent itself from disease and regain health if unhealthy.
5. In Nature cure, it is not the disease but the entire body of the patient which is caused and is renewed.
6. Naturopathy cures patients suffering from chronic ailments are also treated successfully in comparatively less time by Naturopathy.
7. In Nature cure, the suppressed diseases are brought to surface and are removed permanently.
8. Naturopathy treats all the aspects like physical, mental, social and spiritual at the same time.
9. Naturopathy treats the body as a whole.
10. According to Naturopathy, "Food is only the Medicine", no external medications are used.
11. Performing prayer according to one's spiritual faith is an important part of treatment (According to Gandhiji "Rama Nama is the best Natural Treatment".

68.8 UNANI

The Unani system of medicine has a long and impressive record in India. It was introduced in India by the Arabs and Persians sometime around the eleventh century. Today, India is one of the leading countries in so for as the practice of Unani medicine is concerned. It has the largest number of Unani educational, research and health care institutions.

As the name indicates, Unani system originated in Greece. The foundation of Unani system was laid by Hippocrates. The system owes its present form to the Arabs who not only saved much of the Greek literature by rendering it into Arabic but also enriched the medicine of their day with their own contributions. In this process, they made extensive use of the science of Physics, Chemistry, Botany, Anatomy, Physiology, Pathology, Therapeutics and Surgery. Unani Medicines got enriched by imbibing what was best in the contemporary systems of traditional medicines in Egypt, Syria, Iraq, Persia, India, China and other Middle East countries. In India, Unani System of Medicine was introduced by Arabs and soon it took firm roots. The Delhi Sultans (rulers) provided patronage to the scholars of Unani System and even enrolled some as state employees and court physicians. During 13th and 17th century A.D. Unani Medicine had its hey-day in India.

The system suffered a severe setback during the British rule in India. The allopathic system was introduced and gained ground. This retarded the growth of education, research and practice of Unani system of medicine. All the traditional systems of medicine along with Unani System faced almost complete neglect for about two centuries. The withdrawal of State Patronage could not harm much as the masses reposed faith in this system and it continued to be practiced. It was mainly Sharifi family in Delhi, the Azizi family in Lucknow and the Nizam of Hyderabad due to whose efforts Unani Medicine survived during the British period.

68.9 SIDDHA

Siddha system is one of the oldest systems of medicine in India. The term Siddha means achievements and Siddhars were saintly persons who achieved results in medicine. Eighteen Siddhars were said to have contributed towards the development of this medical system. Siddha literature is in Tamil and it is practiced largely in Tamil speaking part of India and abroad. The Siddha System is largely therapeutic in nature.

History of Siddha: The original Home allotted to mankind by the Creator was in the temparate and fertile region of the East and pointedly in India. It is from here that the human race began its culture and career. India may, therefore, be safely stated as that the first country from which human culture and civilization originated and spread. According to Indian history prior to Aryans migration, the Dravidian was the first inhabitant of India of whom the Tamilians were the most prominent. The Tamilians were not only the earliest civilized but also those who may more considerable progress in civilization than any other early people.

The languages of India were divided into two great classes, the northern with Sanskrit as the pre-pondering element and the southern with Dravidian language as independent bases. The science of medicine is of fundamental importance to man well-being be and his survival and so it must have originated with man and developed as civilization. It is, therefore rather pointless to try to determine the exact point of time to which the beginning of these systems could be traced. They are eternal, they began with man and may end with him.

68.10 HOMOEOPATHY

Homoeopathy today is a rapidly growing system and is being practiced almost all over the world. In India, it has become a household name due the safety of its pills and gentleness of its cure. A rough study states that about 10% of the Indian population solely depend Homoeopathy for their health-care needs and is considered as the second most popular system of medicine in the country.

History of Homoeopathy: It is more than a century and a half now that Homoeopathy is being practiced in India. It has blended so well into the roots and traditions of the country that it has been recognized as one of the National System of Medicine and plays a very important role in providing healthcare to a large number of people. Its strength lies in its evident effectiveness as it takes a holistic approach towards the sick individual through promotion of inner balance at mental, emotional, spiritual and physical levels.

CONCLUSION

Alternative medicine practices are used instead of standard medical treatments. Alternative medicine is distinct from complementary medicine which is meant to accompany, not to replace, standard medical practices. Alternative medical practices are generally not recognized by the medical community as standard or conventional medical approaches. Alternative medicine includes dietary supplements, mega dose vitamins, herbal preparations, special teas, massage therapy, magnet therapy, and spiritual healing. Complementary and alternative medicine has never been more popular. Nearly 40 percent of adults report using complementary and alternative medicine, also called CAM for short. Doctors are embracing CAM therapies, too, often combining them with mainstream medical therapies-spawning the term "integrative medicine."

Glossary

1. **Abortion:** Expulsion or removal of a usually nonviable fetus. (a fetus that cannot live outside the uterus at that time).
2. **Accounting system:** The series of tasks and records of an entity by which transactions are processed as a means of maintaining financial records.
3. **Acculturation:** Process of learning norms, beliefs and behavioral expectations of a group other than one's own group.
4. **Active euthanasia:** The ending of another person's life by an aggressive method to end suffering.
5. **Advance directive:** Written document recognized by state law that provides directions concerning the provision of care when a person is unable to make his or her own treatment choices.
6. **Advanced practice nurse:** A master's-prepared nurse with specialization and licensure to practice as a nurse practitioner, nurse anesthetist, nurse midwife, clinical nurse specialist, clinical nurse leader, or other advanced specialist role.
7. **Advocacy:** Acting on the behalf of the client and protecting the client's rights to make his or her own decisions.
8. **Analysis:** The process by which the nurse organizes the data, identifies the client's health needs and problems, and prioritizes those problems.
9. **Analytical procedures:** Consist of the analysis of significant ratios and trends including the resulting investigation of fluctuations and relationships that are inconsistent with other relevant information or deviate from predictable amounts.
10. **Assault:** A deliberate act wherein one person threatens to harm another without consent and the victim feels the attacker has the ability to carry out the threat.
11. **Assessment:** Includes collection of objective and subjective data, organization of data, and statement of the nursing diagnosis.
12. **Audit evidence:** The information obtained by the auditor in arriving at the conclusions on which the audit opinion is based.
13. **Auditing:** A systematic process of objectively obtaining and evaluating evidence in respect of certain assertions about economic actions and events to ascertain the degree of correspondence between those assertions and established criteria and reporting the results to interested parties over a particular period of time.
14. **Auditor:** The person with final responsibility for the audit. This term is also used to refer to an audit firm.
15. **Audit risk:** the risk that auditors may give an inappropriate audit opinion on financial statements.
16. **Audit staff:** The personnel involved in an audit other than the audit engagement partner.
17. **Autonomy:** The concept that patients are to be treated as individuals and informed about procedures to facilitate appropriate decisions.
18. **Belief:** Something accepted as true by a culture.
19. **Beneficence:** The state or act of intentionally doing or producing good. The principle of beneficence involves duties to prevent harm, remove harm, and promote the good of another person. The obligation of healthcare professionals to seek the well-being or benefit of other patients. Duties of beneficence concern the welfare of others.

20. **Career planning:** The process of establishing career objectives and determining appropriate educational and developmental programs to further develop the skills required to achieve short- or long-term career objectives.
21. **Caring:** a function of the whole person in which concern for the growth and well-being of another is expressed in an integrated application of the mind, body, and spirit that seeks to maximize positive outcomes.
22. **Case manager:** A health professional who advocates for the patient to receive the most appropriate treatment with acceptable quality in the most effective manner and appropriate setting at the best price.
23. **Client:** An individual, family, group, population or entire community who requires nursing expertise. In some clinical settings, the client may be referred to as a patient or a resident. In research, the client may be referred to as a participant.
24. **Clinical diagnosis:** Diagnosis based on signs, symptoms, and laboratory findings during life.
25. **Collaboration:** A joint communication and decision-making process with the expressed goal of working together toward identified outcomes while respecting the unique qualities and abilities of each member of the group or team.
26. **Collegial model:** A cooperative method of providing healthcare for the patient involving sharing, trust and the pursuit of common goals. This model may be helpful in addressing patient's emotional needs and engaging their cooperation.
27. **Communication:** A patient has the right of access to people outside of the hospital by means of visitors, and by verbal and written communication when such visitations and communications will not interfere with the patient's treatment.
28. **Community:** Community as a group of inhabitants living together in a somewhat localized area under the same general regulations and having common interests, functions, needs and organizations.
29. **Community health:** Community (public) health is a science and art of preventing disease, prolonging life and promoting health and efficiency through organized effort.
30. **Community health nursing:** Community health nursing is a synthesis of nursing and public health practice applied of promoting and preserving the health of people. The practice is general and compressive. It is not limited to a particular age group or diagnosis, and continuing, not episodic.
31. **Competencies:** Statements about the knowledge, skills, attitudes and judgments required to perform safely and ethically within an individual's nursing practice or in a designated role or setting.
32. **Competent:** A legal concept that describes people who are able to make decisions for themselves. Minors are presumed to be incompetent, except under certain specified conditions. The corollary medical-ethical term is decisional capacity.
33. **Complaint:** The written allegation of wrong doing filed to initiate a lawsuit. It also may called a claim or petition, depending on the court in which it is brought.
34. **Concept:** Concepts are the elements or components of a phenomenon necessary to understand the phenomenon and derived from impressions the human mind receives about phenomena through sensing the human environment.
35. **Confidentiality:** The duties owned by health are providers to protect the privacy of patient information.
36. **Consent:** Except in emergencies, a patient has the right to receive from his/her healthcare provider information in nonclinical terms necessary to give informed consent prior to the start of any procedure or treatment. Such information should include, but not necessarily be limited to, the specific procedures or treatment; the medically significant complications, and benefits, or when the patient requests information concerning medical alternatives. The patient has the right to be advised if the hospital proposes to engage in or perform human experimentation

affecting his/her care or treatment. The patient has the right to refuse to participate in such research projects.

37. **Consent forms:** Useful tools to help inform patients about procedures and document consent.
38. **Consequentially:** An ethical school of thought in which decisions are based on the consequences or outcomes of a given act; the good of an activity is evaluated based on whether immediate harm is balanced with future benefits.
39. **Continuous quality control:** The aspect of quality assurance that monitors technical equipment to maintain standards.
40. **Contractual model:** A healthcare model that defines healthcare as a business relationship between the provider and patient. a contractual arrangement serves as the guideline for decision-making and provision of services.
41. **Criterion:** A criterion is the value free description of variable believed to an indicator of patient care quality.
42. **Critical thinking:** A purposeful, disciplined and systematic process of continual questioning, logical reasoning and reflecting through the use of interpretation, inference, analysis, synthesis and evaluation to achieve a desired outcome.
43. **Cultural assimilation:** Process by which individuals from a minority group absorbed by the dominant culture and take on the characteristics of the dominant culture.
44. **Cultural competence:** The acquisition of knowledge, understanding and appreciation of a culture that facilitates the provision of culturally appropriate healthcare.
45. **Cultural diversity:** The differences among groups of people, the result from ethnic, racial and cultural values.
46. **Cultural imposition:** The tendency to impose one's own belief, values and patterns of behavior on individuals from another culture.
47. **Culturally diverse nursing care:** An optimal mode of healthcare delivery; it refers to the variability of nursing approaches needed to provide culturally appropriate care that incorporates an individual's cultural values, beliefs, and practices including sensitivity to the environment from which the individual comes and to which the individual may ultimately return (Leininger).
48. **Cultural values:** The individual's desirable or preferred way of acting or knowing something that is sustained over a period of time and which governs actions or decisions.
49. **Culture:** Refers to norms and practices of a particular group that are learned and shared and guide thinking, decisions, and actions.
50. **Culture shock:** A disorder that occurs in response to transition from one cultural setting to another.
51. **Deductive reasoning:** Reasoning from the general to the specific
52. **Deontology:** An ethical school of thought that bases decision-making on individual motives and morals rather than consequences and examines the significances of action themselves. Deontological problem solving uses personal rules of right and wrong derived from individual actions, relationships of all kinds and society.
53. **Differential diagnosis:** The determination of which one of several diseases may be producing the symptoms.
54. **Diversity:** Differences rooted in culture, age, experience, health status, gender, sexual orientation, racial or ethnic identity, mental abilities, and other aspects of sociocultural description and socioeconomic status.
55. **Documentation:** Standardized recording information necessary for continuity of patient care and to protect from medical negligence litigation risks.
56. **Durable power of attorney for healthcare:** An advance directive that goes into effect in the event that a patient who has completed such a document loses decisional capacity. Allows an individual to name a person(s) who is empowered to make healthcare decisions when the individual becomes incapacitated.

57. **Emancipated minor:** A teenaged minor, who is legally, independent of parental control and who can thus give informed consent to medical treatments.
58. **Empathy:** Intellectual and emotional awareness and understanding of another person's thoughts behaviors and feelings.
59. **Engineering model:** A healthcare model that identifies the healthcare provider as a scientist concerned with facts and defines the patient as a condition or procedure, not a person. A healthcare professional using the engineering model tends to view a patient as a collection of body system.
60. **Environment:** Internal and external surroundings that affect the client.
61. **Ethics:** Refer to the study of philosophical ideas of right and wrong behavior.
62. **Ethics committees:** An interdisciplinary group that deals with conflicts of values in patient care in acute and long-term settings. Such committees discuss policy issues (e.g. regarding withholding and withdrawing of life-sustaining treatments).
63. **Ethnic:** Relates to large groups of people classified according to common traits or customs.
64. **Ethnocentrism:** An assumption of cultural superiority and an inability to accept the ways of another culture.
65. **Ethnography:** The study of a culture. The methodological approach of ethnographic research central to the nurse's ability to develop a heightened awareness of culturally diverse needs of individuals is to define a field for observation for study of the environment and its people as well as the reciprocal relationship that exists between the two.
66. **Euthanasia:** The act of either permitting a person to die or intentionally ending a person's life generally rooted in motives of mercy, beneficence, or respect for patient dignity.
67. **Evaluation:** Consists of measuring the outcomes of therapeutic nursing interventions and the effectiveness of nursing care in relation to established criteria. The client's progress in relation to the achievement of established goals indicates whether optimal health has been attained or revisions in the plan need to occur.
68. **Expanded role:** Expanded role of nursing means enlargement of nurse with the bonders of nurse.
69. **Goodwill:** The difference between the value of a business as a whole and the aggregate of the fair values of its separable net assets.
70. **Governance:** Describes the role of persons entrusted with the supervision, control and direction of an entity by ensuring that the entity achieves its objectives, financial reporting, and of reporting to interested parties.
71. **Health:** A state of physical, mental and social well-being and the absence of disease or other disorders. It involves constant change and adaptation to stress.
72. **Holistic:** Approach that takes into account the client as a physical, mental, emotional, and spiritual being.
73. **Hospital charges:** A patient has the right to examine and receive a detailed explanation of his/her total bill, regardless of source of payment.
74. **Hospital rules and regulations:** A patient has the right to be informed of the hospital rules and regulations that relate to visitor and patient conduct. Patients are entitled to information about the hospital's mechanism for the initiation, review and resolution of patient complaints.
75. **Identity:** A patient has the right to know, at all times, the identity, professional status, and professional credentials of healthcare personnel, as well as the name of the healthcare provider primarily responsible for his/her care.
76. **Implementation:** It is the operationalization of selected nursing interventions. In addition to providing nursing care and/or management activities, in includes continued collaboration with the client to validate the plan of care and processing new information through continued data collection.
77. **Incoming auditor:** The auditor who is to take over from the current auditor and did not audit the prior period's financial statements.

78. **Independent audit:** Providing reasonable assurance that published audited financial reports are free from material mis-statement and are in accordance with legislation and relevant accounting standards.
79. **Inductive reasoning:** Forming generalizations from a set of facts or observations.
80. **Informed consent:** The legal and ethical requirement that no significant medical procedure can be performed until the competent patient has been informed of the nature of the procedure, risks and alternatives, as well as the prognosis if the procedure is not done. The patient must freely and voluntarily agree to have the procedure done.
81. **Internal audit:** An appraisal or monitoring activity established by management and the directors for the review of the accounting and internal control systems as a service to the entity.
82. **Law:** A system composed of general rules governing conduct and procedures for resolving disputes when rules are not followed.
83. **Malpractice:** Failure to meet the standards of acceptable care, which results in harm to another person.
84. **Medical care:** A patient has the right to quality care and treatment consistent with available resources and generally accepted medical standards. The patient has the right to that care and treatment in a safe environment.
85. **Medical diagnosis:** Diagnosis based on information from sources such as findings from a physical examination, interview with the patient or family or both, medical history of the patient and family, and clinical findings as reported by laboratory tests and radiologic studies.
86. **Minority group:** An ethnic, cultural, racial or religious group that constitutes less than a numerical majority of the population.
87. **Model:** A model is a phenomenological analogy used to describe something that cannot be directly observed and about which deeper understanding is sought.
88. **Models:** Models are graphic or symbolic representations of phenomena that objectify and present certain perspectives or points of view about nature or function or both.
89. **Negligence:** Failure to provide care that a reasonable person ordinarily would use in similar circumstances.
90. **Nonmaleficence:** The state of not doing harm or evil; see also beneficence.
91. **Norm:** A norm is the current level of performance of a particular criterion, as determined by description study of the target population.
92. **Nurse anesthetics:** A nurse who completed the course of study in an anesthesia school and carries out preoperative status of clients.
93. **Nurse midwife:** A registered nurse who has advanced education and certification to practice uncomplicated obstetrical care, including normal spontaneous vaginal delivery, without direct physician supervision.
94. **Nurse practitioner:** A registered nurse who has advanced education and certification to carry out expanded healthcare evaluation and decision-making regarding patient care; boundaries of independent practice are set by state laws.
95. **Nursing:** Nursing is an art, science and profession by which we render, serve to human being to help him to regain or to keep a normal state of body and mind and when it cannot accomplish this, it help him for the relief from physical pain, mental anxiety or spiritual discomfort.
96. **Nursing audit:** Nursing audit is the process of analyzing data about the nursing process or patient outcomes to evaluate the effectiveness of nursing intervention.
97. **Nursing diagnosis:** A clinical judgment about an individual's mental or physical condition to determine whether the condition can be improved or resolved by appropriate interventions of the registered nurse to achieve outcomes for which the registered nurse is accountable.
98. **Nursing order:** A nursing order is a prescribed action issued in the form of a command by one nurse to other nursing personnel.

99. **Nursing problem:** A nursing problem is difficult situation encountered by care giver in pursuing nursing goal.
100. **Nursing process:** A system of assessing patients, diagnosing individual nursing care needs, planning care, implementing plans, and evaluating care.
101. Nursing roles competencies and skills performed by nurses in response to current and anticipated health needs of the client.
102. **Nursing science:** Knowledge (e.g. concepts, constructs, principles, theories) of nursing derived from systematic observation, study and research.
103. **Objective:** An objective is a concrete statement of intention, an external goal towards which effort is directed.
104. **Objective data:** Signs that are detectable by an observer or can be tested against an accepted standard
105. **Optimal health:** The highest potential degree of physical, psychosocial, and spiritual well-being that is within the client's capacity.
106. **Patient problem:** A patient is an active or potential need, condition or complication that derives from the patient diagnosis or care and indicates needs for intervention.
107. **Patient's bill of right:** The rights and responsibilities of clients receiving care.
108. **Philosophy:** A philosophy is statement of belief and values about human being and their world.
109. **Physical diagnosis:** Diagnosis based on information obtained by inspection, palpation, percussion, and auscultation.
110. **Planning:** It is based on analysis of data, is the development of individualized nursing care. It includes collaboration with the client for determining client/nursing goals, setting priorities, and selection of therapeutic nursing interventions.
111. **Principal auditor:** The auditor with responsibility for reporting on the financial statements of an entity when those financial statements include financial information of one or more components audited by other auditors.
112. **Privacy:** A patient has the right to privacy concerning his/her own medical care program. Case discussions, consultation, examination, and treatment are confidential. Those not directly involved in the patient's care must have the patient's permission to be present.
113. **Privileged communication:** Information communicated to an attorney, physician, spouse, or counselor that may not be revealed, even in court, without the consent of the person who made the statement.
114. **Profession:** A profession is an occupation with moral principles that are devoted to the human and social welfare. The service is based on specialized knowledge and skill developed in a scientific and learned manner.
115. **Professional conduct:** Professional conduct is behaving with a real sense of dignity and respect for the service given for the patient and for theses with which one works.
116. **Proxy consent:** Voluntary informed consent given on behalf of another who is for some reason incapable of giving it for himself or herself.
117. **Quality improvement:** A quality improvement is the process or establishing optimum standards of nursing practice and planning or providing care that meets those standards.
118. **Race:** A term related to biology, since members of the same group share distinguishing physical features such as skin color, bone structure, and blood group.
119. **Racism:** Discrimination directed towards individuals or group who are perceived to be inferior because to biological differences, often accompanied by oppression.
120. **Refusal of treatment:** A patient has the right to refuse treatment to the extent permitted by law and existing government regulations, and to be informed of the medical and administrative consequences of his/her refusal.

121. **Respect and dignity:** A patient has the right to considerate and respectful care, with recognition of his/her personal dignity.
122. Settings Geographical and/or situational environments where nurses practice. Settings may be traditional in which policies, procedures, and protocols for providing healthcare may be established or nontraditional where policies, procedures, and protocols are implied.
123. **Stereotyping:** An expectation that all people within the same racial, ethnic or cultural group act alike and share the same beliefs and attitudes.
124. **Subculture:** A group of people with characteristic patterns of behavior that distinguish the group from the larger cultural or society.
125. **Subjective data:** Symptoms; facts, perceptions, or sensations apparent only to the person affected.
126. **Sympathy:** Is balancing someone's feeling especially in his sorrow or trouble.
127. **Theories:** Ways of looking at a discipline—such as nursing—in clear, explicit terms that can be communicated to others.
128. **Theory:** It refers to a set of logically interrelated concepts, statement, proposition and definitions which have been derived from philosophical beliefs of scientific data and from which questions or hypothesis can be deduced, tested and verified.
129. **Therapeutic communication skills:** The application of a dynamic process between two or more persons, in which there is an exchange of information, thoughts, and feelings. The skills involved are accurate perception, interpretation and expression, in a style sensitive to the purpose and context of the interaction. This interaction may occur in various formats including: verbal, nonverbal, tactile, artistic creations, test base, or information technology.
130. **Therapeutic nursing interventions:** Holistic nursing actions that are implemented in an accurate, safe manner according to national standards and practice guidelines.
131. **Transcultural nursing:** A humanistic and scientific area of formal study and practice in nursing which is focused upon differences and similarities among cultures with respect to humancare, health, and illness based upon the people's cultural values, beliefs, and practices, and to use this knowledge to provide cultural specific or culturally congruent nursing care to people (Leininger).
132. **Transfer and continuity of care:** A patient has the right to expect reasonable continuity of care. The patient has the right to know in advance what appointment times and healthcare providers are available and where. Following discharge, the patient has the right to expect that the hospital will provide a mechanism whereby he/she is informed by his/her provider or a delegate of the provider of the patient's continuing healthcare requirements.
133. **Values:** Beliefs and attitudes that may influence behavior and the process of decision-making.

Index

B

C

D

F

G

H

I

J

K

L

M

N

S

T

U

V

W

X

Y

Z